- how rigidly we hold
  to our illusions
- when we're young

- how tightly we hold is a fx of
  our parents?

Relational Concepts in Psychoanalysis

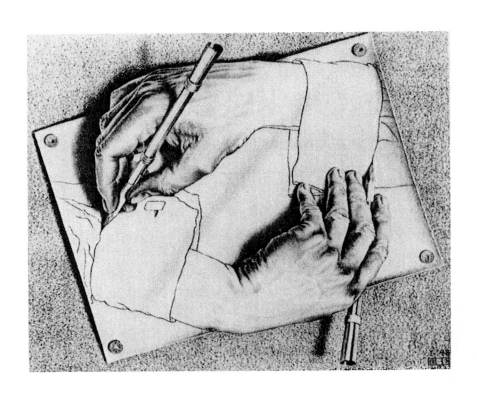

Relational Concepts in Psychoanalysis
An Integration

Stephen A. Mitchell

Harvard University Press
Cambridge, Massachusetts, and London, England

Frontispiece: M. C. Escher's *Drawing Hands*. © 1988
M. C. Escher c/o Cordon Art, Baarn, Holland.

Portions of Chapters 6, 7, and 9 appeared in the following articles:
"Object relations theories and the developmental tilt," "The wings
of Icarus," and "The problem of the will," in *Contemporary Psychoanalysis* 20 (1984) and 22 (1986).

This book is printed on acid-free paper, and its binding materials
have been chosen for strength and durability.

Library of Congress Cataloging-in-Publication Data

Mitchell, Stephen A., 1946–
    Relational concepts in psychoanalysis: an integration / Stephen
A. Mitchell.
            p.   cm.
        Bibliography: p.
        Includes index.
        ISBN 0-674-75411-5 (alk. paper)
            1. Psychoanalysis.   2. Object relations (Psychoanalysis)
3. Interpersonal relations.   4. Motivation (Psychology)
5. Freud, Sigmund, 1856–1939.   I. Title.
        [DNLM: 1. Psychoanalysis. 2. Psychoanalytic Theory.
WM 460 M682r]
BF175.5.O24M58 1988
150.19'5—dc19
DNLM/DLC
for Library of Congress   88-11168
                                                    CIP

This book has been digitally reprinted. The content
remains identical to that of previous printings.

For Margaret

Preface

The most pressing questions in contemporary psychoanalytic theory and practice are, What do the vast array of different psychoanalytic schools and traditions have to do with one another? Do they fit together? If so, how? If not, why not? In one fashion or another, these questions haunt (and often excite) every member of the psychoanalytic community, from the beginning candidate to the most seasoned theoretician and clinician. The two most popular approaches for dealing with the burgeoning heterogeneity of psychoanalytic schools have been the adoption of a single theory—classical, neoclassical, or contemporary—to the exclusion of the rest, or the retention of all theories in a broadly encompassing eclecticism.

Orthodoxy (of whatever denomination) rests on the fiat that there is one true psychoanalytic path; all others are, by some arbitrary definition, excluded. Eclecticism rests on the fiat that all theories are true or useful and that it is possible simultaneously to maintain belief in and employ different theories for different patients, or different theories for the same patient at different times. The advantage of the single-theory approach is its continuity and simplicity; the disadvantage is the loss of richness and cross-fertilization with other traditions. The advantage of eclecticism is its inclusiveness; the disadvantage is its lack of conceptual rigor.

We are all dealing with the same reality, the eclectic argues, but with different pieces of it from different perspectives. Various psychoanalytic theories are like so many blind men exploring different parts of the elephant. Each report is right; all can be contained in a larger framework. This outlook can be very misleading. Reality is not simply discovered, but is partially created by theoretical presuppositions. There are lots of blind men out there, but they are not all operating on the same premises, within the same reality; they are not all exploring elephants. Some may be grappling with giraffes. To try to contain all reports within the same framework may lead to strange hybrids: four stout legs; a long, graceful neck; four thin legs; a long trunk; and so on.

A third, less frequent approach to psychoanalytic heterogeneity—the one that characterizes this volume—entails an effort at *selective integration*. From this perspective, different theories and traditions are seen as enriching the field of analytic inquiry and providing valuable contributions, in some areas compatible with one another, in some areas mutually exclusive. What is called for is not simply the retention of these various contributions in an overarching ecumenicism, but a critical integration of them. Around what issues can different theories be fitted together? Around what issues do the different concepts require a new and broader framework to house them? Around what issues are they incompatible?

Amid the apparent conceptual disarray in contemporary psychoanalysis are two broad, competing perspectives, *Freud's drive theory* and a cluster of theories (including British object-relations theory, interpersonal psychoanalysis, and self psychology) which derive from a set of premises that Jay Greenberg and I have termed the *relational model*. Drive theory is unified, comprehensive, and outdated. It is preserved as a loyally maintained belief system around which innovative thinking is arranged, fitted in so as not to dislodge traditional principles. This process tends to inhibit and distort innovation, and to keep theory at some distance from the way most contemporary clinicians think and work.

On the other hand, relational theory is fragmented, diffuse, and developed by psychoanalytic schools that regard themselves as competing with, rather than complementing, one another. Although relational theory is much more consistent with the way most clinicians practice psychoanalysis and psychoanalytic therapy, it has never been developed into a coherent, comprehensive theoretical framework. This book aims at such a unification, by considering the major domains of psychoanalytic inquiry—sexuality, early development, fantasy and illusion, continuity and change—from an integrated relational perspective.

Part of what makes psychoanalysis such an exciting discipline is its heterogeneity and the infinite possibilities for integrating the diversity of its traditions into one's own personal view and clinical style. In that sense, this book represents my own unique vision. Yet the world of psychoanalysis is also a community of rich and complex relationships spanning different traditions and generations. No psychoanalytic position develops in a vacuum; each is in some sense a crystallization of many influences, some known, many unknown.

I want to give special thanks to my many patients, students, and supervisees, necessarily anonymous, who have stimulated and helped me refine much of the thinking found here.

Many colleagues have read and critically reacted to different portions of this book over the years of its development. They include Lewis Aron, David Brand, Peter Casey, Harold Cook, Emmanuel Ghent, Ruth Gruenthal, Susan Knapp, Joseph Newirth, Susan Robertson, Dennis Schulman, and Charles Spezzano. I want to express particular thanks to Margaret Black, Philip Bromberg, Jay Greenberg, and John Schmerler, all of whom read numerous versions of these ideas and cared enough to tell me when they thought I was barking up the wrong tree. I also want to express deep gratitude to Merton Gill, who repeatedly and incisively challenged this material, and in whose own work I have found a deep passion for ideas and an intellectual integrity which has served as inspiration for me.

Contents

Relational Concepts in Psychoanalysis

Introduction

The "Preliminary Communication" coauthored by Freud and Breuer in 1893 is generally considered the first truly "psychoanalytic" publication; thus, the history of psychoanalytic ideas now spans nearly a century. The first half of that century was dominated by Freud's fertile and monumental genius. Once the early collaboration with Breuer was ruptured, Freud seems to have cherished the solitary development of his ideas, his "splendid isolation" (1914a, p. 22), and even after he had attracted a vast following, he was only minimally affected by the contributions of others. No comparable intellectual discipline in our culture has been so nearly single-handed. Freud's psychoanalytic theory clearly represents one of our culture's inspiring individual intellectual achievements.

The theory of instinctual drive is the conceptual framework which houses all of Freud's ideas: theoretical postulates, clinical insights, technical recommendations. Freud characterized the drive theory as part of his "metapsychology"—which suggests that it is the most abstract level of his theorizing, the furthest from clinical experience. Nevertheless, it would be a mistake to think of Freud's metapsychology as merely of philosophical interest, separate and detachable from clinical theory, capable of being peeled back to reveal clinical concepts undisturbed within. As Kuhn (1962) has demonstrated in his history of scientific revolutions, paradigmatic frameworks and broad models shape the entire scientific enterprise which operates within them. Freud's drive-theory metapsychology informs and impacts in varying and complex ways on all areas of his thinking, from the most abstract speculations to the most minute clinical observations.

Freud's drive theory provides a powerful and compelling vision of human nature and experience. We are portrayed as a conglomeration of asocial, physical tensions represented in the mind by urgent sexual and aggressive wishes pushing for expression. We live in the clash between these wishes and the secondary, more superficial claims of social reality; our very thought itself is derivative of, a transformation of, these primitive, bestial energies. Mind is composed of complex and elegant compromises between the expression of impulses and the defenses which control and channel them. Classical analytic inquiry entails an uncovering and eventual renunciation of infantile instinctual impulses. In its first half-century this vision dominated the generation and development of psychoanalytic ideas.

Despite Freud's remarkable achievement, the past several decades have witnessed a revolution in the history of psychoanalytic ideas. Recent psychoanalytic contributions have been informed by a different vision: *we have been living in an essentially post-Freudian era.* Yet because of the enormous shadow cast by Freud's genius and authority, and because theory has been developed by so many different authors (who generally do not acknowledge the contributions of others), it is often not appreciated how different from Freud's initial vision psychoanalysis has become. The "big ideas," the most important influences on theory building and clinical practice, have not come from within the drive model, which Freud himself elaborated to a considerable complexity and refinement. The most creative and influential contributions derive from what Greenberg and I (1983) have termed the relational model, an alternative perspective which considers relations with others, not drives, as the basic stuff of mental life. Some of these contributions have come from authors who maintain a general allegiance to the drive model, but have developed perspectives which largely supplant it (Mahler, for example). Some have come from authors who write in drive-model language but redefine all the key terms and rederive all the basic structural components, resulting in a vision which is relational in all major respects (for instance, Winnicott and Loewald). Other significant contributions have come from authors who have explicitly broken with drive theory (as Sullivan, Fairbairn, and Kohut).

The relational-model theories which have dominated the psychoanalytic thinking of the past several decades are varied and heterogeneous—they differ from one another in many significant respects. Yet they draw on a common vision quite different from Freud's and, taken together, have changed the nature of psychoanalytic inquiry. We are portrayed not as a conglomeration of physically based urges, but as being shaped by and inevitably embedded within a matrix of relationships with other people, struggling both to maintain our ties to others and to differentiate ourselves from them. In this vision the basic unit of study is not the individual as a separate entity whose desires clash with an external reality, but an interactional field within which the individual arises and struggles to make contact and to articulate himself. *Desire* is experienced always *in the context of relatedness,* and it is that context which defines its meaning. Mind is composed of relational configurations. The person is comprehensible only within this tapestry of relationships, past and present. Analytic inquiry entails a participation in, and an observation, uncovering, and transformation of, these relationships and their internal representations. In this perspective the figure is always *in* the tapestry, and the threads of the tapestry (via identifications and introjections) are always in the figure.

MANY CONTEMPORARY authors retain the term "drive" (or "instinct") but alter its meaning to enable them to employ and develop relational-model concepts (Winnicott and Loewald, for instance). This tends to confuse efforts to ascertain what of Freud's understanding has been preserved and what has been fundamentally changed. Further, much of the rhetoric within psychoanalytic controversies involves what are essentially disputes over language, in which different words are embraced or vilified, depending on one's political persuasion: "drive," "interpersonal," "intrapsychic," "social," and so on.

This book is based on the belief that there is a fundamental distinction between *Freud's* drive theory and the major trends within *contemporary* psychoanalytic thinking (some of which retain the language of "drive"). Freud views mind as fundamentally monadic; something inherent, wired in, prestructured, is pushing from within. Mind for Freud emerges in the form of endogenous pressures. Relational-model theories view mind as fundamentally dyadic and *interactive*; above all else, mind seeks contact, engagement with other minds. Psychic organization and structures are built from the patterns which shape those interactions.

These two theoretical perspectives are not discretely dichotomous—they overlap considerably. Persuasive monadic theories like Freud's are not naively sollipsistic. They regard mind as seeking expression *within* an environment, and inherent pressures as necessarily finding gratifications, impasses, channelization, in interactions within that environment. The resolution of the conflicts created by these internal pressures may include selective internalization of the interpersonal world through identifications, introjects, and so on.

Similarly, relational theories are not naively environmental. Experience is understood as structured through interaction, but the individual brings a great deal to that interaction: temperament, bodily events and processes, physiological responsivity, distinctive patterns of regulation and sensitivity. Within the relational model, psychological meanings are not regarded as universal and inherent; bodily experiences and events are understood as evoked potentials which derive meaning from the way they become patterned in interaction with others. From this viewpoint *what is inherent is not necessarily formative;* it does not push and shape experience, but is itself shaped by the relational context. The mind employs what anatomy and physiology supply, but the *meanings* of those body parts and processes, the underlying structure of experience and its deeper meanings, derive from relational patterns—their role in the struggle to establish and maintain connections with others.

The distinction between the drive model and the relational model is *not* equivalent to the distinction between biology and culture, or between the body and the social environment. Both the drive model and the relational model contain considerations of biology *and* culture, the body *and* the social environment. What is different is the way they conceive of the interaction between these factors. In the drive model, "anatomy is destiny" (Freud, 1924b, p. 178); social factors are shaped by inherent, underlying drive pressures. In the relational model, biology and interpersonal processes constitute perpetual cycles of mutual influence. Human evolution has generated an animal whose need for and enormous capacity for cultural development redefines his very biological nature. The body houses mental processes, which develop in a social context, which in turn defines the subjective meanings of body parts and processes, which further shape mental life. Escher's image *Drawing*

Hands, which serves as the frontispiece of this book, vividly captures the nature of such a cycle of mutual influence. Each hand is both the product and the creator of the other. Human biology and human relatedness both generate and are the creation of each other.

The distinction between a monadic theory of mind and an interactive, relational theory of mind (sometimes characterized as a one-person rather than a two-person psychology; see Rickman, 1957; Modell, 1984) is crucial in sorting out differences among psychoanalytic concepts, in defining what is *new* in contemporary theorizing and how it differs from what has gone before. What these theories are called does not matter much; what does matter is the underlying premise, the operational metaphor of mind beneath the language. Although all psychoanalytic theories contain both monadic and dyadic features, each theory necessarily breaks on one side or the other of this dichotomy in assigning the source of the structuralization of experience, the shaping of meaning, and this choice is fundamental. Either interaction is viewed in the context of the expression of preformed forces or pressures, *or* mental content is viewed as expressed and shaped in the context of the establishment and maintenance of connections with others. Psychological meaning is either regarded as inherent and brought to the relational field, *or* as negotiated through interaction. The various relational-model theories (often employing different terminologies) draw on a common interactive vision, leading to an approach to virtually every domain of psychoanalytic theorizing different from that provided by Freud's drive theory.

IF SO MANY of the most influential thinkers in contemporary psychoanalysis draw on and are developing similar, essentially compatible visions, why is there so little apparent consensus? Why has psychoanalysis in recent years seemed to spawn one theoretical system after another, each with its own language, devotional following, and deep conviction of proceeding on the only true path? In fact, psychoanalysis appears to be more diffuse and divided than any comparable intellectual or professional discipline. The major problem lies in the claim of each proponent of the new model to sole ownership of the new paradigm.

It is difficult to think of another figure in the Western intellectual tradition who has had more impact than Freud on the way people have come to understand themselves. Only Darwin and Marx seem to have had comparable influence. Further, Freud had so much to say about so many things. The twenty-three volumes (plus index) which contain his writings are breathtaking in their range, often scintillating in their argumentation, and lovely in their literary style. Therefore, the abandonment of Freud's drive theory creates an enormous conceptual vacuum. Most of the would-be successors to the architect of drive theory have attempted to fill this void by substituting new systems of their own design. None of these models, in itself, has been up to the task—each has been stretched too thin. There is not enough substance to fill the same space or attain the depth and scope of Freud's drive theory. The result has been a series of partial solutions, each important in its own right and perhaps closer to the clinical data than classical drive theory, but not as rich, comprehensive, or compelling to large numbers of practicing analysts.

Each of the rival would-be successors tends to portray his own work as a singular line of descent, and any acknowledgment of closely related contemporary authors is only minimal. Each major theorist establishes a new perspective around a particular issue, which he sees as *the* crucial failure of classical theory. The treatment of this new issue then becomes the rallying point for a new metatheory; all other critiques of classical theory are seen as incomplete, not quite radical enough, ventures in the same direction. In the 1930s and 1940s, Sullivan, Melanie Klein, Fromm, Fairbairn, and Horney took scant notice of the areas of striking overlap in their efforts. More recently, Winnicott, Mahler, Loewald, Kohut, Gedo, and Schafer, when they do remark on the closely related work of the others, do so by regarding it as a series of incomplete way stations on the road to the final destination—their own system.

Thus, much of the apparent fragmentation of the discipline known as psychoanalysis is an artifact of its history. Psychoanalysis was created by an individual intellect of towering genius. Freud's system, like all intellectual constructions, has been inevitably outgrown, but the singularity of his achievement became the model followed by his successors, who tend to present their contributions not as partial replacements or solutions to particular features which Freud addressed, but as alternative, comprehensive systems. Consequently, they overlook the similarity and compatibility of their efforts and call for exclusive loyalty, which is neither compelling nor necessary.

A second and closely related historical cause of the apparent fragmentation within psychoanalytic theories is the heavily political nature of the psychoanalytic movement from the very beginning of Freud's relationships with his early followers. Freud saw psychoanalysis not just as an intellectual discipline and a method of treatment, but as a highly provocative and personally disturbing set of truths about human nature. With considerable justification, he rated himself third (chronologically) behind Copernicus and Darwin as the bearer of humbling tidings to mankind. Based on his own experience with patient resistance, he anticipated massive general opposition to psychoanalytic ideas and methods.

Thus, from early on, Freud regarded psychoanalysis as a "movement"; its successes and failures, its adherents and detractors, were thought about in a quasi-religious, quasi-political frame of reference. It was not without justification that psychoanalysts began to feel that psychoanalytic concepts could only be evaluated meaningfully by the initiated— those having undergone a personal analysis. A change of conviction in those who had already been analyzed became prima facie evidence of "unanalyzable" psychopathology. It was a hallmark of Freud's genius that he was extraordinarily willing to change his mind, and many of the most fruitful avenues of his theory followed the realization that a prior direction had been misguided. Freud's openness toward changes in his own mind, however, did not extend to a toleration of change in the minds of his followers. And with Freud's death, the possibility of any *openly acknowledged* shifts in basic premises within traditional Freudian circles was virtually eliminated.

Thus, intellectual beliefs tend to become blurred with accusations and counteraccusations hurled in both directions by loyalists and dissidents. A key factor in these controversies is the designation "psychoanalytic." Freud characterized different features of his theory at different times as being the essence of psychoanalysis. Nevertheless, those who broke from orthodoxy, even if they retained a belief in many of Freud's ideas, were accused of no longer representing psychoanalysis. The claim to direct conceptual lineage to Freud became the psychoanalytic equivalent of possession of the royal scepter, and many psychoanalytic papers begin by claiming that some obscure passage from Freud's opus reveals a hidden meaning suggesting Freud's belief in whatever argument the author then proceeds to make. Political loyalties and fears have had a major impact on the way in which innovative psychoanalytic concepts are presented and positioned, often obscuring both their distance from classical psychoanalytic thought and their similarities to one another. A major consequence has been widespread failure to grasp how compatible many of the different contemporary psychoanalytic schools are and how far they have moved from the basic premises of Freud's drive theory.

The traditions that have been most important to me in terms of contributing to a comprehensive conceptual framework based on the premise of interaction are interpersonal psychoanalysis, British-school object-relations theories, and various psychologies of the self (including existential psychoanalysis). These different schools, I will demonstrate in the chapters that follow, complement one another in interesting and useful ways. It will become apparent that I do not regard any of these traditions as complete or sufficient in its own right; each has been both enhanced and constrained by its history and particular perspective, which is what makes it compelling to draw on them in an integrated fashion. I regard them as valuable correctives for one another.

Taken together, these traditions make it possible to view all psychodynamic phenomena within a *multifaceted relational matrix* which takes into account self-organization, attachments to others ("objects"), interpersonal transactions, and the active role of the analysand in the continual re-creation of his subjective world. The basic features of the integrated relational approach described in the following chapters were not constructed from these theoretical traditions and then applied to clinical work. Rather, they were *discovered* in the process of doing analysis, supervision, and teaching. I began to realize that what I had gained from these traditions had infused my clinical work and understanding, my own practice of analytic inquiry, in an integrated fashion.

Freud's opus frequently has been neatly bifurcated into his *clinical theory* and his *metapsychology* (in which the drive theory plays the central role). Although, as we shall see, this distinction is often trickier and less easily drawn than one might suppose, many of Freud's clinical insights *can* be disentangled from drive-theory metapsychology and *translated,* recast within the context of a relational matrix. Freud opened hitherto unexplored paths that allowed the exploration of unconscious processes, identifications, and powerful conflictual passions within dyadic and triangular familial constellations. Much of Freud's wisdom is the stock-in-trade of all practicing analysts, no matter where they position themselves vis-à-vis drive theory, and many of Freud's contributions and those of contemporary "Freudians" (particularly Loewald and Schafer) find a prominent place in the synthesis developed here.

*   *   *

I USE the term "relational matrix" in an effort to transcend the unfortunate tendency to dichotomize concepts like interpersonal relations and "object" relations, or the interpersonal and the intrapsychic, as if a focus on either side necessarily implies a denial or deemphasis of the other. I do not believe that interpersonal interactions are merely an "enactment" of a more psychologically fundamental world of internal object relations or "representations"; nor do I believe that subjective experience is merely a recording of actual interpersonal transactions. *The most useful way to view psychological reality is as operating within a relational matrix which encompasses both intrapsychic and interpersonal realms.* The mind operates with motivations concerning self-regulation as well as regulation of the relational field. Like Escher's *Drawing Hands,* the interpersonal and the intrapsychic realms create, interpenetrate, and transform each other in a subtle and complex manner.

Drive theory, in conceiving of mind as essentially monadic, has necessarily tended to minimize the generation of personal meaning through interaction. What is crucial is what is given a priori and the individual's internal psychological economy; interpersonal relations provide the raw material for the inborn drives and the universal, primal fantasies to shape experience according to the constitutional design of the drives, their pressures and their restraints. Relational-model theories most closely linked to drive theory (Freudian ego psychology, self psychology), even when they drop the concept of drive itself, often preserve some aspects of this monadic view of mind. They tend to retain a stress on the "self" dimension of the relational matrix. Even though they derive the self from interaction, once established, the self is often viewed as existing and operating more or less independently of interactions with others. Thus, these theories emphasize self-organization, ego functions, homeostatic regulation of affects, developmental needs, a true or nuclear self, and so on. This version of the relational model, in which *past* interactions are regarded as formative but *present* interactive properties of mind are minimized, underlies what has been termed the developmental-arrest concept of the therapeutic action of psychoanalysis.

The most important contribution of both Fairbairn's theory of object relations and American interpersonal psychoanalysis has been to add a deeper and more consistent consideration of the "other," both as an actual interactional presence (in interpersonal psychoanalysis) and as an intrapsychic, internal presence (in the British school). I regard this emphasis not as an alternative to considerations of self-organization and internal needs, but as providing a more fully interactive, broader context for understanding self-organization and the individual's psychic economy. Thus, one of the larger aims of this book is to develop a broad perspective on problems of psychoanalytic theory and technique, which offers a *third option* to the drive model and the developmental-arrest model.

The drive model places great importance on *conflict,* between instinctual impulses and defenses, and, in the later structural theory, among the psychical agencies of id, ego, and superego. The developmental-arrest model tends to deemphasize the importance of conflict, stressing instead the expression of developmental needs and environmental provisions understood to be prerequisites for psychological growth. The third option, developed in these chapters, is a *relational-conflict model.* Like the drive model, it regards the central psychodynamic struggle in human experience as involving conflicts among powerful desires, wishes, and fears. Yet, like the developmental-arrest model, it considers the basic ingredients of mind to be relational configurations, not drive derivatives. In the relational-conflict model, the antagonists in the central psychodynamic conflicts are relational configurations; the inevitable conflictual passions within any single relationship; and the competing claims, necessarily incompatible, among different significant relationships and identifications.

THE PARTS of this book are organized in pairs of chapters—the first chapter is largely theoretical; the second, largely clinical.

Part One presents the various strategies, options, and terminology which relational-model theorists have developed in their efforts to establish relatedness as the primary psychological unit of emotional life and to position relational concepts vis-à-vis prior tradition.

Part Two explores Freud's drive model and its limitations by considering the nature of sexuality, the keystone of the classical theory of mind as structured from within through the expression of internal forces. According to this view, since we are in fact animals, our bestial nature, honed over millennia of evolution for purposes of survival, is wired into our very bodies, pushing for expression. Yet if one begins with the premise that the basic thrust of mind is engagement, and that psychological meaning is not provided a priori in bodily urges but shaped by inevitably conflictual patterns of interaction, the domain of sexuality is understood quite differently. The intense physiology and phenomeno-

logical power of sexuality as evoked potentials within intensely conflictual relational contexts make bodily and sexual experiences the
medium par excellence for the experience of self in interaction with
others.

Part Three explores the way in which developmental "history" and
images of the "baby" are used in classical drive theory and the new
variety of "infantilism" that has emerged within the developmental-
arrest model. Whereas Freud regarded sexuality as made up of *phylogenic*
vestiges pressing for release, modern developmental theorists regard
unmet infantile longings and relational needs as *ontogenic* vestiges pressing for release. This has resulted in a skewing of the relational matrix, in
both analytic theory and technique, in a way that underemphasizes
conflict, overemphasizes the emergence of the past (especially the earliest relationship between mother and child), and portrays the analysand
as essentially passive.

Part Four explores psychoanalytic approaches to the key theoretical
and technical problems concerning the nature of narcissism. I consider
the monadic premise in both the traditional approach to narcissistic
illusion as defense and the developmental-arrest approach to illusion as
the vital core of the self. I then develop a more balanced, relational
conflict perspective, in theory and technique, which takes into account
both the defensive and the growth-enhancing features of illusion.
Viewed from an interactive perspective, compulsive illusions are understood as operating within a relational matrix to preserve attachments to
old objects and repetitive interpersonal patterns.

Part Five explores continuity (the regeneration of the analysand's
relational world) and the nature of analytic change. I consider the
deterministic assumptions underlying all psychoanalytic theories, and
the existential critique of these assumptions. I then explore and extend
contemporary contributions, which enable us to transcend this dialectic
by regarding the relational matrix as something both experienced and
loyally constructed. In the final chapter the clinical implications of this
perspective are more fully developed, and a sketch of an interactional,
"relational-conflict" model of the therapeutic action of psychoanalysis is
presented and contrasted to the classical drive model and the developmental-arrest model. The differences in understanding the nature of the
psychoanalytic situation and the contributions of the participants highlight the contrast between a view of the mind as monadic and a view of
the mind as interactive.

Clinical examples of varying length and complexity appear throughout the book. The more extended examples are not drawn from work with any single patient. To preserve confidentiality, the cases are disguised composites of work (my own and that of colleagues) with different analysands having similar psychodynamic configurations and posing similar theoretical questions and technical problems. This material is offered not as evidence, but for purposes of illustration—to demonstrate what the theoretical concepts and integration presented here look like when applied to actual clinical material.

The larger purpose of this book is to demonstrate that current traditions of psychoanalytic thought are not isolated conceptual islands but are, in principle, often integratable, and that it is interesting, clinically useful, and fun to integrate them. A great deal of confusion is generated by the claim that all contemporary psychoanalytic innovations are merely extensions of drive theory, which they are not; similarly, much precious opportunity for cross-fertilization is lost in the claim that one among the various contemporary schools of thought has exclusive rights of descent, which it does not. The maturity of psychoanalysis as a discipline depends on our recognition of how far we have come, and the exciting interplay among the routes we have taken.

Part One

Boundaries

THEORIES are not facts, observations, or descriptions—they are organizational schemes, ways of arranging and shaping facts, observations, and descriptions. Why choose, the eclectic asks? Why not retain all theories as potentially useful? Adding observations enriches one's vision; adding new ways of arranging them may or may not, depending on the compatibility of the organizational schemes. Mixing theories can result in greater richness, subtlety, and complexity, or in a jarring assembly of fragments, in partial perspectives which do not lend themselves to a cohesive, larger vision. Choice, although difficult, is sometimes essential.

In the first chapter I establish the "relational matrix" as an organizing framework for assembling and integrating apparently diverse relational-model theories into a fuller, more comprehensive perspective. In Chapter 2 I consider whether drive theory too can be contained within this framework. Freud's development of drive theory and his struggle (and those of contemporary theorists) to locate relational concepts within the drive model sheds light on what is at stake in the choice of whether or not to combine the drive and relational models.

*It could be said that with human beings there can be no separation,
only a threat of separation.* ·   —D. W. WINNICOTT

1 The Relational Matrix

Psychoanalytic theories of the past several decades have undergone what
Kuhn, in his depiction of the evolution of theories in the natural sciences, calls a paradigm shift. The very boundaries around the subject
matter of psychoanalysis have been redrawn, and that broad reframing
has had profound implications for both theory and clinical practice.
*Mind has been redefined from a set of predetermined structures emerging
from inside an individual organism to transactional patterns and internal
structures derived from an interactive, interpersonal field.*

As a social theory of mind, the relational model is by no means the
exclusive province of psychoanalytic theorizing. Interpersonal theory
and object-relations theory are part of a larger movement in the direction of social theories of mind in several closely related disciplines.
Although a full substantiation of this claim would lead us too far astray,
let us briefly consider two parallel shifts.

Late-nineteenth-century and early-twentieth-century anthropologists
assumed that humans evolved at a single point, all of a piece. It was
thought that physical attributes, most notably the human brain, evolved
because they were adaptive for physical survival, and that this increased
cognitive capacity then allowed the possible development of culture and
other features of social interchange. In the last several decades, mostly
because of recent fossil discoveries, we have come to believe that various
human attributes evolved sequentially over time, and that cultural rela-

17

tions are not just a *consequence* of increased brain size, but a major factor in *selecting* for increased brain size. That is, protohumans gradually became involved in social interchanges such as sharing, mutual sensitivity, perhaps empathy, and so on, and these social skills provided a selective advantage which made larger brains more adaptive. As Clifford Geertz put it:

> In a sense the brain was selected by culture. It is not that the human brain came first and culture, or rather man's capacity for culture, emanated from it; and this carries the additional implication that the human brain probably could not effectively function outside of culture, that it would not work very well if indeed it would work at all. (in Miller, 1983, p. 195)

Human beings did not evolve and then enter into social and cultural interactions; the human mind is, in its very origins and nature, a social product.

A very similar shift has taken place in the field of linguistics. Earlier theories regarded language as essentially separable from and secondary to experience. The individual lives in a world of experience, which is then translated into language as a social medium and vehicle of interaction. The separability of language from experience is now generally questioned; experience is understood to be structured *through* language, making experience essentially and unavoidably social and interactive in nature. Preverbal experiences developmentally antedate the emergence of language, and nonverbal communication can be extremely important in adult relationships. Once a semiotic matrix is established, both preverbal and nonverbal dimensions of experience can be retrieved, experienced, and expressed only within a socially shaped system of linguistic meanings.

> The hallmark of the "linguistic revolution" of the twentieth century, from Saussure and Wittgenstein to contemporary literary theory, is the recognition that meaning is not simply something "expressed" or "reflected" in language: it is actually *produced* by it. It is not as though we have meanings, or experiences, which we then proceed to cloak with words; we can only have the meanings and experiences in the first place because we have a language to have them in. What this suggests, moreover, is that our experience as individuals is social to its roots; for there can be no such thing as a private language, and to imagine a language is to imagine a whole form of social life. (Eagleton, 1983, p. 60)

The relational model within psychoanalysis is a social theory of mind in a similar sense. Sullivan and Fairbairn, its purest representatives, felt that Freud had established the wrong unit for study of emotional life by focusing on the individual mind, the psychic apparatus, rather than on the interactional field. Freud, like the nineteenth-century anthropologist and the nineteenth-century linguist, portrayed the human being with mental content outside of and prior to social experience. Meaning is inherent in man's physiology, his biological equipment. Thus, the individual mind has a priori content, which seeks expression within the larger social environment, either in absorbing the culture, learning a public rather than a private language, or in taming and channeling drives. For relational-model theorists, as for the modern anthropologist and the modern linguist, the individual mind is a *product* of as well as an interactive participant in the cultural, linguistic matrix within which it comes into being. Meaning is not provided a priori, but derives from the relational matrix. The relational field is constitutive of individual experience.

In the more radical statements of the relational position, the very notion of a single mind as a meaningful unit for study is called into question. From the earliest days of infancy the individual is in continual interaction with others; his very experience is in fact built up out of these interactions. The representation of self which each of us forms is a secondary construction superimposed upon this more fundamental and fluid interactional reality. "We organize our acquaintance with the world," Sullivan suggests, "in order to maintain necessary or pleasant functional activity within the world with which, whether the objects be manageable or unmanageable, remote or immediate, one has to maintain communal existence—however unwittingly" (1940, p. 34). Similarly, Stern's synthesis of infancy research leads him to the view that "the infant's states of consciousness and activity are ultimately socially negotiated states" (1985, p. 104). Furthermore, "the infant's life is so thoroughly social that most of the things the infant does, feels and perceives occur in differing kinds of relationships . . . In fact, because of memory, we are rarely alone, even (perhaps especially) during the first half-year of life . . . The notion of self-with-other as a subjective reality is thus almost pervasive" (p. 118).

Establishing the relationship as the basic unit of study does not eliminate the "nature" in contrast to the "nurture" dimension of things. On the contrary, it makes it possible to view nature and nurture less dichotomously. Social relations are not regarded as a secondary addition, an overlay upon more basic and primary biological functions such as sexuality and aggression. Social relations are regarded as themselves biologically rooted, genetically encoded, fundamental motivational processes. Thus, sexuality and aggression are understood not as preformed instincts with inherent meanings, which impinge upon the mind, but as powerful responses, mediated physiologically, generated *within* a biologically mandated relational field and therefore deriving their meaning from that deeper relational matrix.

None of the major relational theorists regards the child as a blank slate onto which are imposed external events and qualities of significant others. Early relationships, like later relationships, are multiple and complex. They are not simply registered, but experienced *through* physiological response patterns, constitutional features of temperament, sensitivities, and talents, and worked over, digested, broken down, recombined, and designed into the new, unique patterns which comprise the individual life. The work of Bowlby and a great many of the data from infancy research suggest that relationships are best understood not as wholly externally derived, but as grounded in the genetics and physiology of human experience and therefore transcending the nature-nuture dichotomy. The study of cognitive development, the ways in which infants and children think and organize experience, continues to yield increasing understanding of the ways in which early relational experience is processed and reorganized.

Why are relations with others the very stuff of human experience? What is the nature of personal relatedness? Why are we so much entangled with other people? Why are our earliest relationships with others so crucial that we are actually composed of these relationships—"precipitates," as Freud (1923) put it, of our earliest attachments?

There is no consensus on these questions; the past several decades in the history of psychoanalytic ideas have been characterized by exploration of a variety of possible answers. The political heterogeneity of the field results from the fact that these avenues of theory building have been regarded as unrelated, or perhaps mutually exclusive. Their conceptual interfaces, their rich compatibilities, however, are actually quite striking. To illustrate this overlap, I consider some of the major relational-model theorists, neither chronologically nor in terms of political groupings, but in terms of conceptual angle, the manner in which they establish relational primacy within human experience. The three basic strategies into which most relational-model theorizing can be grouped represent different angles of approach to this common puzzle—the relational nature of human experience. In what follows, I consider these various efforts not in the fullness of their argumentation and evidence, which would require a volume in its own right, but in an effort to highlight the key premises and strategies and to explore their interpenetrability. I have made no effort to be comprehensive or representative of the entire range of analytic literature; I have chosen the theories that are most influential or illustrate most clearly a particular conceptual strategy.

Relational by Design

The first general strategy for addressing the question of the origins and motivations of personal relatedness might be characterized by the answer, *because we are built that way*. People are constructed in such a fashion that they are inevitably and powerfully drawn together, this reasoning goes, wired for intense and persistent involvements with one another. This strategy has been developed in various forms, differing in their levels of abstraction and the kinds of mechanisms proposed.

Bowlby's concept of "attachment" represents an extended attempt to place human relatedness on a primary footing of its own. Bowlby was concerned with preserving a biologically rooted explanation for motivation and, like Freud, draws heavily on Darwinian theory as a frame of reference. Yet Bowlby felt Freud had construed the baby's built-in survival mechanisms too narrowly. The infant's survival is contingent on more than just specific physical needs like eating, temperature regulation, and so on. For the infant to survive, the mother's more or less constant proximity and attention is necessary—the infant's *need for the mother* is the most important, pressing need, as a precondition for the satisfaction of all other needs. Therefore, argues Bowlby, the infant is powerfully drawn to and involved with the mother from the very start. Much as the young of other species at an early "critical period" become forever imprinted on their caretaker in a powerful, automatic, and irreversible fashion, the human infant intensely and automatically attaches itself to its caretaker, both behaviorally and emotionally. The mother need not *do* anything in particular. She need not earn her importance through gratifying the infant's needs. In effect, she simply has to be there.

Bowlby draws on ethological studies of instinctive behavior in other species to argue that species survival necessitates complex systems of behaviors, hierarchically organized through internal control and feedback mechanisms. Attachment in humans is mediated, he suggests (1969), through five component instinctive responses: sucking, smiling, clinging, crying, and following, which collectively serve to establish a powerful bond between mother and infant, ensuring the former's proximity to the latter and thus maximizing chances for survival. These responses directly mediate the child's attachment to the mother, in contrast to the traditional psychoanalytic concept of orality, which is prior to, and separate from, the later development of any affectional bonding.

Since children under the care of the mother are less vulnerable to predators and other threats to survival, Bowlby sees the child's attachment to the mother as representing an "archaic heritage," genetically encoded, from the earliest beginnings of the human species. Attachment is not, as in the drive model, derived from more basic biological needs; attachment is itself a basic biological need, wired into the species as fundamentally as is nest-building behavior in a bird.

Bowlby (1969, 1973, 1975) draws on a wide range of empirical evidence, both animal studies and observations of the effects of separation on children, to support his claim that attachment is primary in its own right, rather than becoming established secondarily through the gratification of physical needs such as orality. Some of the most dramatic evidence, however, for the biological, physiological, and psychological primacy of the early relation of the child to its caretakers has emerged from another field entirely—infancy research.*

If personal relatedness were a vicissitude of more basic drive processes, the infant would necessarily have to *learn* to relate to the mother. Mechanisms for need gratification (feeding mechanisms, sucking reflexes, and so on) would be wired in, but the infant would only slowly become aware that needs were being satisfied by an external human figure, who would only then become interesting in her own right. From this perspective, that of the drive model, personal relatedness is less "natural" than drive pathways, social relations being an overlay necessitated by the exigencies of reality. But over the past two decades the increasingly sophisticated field of infancy research has yielded an im-

---

* A great deal of contemporary psychoanalytic thinking about infants derives from empirical studies of mothers and babies. Although much of this research is very persuasive, I am not presenting it *as fact;* for reasons which will become apparent in subsequent chapters, I would consider it a mistake to do so. Current thinking about infants, like all psychoanalytic ideas, is a blend of facts and theories and is presented here as an example of a way of thinking, a conceptual strategy, not as incontrovertible truth.

pressive array of data suggesting that the infant is capable of and in fact seeks out an extremely personal kind of interrelatedness from the earliest days of life.

Contrary to the traditional image of the infant's beginning life in an autistic blur (James's "blooming, buzzing confusion") and only gradually becoming oriented to the external social world, it now appears that all of the perceptual systems of the infant are functional at birth. Further, what is most interesting to the infant, even in the moments after birth, is other human beings. The human voice is the auditory stimulus most likely to capture the infant's attention, and studies have shown that babies move in distinctive rhythms to human speech patterns (Condon and Sandler, in Tronick and Adamson, 1980, p. 137). The human face is the visual stimulus most compelling even to the newborn. A study of infants in the delivery room uncovered a preference for the visual configuration of the human face even before the newborn had seen real human faces (that is, without surgical masks; Goren, in Tronick and Adamson, 1980, pp. 59–60). For the first several weeks of life, the infant's eyes converge not immediately in front of him, as one would expect if feeding at the breast were the major, predetermined object of his concern, but eight inches from his face, the distance of the mother's face in the normal nursing posture (Stern, 1977, p. 36). Observers are continually impressed with the quantity and the complexity of the infant's interactions with other people, both in response to their initiative and as actively initiated by the baby himself. "Very clearly then, by 3 months at least, the infant is well equipped with a large repertoire of behaviors to engage and disengage his caregivers. All of his behaviors—the simple motor patterns; the more complex combinations of these simple patterns into integrated units; and the patterned sequences of these units—have a strong innate predisposition" (pp. 48–49).

In addition to being active and responsive to people in general, the infant very quickly learns to discriminate the most significant people in his life from one another and from strangers. By the end of the first week, the mother's face has become a familiar perceptual gestalt, so that the mother's face obscured by a mask, or paired with a different voice, becomes disturbing (Tronick and Adamson, 1980, p. 141). By the eighth day he can discriminate pads soaked with his mother's milk from pads soaked with the milk of other nursing women, and he prefers the smell of his own mother. By four weeks the baby moves hands and feet in distinctive patterns, one for the mother, a different one for the father.

Lichtenberg, in reviewing this research, concludes, "Study after study documents the neonate's preadapted potential for direct interaction—human to human—with the mother" (1983, p. 6). The phrase "preadapted potential" is crucial here. The evidence seems overwhelming that the human infant does not *become* social through learning or conditioning, or through an adaptation to reality, but that the infant is programmed to be social. Relatedness is not a means to some other end (tension reduction, pleasure, or security); the very nature of the infant draws him into relationship. In addition, relatedness seems to be rewarding in itself. Babies seek human contact, and many studies have shown that simple human contact or the opportunity to observe human activity is itself a powerful inducement for infants to solve puzzles or do work of various sorts.

This line of infancy research complements Bowlby's theory of attachment by uncovering and charting some of the built-in, physiological equipment and newborn-to-mother patterning which mediate attachment. Bowlby's hypotheses derive from data on separation and psychopathology in older children and adults, and macrocosmic considerations concerning species survival; the infant research provides a microcosmic analysis of the infant's capacities for, intricate mechanisms for, and powerful interest in interactions with other people.

Is it not true that Bowlby and theorists drawing on infancy research (perhaps all relational model authors) are in effect establishing "attachment" as a "drive," with the same sort of inherent properties as Freud's "libido"? Yes and no. Of course, any positing of attachment or relatedness as primary suggests that it has motivational properties *within* the organism and might meaningfully be considered a "drive." But because "attachment" is by definition interactional, this is a concept of motivation very different from Freud's "drive." The latter presupposes motives and meanings in the individual a priori, in the tensions in bodily tissues themselves, which are brought to the interaction and which shape the interaction. Bowlby's motive of attachment and the built-in patterns of interaction described by infancy researchers propel the individual to seek *contact qua contact*, interaction in and for itself, not contact as a means of gratifying or channeling something else. This reversal of means and ends (captured in Fairbairn's slogan, "Libido is not pleasure-seeking but object-seeking") is crucial. *Who* the other is, *what* the other does, and *how* the other regards what is going on become much more important.

The other is not simply a vehicle for managing internal pressures and states; interactive exchanges with and ties to the other become the fundamental psychological reality itself. As we shall see in subsequent chapters, this difference has major implications for all facets of psychoanalytic theorizing.

Sullivan's theoretical perspective represents another variant of the principle that humans are inherently structured in relational terms, although his focus is not on genetic coding or perceptual capabilities, but on a theoretical perspective which highlights the way human needs interact and become intertwined with one another in the patterning of human experience.

One of the chief impediments to our self-understanding, Sullivan feels, is our tendency to think of ourselves in concrete, reified terms. People "have" a personality, this way of thinking goes, they "are" a collection of traits or characteristics which they carry around, as if actually located inside them, from situation to situation—like a door-to-door salesman revealing the same product at one home after the next. For Sullivan this way of thinking obscures the extent to which people are responsive to, and in fact take form in, situations involving other people. Human beings manifest themselves not in the same identical performance; the performance varies according to the situation, the audience, the other performers. A personality is not something one has, but something one does. Consistent patterns develop, but the patterning is not reflective of something "inside." Rather, the patterns reflect learned modes of dealing with situations and are therefore always in some sense responsive to and shaped by the situations themselves.

In Sullivan's way of thinking, people are not separate entities, but participants in interactions with actual others and with "personifications" (or "representations") of others derived from previous interactions with actual others. In short, the individual is understandable only in the context of the interpersonal field. Thus, Sullivan also sees people, from infancy through senescence, as inherently social, by design. Their very self-expression draws them into relatedness. By the time the infant has begun to be able to develop an image of himself, to reflect himself to himself, he has long since become embedded in a living web of interactions with others. His needs, his thoughts, his very sense of himself, has taken shape in the context of others' needs, thoughts, and self-understanding.

Relational by Intent

A second broad grouping of approaches to the primacy of relatedness sees human relations less in terms of wiring than of intent. We develop intense attachments because we *crave relatedness,* and this is regarded as a phenomenological fact and an irresistible clinical deduction. Patients seek and maintain relatedness at any price. Fairbairn's object-relations theory is the most developed exploration of this point of view.

Fairbairn dated the beginnings of the development of his innovative theorizing to his encounter with the puzzling phenomenon of the loyalty of abused children to their abusing parents. According to classical drive theory, people are essentially hedonistic, seeking to maximize pleasure and minimize pain. Fairbairn encountered children whose relationships with their parents were extremely painful; yet when offered alternative caretakers, they uniformly declined and expressed great devotion to their natural parents. If libido is primarily pleasure seeking, Fairbairn reasoned, libidinal objects ought to be more exchangeable.

Further reflection leads to the realization that this is a problem not just with abused children, but with psychopathology in general. Psychopathology, throughout its entire spectrum, may be defined in its broadest terms as the tendency of people to do the same painful things, feel the same unpleasant feelings, establish the same self-destructive relationships, over and over and over. How is this pattern reconcilable with the hedonistic premise of the pleasure principle? If people operate on the basis of pleasure seeking, why are unpleasant experiences, early conflicts, and traumas not simply dropped and forgotten rather than restructured so systematically and persistently throughout life?

Freud was not unmindful of this problem and struggled with several possible solutions. He spoke of the "adhesiveness" of the libido in its tenacious loyalty to early object relations, even if painful, and the "repetition compulsion," the continual re-creation of earlier traumas. Freud initially attempted to account for these phenomena *within* the framework of the pleasure principle: the suffering in psychopathology represents punishment for forbidden wishes (1900); the libido picks up "clichés" of loving, which remain attached to it throughout later life (1912b); suffering itself is inherently sensually pleasurable (1924a); and so on. Freud himself, however, considered these attempts to account for the repetition compulsion within the framework of the pleasure principle to be insufficiently persuasive, and he argued (1920a) that the repetition of painful early experiences operates "beyond the pleasure principle" and is an instinctual characteristic of mental functioning, derivative of the death instinct. This explanation has not been very persuasive to most analysts, and there have been numerous attempts since to reexplain painful repetitions *within* the pleasure principle.

FOR FAIRBAIRN, a basic shift in premises leads to a much more economical explanation, neither within nor beyond the pleasure principle. Libido is not pleasure seeking, he argues, but object seeking. The superordinate need of the child is not for pleasure or need gratification, but for an intense relationship with another person. If the caretakers provide opportunities for pleasurable experiences, pleasure is sought, not as an end in itself, but as a vehicle for interaction with others. If only painful experiences are provided, the child does not give up and look for pleasurable experiences elsewhere, but seeks the pain as a vehicle for interaction with the significant other. It is the contact, not the pleasure, which is primary. In Fairbairn's view, the central motivation in human experience is the seeking out and maintaining of an intense emotional bond with another person. If we start with this premise, the adhesiveness of early relationships and modes of gratification and the ubiquity of the painful redundancies of the repetition compulsion seem less puzzling. Painful feelings, self-destructive relationships, self-sabotaging situations, are re-created throughout life as vehicles for the perpetuation of early ties to significant others.

The child learns a mode of connection, a way into the human family, and these learned modes are desperately maintained throughout life. In some families, sensuality is the preferred mode of emotional contact; in others, it is rageful explosions; in others, depressive longing. In Fairbairn's system, it is precisely the parents' character pathology to which the child becomes most compulsively connected and which he internalizes, because it is there that he feels the parents reside emotionally. By becoming like the depressed, masochistic, or sadistic parents, he preserves a powerful bond to them. Thus, in Fairbairn's system, at the core of the repressed is not a trauma, a memory, or an impulse, but a relationship—a part of the self in close identification with a representation of the actual caretakers—which could not be contained in awareness and in continuity with other experiences of the self. Psychopathology for Fairbairn is structured around conflicts, not between drives and defenses, but concerning split loyalties to different others and to different dimensions of one's relations with others.

To abandon these bonds and entanglements is experienced as the equivalent of casting oneself off from intense human contact altogether, an impossible option. Thus, patients in analysis who are beginning to sense the possibility of living and experiencing themselves and their worlds in a different way, are generally terrified of profound isolation. To be different, even if that means being open to joyfulness and real intimacy with others, means losing ties to internal objects which have provided an enduring sense of belonging and connectedness, although mediated through actual pain and desolation.

Fairbairn regards object seeking as innate, and his approach is closely related to and complements Bowlby's notion of attachment. Bowlby portrays attachment as an automatic mechanism, the product of instinctive, reflexive behavioral subsystems, and he focuses for the most part on physical proximity; Fairbairn adds a consideration of intention and emotional presence or absence, and thereby highlights the longing, the hunger for contact and connection, that propels human relationships.

Fairbairn's concept of object seeking similarly complements Sullivan's notion of the interpersonal field. For Sullivan, the child is object related more by design than by emotional intent, drawn into relatedness by virtue of the form and nature of his various needs. The child does not *seek* caring connections with others; rather, the very structure of his needs for satisfactions and his responsiveness to anxiety in others pulls him into those connections. An intense longing for contact appears in Sullivan's scheme of development only in preadolescence, in the first truly loving relationship with the "chum," which Sullivan describes with lyric intensity, as an antidote to the warping effects of earlier relationships and the threat of isolation. Sullivan takes pains to argue that only at preadolescence does the child begin to seek intimacy and really care about others. Parents who see caring in their child's egocentricity are, Sullivan suggests, sadly if perhaps necessarily deluded. Fairbairn, on the other hand, sees this longing for connection and intimacy in the earliest relationship of the infant to the mother.

There are also striking similarities between Fairbairn's theory and the variant of interpersonal theory developed by Erich Fromm. The latter regarded the dread of social isolation as the major dynamic factor in the development of all forms of psychopathology, which he saw as regressive efforts to escape the existential rigors and terrors of the human condition. People take on cultural and familial roles and identities so as not to face the realities of their independent existence. Fairbairn's perspective, although less philosophical in language and concern, has a similar implication. The overwhelming motivational priority is entry into the human community, intense ties with others, and these are established and preserved at all cost.

Melanie Klein's concept of reparation (1935, 1940) should be noted in this context. Her focus on aggression and envy often obscures the extent to which love and gratitude also play a central role in her theorizing. The infant, Klein posits, feels a deep sense of appreciation for the good breast and the loving object, and an intense regret at the fantasized damage he fears he has caused them in his destructive, vengeful reveries. The urge for reparation expresses a longing to repair, to console, to make amends. Envy becomes such a powerful dynamic in Klein's account precisely because the uncontrollable other is so important that love and gratitude become painful.

Klein developed her concept of reparation in the context of her theoretical emphasis on constitutional forces and fantasy. However, her depiction of the struggle between gratitude and reparation on the one hand and envious spoiling and manic triumph on the other is usefully relocated and translated into the interactional matrix of Fairbairn's metapsychological framework, rooted in a consideration of parental character and actual transactions. The urge for reparation can be understood as emerging not as a reaction to fantasized damage, but to the other's real sufferings and characteristic pathology. Envious spoiling can be understood not as an excess of constitutional aggression, but as an attempt to escape from the painful position of loving and desiring a largely absent or damaged parent, or, particularly, an inconsistent parent. The central dynamic struggle throughout life is between the powerful need to establish, maintain, and protect intimate bonds with others and various efforts to escape the pains and dangers of those bonds, the sense of vulnerability, the threat of disappointment, engulfment, exploitation, and loss.

Relational by Implication

Philosophers have traditionally distinguished human from other forms of animal consciousness on the basis of its reflexivity; human beings are *self*-conscious. We develop and maintain a self-awareness, self-images, self-esteem, and these play a significant role in the way we experience and record our encounters with the external world and other people, and the choices we make throughout our lives. It is often assumed that a sense of self is easy to come by, that it unfolds maturationally or is just provided to us by experience, like our body parts or perceptual functions. But psychoanalysts have come to regard the development of a sense of self as a complex process, an intricate and multifaceted construction, that is a central motivational concern throughout life and for which we are deeply dependent on other people. Some relational-model theorists regard the establishment and preservation of a sense of identity or selfhood as *the* primary, superordinate human motivation, which also posits certain kinds of interpersonal relations, those crucial for reflexivity, as key psychological building blocks.

Two features of human consciousness contribute greatly to the difficulties involved in developing a sense of self—its temporal quality and its complexity. Human consciousness operates in time, it is a stream of thoughts, feelings, sensations, and desires in continual flux. Anything that is constantly changing is necessarily at any particular moment incomplete. As soon as you have grasped it and characterized it, it has shifted within your grasp and is now something different. This quality of ineffable, continual change has always been problematic for humankind, both historically in the evolution of cultures and developmentally in the life of each individual. Plato's theory of forms is probably the most elegant effort to establish a static superstructure, to fix an atemporal frame of reference, a world of Being outside the flow of human consciousness. But the need to establish fixed reference points is also a need within the life of each individual, to find a way of ordering experience that transcends its shifting discontinuities.

The child's gradually dawning grasp of who or what he is amid the temporal flux and complexities of consciousness is no simple process. All of the hallmarks of healthy mental life—durable and integrated self-representations, object constancy, and resilient self-esteem regulation—are slowly acquired. If experience does not just provide us with an organized mental life and reflexivity, how is it attained? According to most contemporary psychoanalytic theorists, it is attained at least in part through relationship. The child's organization of his experience is mediated through the mother's experience. Individual cognition grows out of *re*cognition, whereby the child learns to know himself, finds himself, in the mother's eyes and words. Thus, the self as a phenomenological entity is a developmental achievement. In this line of relational-model theorizing, the pursuit and maintenance of reflexive stability, a sense of self, is innate and motivationally central, and powerfully and inevitably draws us into relation with others.

This approach to the primacy of relatedness has been a central theme in Freudian ego psychology. In the work of both Mahler and Loewald, for example, the infant's ego is seen as dawning within a psychic merger with the other. For Mahler, the development of a healthy sense of self is contingent upon the mother's provision for the infant of adequate experiences of symbiotic fusion, gradual self-articulation and differentiation, and continual, periodic returns and reimmersions. (See Mahler, Pine, and Bergman, 1975.) Loewald (1960a) stresses the parental organization and processing of the child's experience, which the child gradually learns, through identifications, to do for himself. Parental secondary process, applied to the child's more fluid, primary process experience, eventually results in a secondary process of the child's own. (Bion, 1957, has characterized the mother's holding and organizing functions relative to the child's inchoate early experience in terms of the metaphor of the "container.")

The two contemporary theorists who have addressed the development of the self most directly and comprehensively (and in remarkably similar fashion) are Winnicott and Kohut.

Winnicott came to regard the establishment of a solid sense of self as the central achievement of normal early development. Some patients only *seem* to be persons, argues Winnicott. They lack an experience of themselves as real, as actually existing over time—as opposed to something fashioned de novo, differently for each interpersonal occasion. How does this happen?

Winnicott portrays the infant as becoming aware of spontaneously arising needs. The key feature of the necessary "facilitating" environment provided by the mother is her effort to shape the environment around the child's wishes, to intuit what the child wants and provide it. The infant's experience is one of scarcely missing a beat between desire and satisfaction, between the wish for the breast and its appearance, for example. The infant naturally assumes that his wishes produce the object of desire, that the breast, his blanket, in effect his entire world, is the product of his creation. The mother's provision and perfect accommodation to the infant's wish creates what Winnicott terms the moment of illusion. Thus, in the earliest months of life, Winnicott's "good-enough mother" is invisible, and it is precisely her invisibility which allows the infant the crucial megalomaniacal, solipsistic experience which Winnicott characterizes as the state of "subjective omnipotence." In his view, a relatively prolonged experience of subjective omnipotence is the foundation upon which a healthy self develops.

Early in life, says Winnicott, the infant is almost oblivious to the mother as a person; she "brings the world to the infant" and is the invisible agent of his needs. Later, the infant becomes more aware of her as a presence, but a key aspect of her role is reflecting back to the child his own appearance, his own being. The capacity to experience and hold a sense of one's own being as real depends on the mother's doing so first, mirroring back to the child who he is and what he is like. Thus, in Winnicott's system the first developmental task is the establishment of a sense of self. The caretaker must perform certain kinds of roles for this to happen, provide certain kinds of experiences.

Kohut's thinking developed along similar lines. Certain kinds of patients suffer not from conflicts concerning drives and defenses, but from deficiencies in their sense of self—experienced as brittle, lacking in cohesion or integrity, vulnerable to sudden plunges in self-esteem. Like Winnicott, Kohut moved from clinical observation to developmental questions. How does a healthy, cohesive, stable sense of self develop? How does this process get derailed? In Kohut's view, the self develops out of certain key relationships, which he terms self-object relationships, in which the parents serve not just as objects of the child's needs and desires, but as providers of certain "narcissistic" functions. Kohut's early formulations (1971) emphasized two distinct self-object functions, "mirroring" of the child's spontaneously arising grandiosity (this concept is closely related to Winnicott's notion of the parent's providing the moment of illusion), and allowing the child to idealize the parent. The sense of self as stable and valuable grows out of these "narcissistic" experiences, reasoned Kohut, in which either the child is seen as perfect by the admiring parent or the parent is seen as perfect and linked to an admiring child.

Little by little the narcissistic glow of these experiences is consolidated into a more realistic, abiding sense of self as valuable. Kohut's later formulations and those of subsequent authors within or influenced by the self-psychology tradition have emphasized the self objects' general "empathic" function, from earliest infancy on, "attuning" themselves to the child's subjective experience, resonating with it and reflecting it back. From this perspective, like Winnicott's, it is as if the child's experience comes to take on a subjective sense of reality only when it is mediated through the mother's consciousness. From the self-psychological point of view, relational issues are primary because the analysand suffering disorders of the self seeks out and uses self-objects to supply the crucial parental functions that were missed in childhood. A shaky sense of self is bolstered or a low sense of self-esteem is raised through the establishment of relationships with mirroring or idealized self objects. Thus, for Kohut, as for Winnicott, the establishment of reflexive stability is the central motivational thrust in human experience, and relations with others and the roles they play in this pursuit is the primary context for human experience.

A Multiplicity of Voices

The relational model rests on the premise that the repetitive patterns within human experience are not derived, as in the drive model, from pursuing gratification of inherent pressures and pleasures (nor, as in Freud's post-1920 understanding, from the automatic workings of the death instinct), but from a pervasive tendency to preserve the continuity, connections, familiarity of one's personal, interactional world. There is a powerful need to preserve an abiding sense of oneself as associated with, positioned in terms of, related to, a matrix of other people, in terms of actual transactions as well as internal presences.

The basic relational configurations have, by definition, three dimensions—the self, the other, and the space between the two. There is no "object" in a psychologically meaningful sense without some particular sense of oneself in relation to it. There is no "self," in a psychologically meaningful sense, in isolation, outside a matrix of relations with others. Neither the self nor the object are meaningful dynamic concepts without presupposing some sense of psychic space in which they interact, in which they do things with or to each other. These dimensions are subtly interwoven, knitting together the analysand's subjective experience and psychological world.

Theorists emphasizing *relatedness by design* have contributed tools for understanding the specific interactions which transpire between self and other, focusing not so much on either pole, but rather on *the space between them*. Thus, developmentalists such as Stern who have studied the "interpersonal world" of the infant have focused on the highly subtle interactions and mutual regulation of caretakers and babies. Similarly, interpersonal psychoanalysis tends to highlight actual transactions between the analysand and others, to make a detailed inquiry into what actually took place in early family relations, into what currently takes place between the analysand and others, and into the "here and now" perceptions and interactions in the analytic relationship. What does the analysand actually *do*? What takes place between him and actual others? The central question for the interpersonal analyst, as Levenson (1983) has put it, is What's going on around here?

Theorists emphasizing *relatedness by intent* have contributed tools for exploring and understanding the *object pole* of the relational field, the manner in which various kinds of identifications and ties to other people serve as a latticework, holding together one's personal world. Thus, Klein regards moods and self experience as determined by unconscious fantasies regarding various kinds of internal objects, and Fairbairn sees ties to "bad objects" as determining the latent structure of personality. The self is always at least implicit in these formulations. Klein's psychodynamic descriptions imply different ego states corresponding to different fates of internal objects, and Fairbairn sees particular aspects of the self fragmenting to retain specific dynamic configurations in their ties to various internal objects. Nevertheless, the focus, the clinical highlight, is on the object images themselves largely as internal presences. What are the residues of the analysand's earlier experiences with others? What does he experience, consciously and unconsciously, when he does what he does with other people?

Those theorists emphasizing *relatedness by implication* have contributed tools for exploring and understanding the *self pole* of the relational field. Thus, Winnicott focuses on the internal fragmentation and splits in self experience and the presence or absence of a sense of authenticity and reality. Kohut stresses the superordinate need of the "self" to preserve its continuity and cohesion, and the complex intrapsychic and interpersonal processes through which this is accomplished. "Others" are always at least implicit in these systems. Throughout, Winnicott emphasizes the function of the mother in providing experiences which make possible a sense of vitalization and realization, and Kohut's "self" is always embedded within and buoyed up by a supporting cast of "self objects." Nevertheless, the focus, the clinical highlight is on the nature and the subtle textures of self-reflective experience.

The process involved in the preservation of one's personal psychological world might be compared to the factors involved in maintaining the structural cohesion of the human body. To assign priority to sense of self, object ties, or patterns of interaction is like trying to decide whether it is the skin, the bones, or the musculature that preserves the body form. The sense of self, like the skin, is generally closer to the surface, nearer to consciousness, and provides a continuous surface and shape in the flow of mental life. Ties to others, like the bones, are often not visible to the naked eye but provide an underlying skeletal framework which holds experience together. Characteristic patterns of interaction, like the musculature, make possible the action in which both self experience and object relations take place. Just as the different dimensions of the physical body contribute simultaneously and interdependently to the preservation of physical existence, so these different dimensions of the relational matrix are indispensable facets of the analytic inquiry.

In this view, human beings are simultaneously self regulating and field regulating. We are concerned with both the creation and maintenance of a relatively stable, coherent sense of self out of the continual ebb and flow of perception and affect, and the creation and maintenance of dependable, sustaining connections with others, both in actuality and as internal presences. The dialectic between self-definition and connection with others is complex and intricate, with one or the other sometimes being more prominent. Self-regulatory and field-regulatory processes sometimes enhance each other and sometimes are at odds with each other, forming the basis for powerful conflicts. The intrapsychic and the interpersonal are continually interpenetrating realms, each with its own set of processes, mechanisms, and concerns.

Schafer (1983) has suggested that different theoretical traditions, like the drive model and the relational model, generate different "story lines." The various theories operating within the relational model, such as interpersonal theory, object-relations theory, and self psychology, generate what is essentially the same story line, but in different voices. These traditions regard mind as developing out of a relational matrix, and psychopathology as a product of disturbances in interpersonal relations. The *differences* among these traditions concern the various kinds of questions they pursue, based on these same fundamental assumptions. They tend to generate complementary interpretations, and the questions they pose and the answers they generate do not provide alternative visions, but instead different angles for viewing the same, consensually acknowledged scene.

A Dream

Consider the following recurring dream, reported after several years of a productive analysis.

> I am on a subway somewhere—it is very chaotic—I feel overloaded, both mentally and physically, carrying several bags and my briefcase—something catches my attention, and for a few seconds I leave my things to explore it—when I get back, the briefcase is gone—I get very angry at myself for having done this—then I feel a great terror.

The dreamer associates the sense of chaos and mental and physical overloading with the pervasive depression and masochistic entanglements in which she began treatment and with which she still struggles. The briefcase is laden with meaning. She carries around in it much that is important to her. Her briefcase represents her identity—to lose it would be terrifying. Yet she experiences herself as overburdened, heavy with excess baggage, shackled by that same identity. The part of the dream in which she goes after something that interests her is associated with the predominant theme of the analysis in the past several months— her difficulty in allowing herself to really want anything unmediated by sacrifice for or submission to another person—an inability to allow herself to spontaneously wish or desire.

This dream, somewhat typical of the middle phase of analysis, represents a central dimension of the analytic process; different ways of understanding a dream like this highlight similarities and differences between various psychoanalytic traditions. (Of course, no analyst of any persuasion would simply interpret the dream as presented without gathering many more associations; I am using it as an exercise to set out differences in approaches.)

What is happening here? The analysand reaches for something new, and something burdensome yet precious is lost. How are we to understand this? Within a relational-model perspective, the dream would be seen as representing the patient's experience of herself, and herself in relation to others, in different sorts of ways: one mediated by the oppressive, compulsive devotion through which she characteristically binds herself to others, the other more spontaneous and yet also risky and dangerous. Can she go after things she spontaneously desires, or will this isolate her from other people, cut her off with no sense of identity, no way to connect with others? From the vantage point of the relational model, this is the central question of the analysis, and change entails her slowly tolerating enough anxiety to gradually redefine herself in relation to others, the analyst included.

The analysand grew up in a family dominated by a depressed, extremely solicitous mother, who had renounced her own ambitions to devote herself to child rearing and intruded into virtually every area of her children's minds and behavior. The analysand entered adulthood with many talents and resources, but experienced the world as an oppressively dangerous place: there is a "right way" to do everything, and finding and remaining on the straight and narrow path is the only reasonable, sane way to live. Pleasure and fun were particularly suspect; devotion to others, "responsibility" and complex systems of obligations, were "sensible" and reassuring. In both the personal and professional realms, she had a knack for getting involved with powerful but extremely insecure figures, who handled their anxiety by proclaiming emphatic certainty about everything, and in particular knew exactly what would be best for her. It was her sense of bondage in these relationships and a pervasive depression and worry that brought her into treatment.

Analytic inquiry revealed how unconsciously dedicated she was to her symptoms, how the submission, depression, and worry were knit together in her experience to secure her in a somber yet familiar feeling of safety. She longed to feel free and effectual, yet became aware of how powerfully the sense of ineffectuality and stagnation drew her, "like a powerful magnetic force," away from "stepping out," from living more vibrantly. She felt bogged down in petty worries. Yet, as the analysis proceeded, she became aware of how preferable the bog was to her anticipations of what would happen if she freed herself of her anxious, depressed morass—a fear of the unknown, of total isolation from meaningful relations with others, a diffusion of her sense of self. Her surrender to the will of others and her self-imposed blinders kept her focused on the next steps. Although she struggled against her constraints, she became increasingly aware of how frightened she was to live without them.

She also approached analysis as a new version of the old pattern, a new variation of the same relational matrix. The analyst had his own ideas about what was "best" for her, but the rules of this game prohibited his opinions from being made explicit. She had to figure it out for herself, from clues and hints supplied by the analyst. Thus, directions relative to doing the "right thing" were given in secret code, and dedication to the analytic path would surely lead to a better life. Failure to follow this path would anger the analyst, whose desires for influence motivate his work, and thereby make continuation of the treatment impossible. Thus, she attempted to replace the mother's "system" with the analyst's "system" in a perpetuation of her characteristic pattern of integrating relationships and maintaining her subjective world. Continued exploration and analysis of these patterns, both within and outside the transference, had begun to yield the beginnings of different sorts of experiences and different kinds of intimacies with others. It was at this point that she reported the recurring dream.

The dream symbolizes the structure of the relational field in which the analysand lives. She is anxious and overburdened, the briefcase representing oppressive obligations and identifications. The events of the dream reflect her anxious clinging to those identifications and obligations, and her fear that neglecting them would isolate and deplete her profoundly.

Self psychologies call our attention here to the self component of the field—the sense of being overburdened, the fear of her own spontaneity, the terror of depletion. The familiar, oppressive briefcase with its obligations and demands represents the self which is seen and mirrored within her family and which, therefore, although distorted, is the only vehicle for self-recognition; the analysand equates losing her briefcase with disintegration, losing her self.

Object-relations theories call our attention to the function of the briefcase as an anchoring internal object, fragmenting and diverting her vitality away from new, richer relationships. The briefcase represents old object ties, and the analysand is reluctant to release her grip on it because to do so would entail an abandonment of her links to her overburdened, depressed parents, provoking an intolerable sense of loss, guilt, and isolation.

Interpersonal psychoanalysis calls our attention to her use of the briefcase—the way she structures situations by creating external demands and obligations to which she devotes herself as a way of diverting attention from more authentic wishes and her terror of ending up alone. The briefcase represents these well-worn ways of operating in the world, and she is reluctant to release her viselike grip on it because she is terrified to be without it. She does not know any other way to be.

These approaches enrich our understanding of the dynamics reflected in the dream, and of the analytic process as well, in which the analyst, for this analysand, inevitably becomes both a burden and a collaborator in less burdensome, more spontaneous ways of living. Thus, the ritualized, constricted behavior symbolized by the briefcase can be viewed alternatively as a security operation in Sullivan's sense, providing familiarity and an escape from anxiety; as a bad-object tie in Fairbairn's sense, providing her with what she believes are her only reliable connections with other people; and as a self object in Kohut's sense, providing her with the only sense of internal cohesion and continuity she can count on.

This greatly encapsulated understanding of the meaning of this dream in the context of the analysand's life cannot be used to evaluate the relevance or utility of different interpretive models; like all analyses, it is itself partially the product of a model. The analyst's theories and habits of thought inevitably become a powerful factor in the collaborative production of analytic data. The point being made here is that the understandings of this analysand's dream generated by various relational-model theories operate within the same conceptual framework—a framework quite different from the drive model, where the analysand's productions are viewed as complex derivatives of a struggle between powerful, body-based impulses and defenses against those impulses.

In the drive model the basic units of analysis are desire and fear of punishment. Relations with other people are important, but not as basic constituents of mind or as contributing meaning of their own; they are vehicles for the expression of drive and defenses. In this dream the anal referent in the underground tunnel, the phallic significance of the train, the castration and vaginal imagery in the *brief*case, the oedipal significance of following ill-fated impulses—all these would be granted motivational priority. Other people are objects of desire; other people are instruments of punishment. But the form of the conflict, the shape of the drama, is inherent in the desire itself, which will inevitably lead to the fear of punishment. Meaning is provided a priori in the inherent nature of desire.

In the various relational-model approaches, the basic units of analysis are the relational bonds and the relational matrix they form. At stake are different forms of relatedness, one mediated through burden and pain, one mediated through activity and spontaneity. Bodily processes, sexuality, aggression, are all important subjects for inquiry, but the conflicts are formed, the drama is shaped, in the interactions between the analysand and others. Different relational theories focus on different facets of the relational matrix, reflecting important terminological differences and often leading to quite different analytic interpretations and interventions; nonetheless, they operate within the same common meta-psychological vision.

The question of boundaries is the first to be encountered; from it all others flow. To draw a boundary around anything is to define, analyze, and reconstruct it.   —FERNAND BRAUDEL

2   "Drive" and the Relational Matrix

Psychoanalytic theorizing and clinical practice operate within a field defined by many dichotomous concepts: drive or relational; intrapsychic or interpersonal, biological or social, inner world or outer world, conflict or developmental arrest, oedipal or preoedipal, psychic reality or actuality, and so on. Various theoretical positions tend to be identified with one as opposed to the other of these complexly related polarities, or with a posture which attempts to transcend one or more of them.

In the previous chapter I delineated an approach to psychoanalytic theory and technique which is based on the concept of a relational matrix whose content includes self, object, and transactional patterns. Where can we locate this relational matrix within the rhetorical dichotomies mapping out the conceptual field of psychoanalytic ideas? It will become apparent in the following chapters that the relational matrix encompasses many of these polarities: intrapsychic *and* interpersonal, biological *and* social, inner world *and* outer world, conflict *and* developmental arrest, oedipal *and* preoedipal, psychic reality *and* actuality. What about drive? Having contrasted the relational model with Freud's drive model, can we find a place for a drive concept within the relational matrix? What are the advantages and costs of doing so?

To answer these questions, we need to go back to the point in the history of psychoanalytic ideas when the drive concept emerged, to explore both its explanatory power and its constraints, which Freud himself struggled with, and to consider how these problems have been dealt with in the major schools of psychoanalytic thought.

From Seductions to Drives

In his earliest accounts, before 1897, Freud regarded the neurotic mind as one which has been subverted *from the outside,* by other people. Otherwise uniform and transparent consciousness has been fractured by infantile seductions operating as pathogenic seeds, lying dormant until puberty, when they germinate into hidden mental recesses of unacceptable memories and affects. Neurotics, Freud discovered, suffer from "reminiscences." Thus, in his early writings Freud portrays the boundary around the human mind as being fatefully permeable, dangerously susceptible to invasion by outside influences, and traumatic experiences with other people are the central etiological force in generating psychopathology. Whereas the healthy mind operates with integrity and transparency, within clear borders, the neurotic mind has lost its autonomy. Intrusions from the social, interpersonal world have generated hidden pathogenic mental fragments.

In 1897 Freud decided that his patients' accounts of infantile seductions were not veridical, but the product of fantasy. The motives for this reversal have become the subject of considerable recent controversy. The "received view" has been that with more and more stories of infantile parental seductions, Freud estimated the possibility of their accuracy to be less and less. His discovery of his own Oedipus complex (in a series of dreams following the death of his father in 1896) and his accompanying wishes for sexual intimacy with his mother seem to have alerted him to the possibility that his patients' accounts were not of events but of wishes similar to his own (see Ellenberger, 1970). More recent authors have pointed to other, more defensive aspects of Freud's reversal: his reluctance to come to terms with some of his own father's secrets and hypocrisies (Levenson, 1983) and what is claimed to have been Freud's dishonest cover-up of the moral failings of upper-middle-class Viennese parents as well as those of the medical establishment (Masson, 1984).

For our purposes, what is significant is not Freud's motives, but the impact of his reversal on the subsequent history of psychoanalytic ideas. If pathogenic material is not introduced into the mind of the child through seductions from outside, the pathogenic material must emerge *from within.* The implications of this idea were enormous. The mind contains *in itself,* Freud was suggesting, the seeds of its own fragmentation. The innocence of childhood was an illusion—children are dominated, independently of precocious and unusual external stimulation, by powerful, sexual passions, inevitably conflictual in nature and unable to be contained within a uniform, transparent consciousness.

In Freud's shift from the theory of infantile seduction to the theory of infantile sexuality, the mind became an infinitely more complex and textured phenomenon, with inevitable internal dramas and secrets. The line between normal and abnormal was forever shaken. The critics of his theory of infantile sexuality often fail to note that the development of this theory brought with it the shift from the overly simplistic and shallow contaminant model of infantile seduction to the view of the mind as intricate, variegated, inevitably torn by passionate conflicts, and actively generating personal meanings—the view that has inspired subsequent decades of psychoanalytic theorizing and clinical psychoanalysis.

The theory of infantile sexuality also brought with it a very different approach to the question of boundaries and motivation. The seduction theory had placed the individual, at least the neurotic individual, in a social context. One could not understand psychopathology simply by looking at the individual—pathogenic ideas and affects needed to be traced to external social influences, the original interpersonal settings from which they arose. With the abandonment of the theory of infantile seduction, other people, the cultural context, recede far into the background. The individual's mind has produced its own fragmentation and difficulties. It is not other people in themselves that are important, but the patient's fantasies about others; and these fantasies are generated from the mind of the individual itself. What actually happened pales in significance beside what the patient *believes* happened, *wishes* had happened, and so on. The individual mind creates its own world out of the material provided by experience, but the composition of that world is preset. Actual experience and events are not unimportant, but they are appropriated for construction of the inevitable, universal longings, fears, and dramas which are extensions of the child's nature. "Wherever experiences fail to fit in with the hereditary schema, they become remodelled in the imagination," Freud suggests (1918, p. 119). Interpersonal experiences are slotted into the categories generated inevitably by the drives and their vicissitudes, like the mosaic artist setting shards and fragments into a predesigned composition. Freud argues:

These events of childhood are somehow demanded as a necessity . . . they are among the essential elements of a neurosis. If they have occurred in reality, so much to the good; but if they have been withheld by reality, they are put together from hints and supplemented by phantasy. The outcome is the same, and up to the present we have not succeeded in pointing to any difference in the consequences, whether phantasy or reality has had the greater share in these events of childhood . . . Whence comes the need for these phantasies and the material for them? There can be no doubt that their sources lie in the instincts. (1916–17, p. 370)

Psychoanalytic theory became a "genetic psychobiology" (Sulloway, 1979), and the unit of study became the individual organism.

In this crucial shift Freud replaced one set of ideas, emphases, and foci with another, establishing two clusters of dichotomous concepts which later became associated with the terms "intrapsychic" and "interpersonal": fantasy vs. perception, psychic reality vs. actuality; inner world vs. outer world, and drive theory vs. a theory of environmental influences. One might argue that Freud's shift in theory in 1897 split the different sides of these dialectics unnaturally from each other, and that we have been trying to heal that split ever since. These contrasts are not strictly parallel, but were grouped because of Freud's global shift in theorizing in 1897, which led in the direction of a theory stressing the "intrapsychic," that is, fantasy, psychic reality, inner world, and instinctual drives. (British-school theorists like Fairbairn and Winnicott illustrate that one can eliminate, or greatly minimize, Freud's drive concept without at all minimizing the importance of fantasy, psychic reality, and inner world.)

THE DRIVE model which emerged from the abandonment of Freud's theory of infantile seduction reached its fullest and purest point of development by 1910. Instinctual drive was established as the basic constituent, the very stuff of mental life. Drives are bodily tensions with psychic representation. The instinctual impulse begins at a "source," a particular body part, and exerts a pressure on the mind to rid that source of its tensions. Excitation is experienced as displeasure, and the overall movement of all instinctual processes is aimed at reducing excitation, thereby generating pleasure. Freud derived all major aspects of psychic life from extremely complex and intricate derivatives of the "organ pleasure" of the drives: all motivations are fueled from the pursuit of drive gratification; the primary shift in the sequence of child development represents a movement from the centrality of one component psychosexual drive gratification to another; the mind structuralizes itself according to the necessity for controlling and regulating modes of drive gratification and defense. Freud portrays the mind as an organism whose nature and morphology is inherent and predetermined, much as the structure and characteristics of any particular bean plant are inherent in the DNA which generates its existence. The interaction between the basic drives "gives rise to the whole variegation of the phenomena of life" (1940, p. 149).

In the enormously productive fifteen years following his abandonment of the theory of infantile seduction, Freud developed and elaborated the drive model and employed it as the guiding framework for clinical practice. The basic underpinnings of all experience, Freud argued, are the array of component drives manifesting themselves through infantile sexuality and, necessarily thwarted by reality, generating defenses, aim-inhibited derivatives, sublimations, and so on. The drives provide the push which creates dreams, neurotic symptoms, sexual perversions, humor, and religion—the entire gamut of human experience. Clinical psychopathology is to be understood and cured by tracing it to derivatives of infantile wishes. Dora's hysterical symptoms are seen as transformations of various sexual longings in relation to Herr K and, ultimately, her father. The Ratman's obsessions are seen as elaborate transformations of his oedipal longings colored by his powerful anal fixation. Thus, for Freud in 1905, the person himself *is* a composite of bodily tensions, their pressured emergence, transformations, and obstructions.

> What we describe as a person's "character" is built up to a considerable extent from the material of sexual excitations and is composed of instincts that have been fixed since childhood, of constructions achieved by means of sublimation, and of other constructions, employed for effectively holding in check perverse impulses which have been recognized as being unutilizable. (1905a, pp. 238–239)

Freud at the Crossroads

In the second decade of the century a different kind of emphasis began to emerge, as Freud started to stress not just the infantile wishes for objects, but the way in which these objects themselves become internalized. In "On Narcissism" (1914b) Freud described a "special psychical agency" which plays a key developmental role in the transition from the stage of primary narcissism to the development of attachments to external objects. In primary narcissism the child experiences himself as perfect and self-sufficient, and the parents' own narcissistic investment in the child helps preserve this experience. As the child grows older, parental expectations and demands increase; the child no longer experiences himself as perfect, but internalizes an image of a perfect creature based partially on parental standards. This "ego ideal" and the processes involved in comparing the child's actual performance with this ideal were to become the basis for Freud's concept of the superego. At this point in the development of his ideas, Freud stayed close to the clinical data in describing inner voices, the workings of "conscience," the residues of parental values, which seem to have taken on a prominence in his clinical work that is beginning to rival the importance of impulses and defenses.

"Mourning and Melancholia" (1917) represents a crucial benchmark in the development of Freud's growing emphasis on internalized object relations. Here Freud describes the self-accusations of the psychotically depressed. The loss of a loved one has precipitated not a normal mourning process, but vicious self-attacks. What is the nature, he asks, of this relentless, pitiless self-abuse? We are tempted, Freud suggests wryly, to accept the accusations at face value, and believe the patient guilty of the crimes he attributes to himself. Closer listening, however, reveals that the accusations make more sense if we understand them as targeted not at the patient himself, but at the lost love object. It is as if the patient is excoriating his lost beloved, but instead of experiencing the other as an external presence, that other has become somehow internalized and confused with the patient's own self. "The shadow of the object fell upon the ego" (1917, p. 249).

This brilliant piece of clinical elucidation left Freud with a metapsychological problem. How and why *does* an external libidinal object become internalized? Prior to the loss, the other is experienced as external to the subject's self; following the loss, the subject has somehow become internalized and the target of attacks. The internalization, Freud reasoned, is the consequence of an abandoned object cathexis. The object is internalized to keep the object cathexis alive, no longer possible in the real, external world, but maintainable through an identification with the lost object sustained as an internal presence. Identification serves the purpose of preserving a channel for drive gratification and regulation.

Why is it that all object losses do not result in identifications? In normal mourning, Freud observed, there is a temporary preservation of the attachment, a denial of the reality of the loss. Over time, however, memories and hopes involving the lost other are evoked and reality intercedes; little by little the cathexis of the object is given up. Freud characterized this painful bit-by-bit relinquishment as the "work of mourning." The lost object is given up because real, available objects offer greater possibilities for pleasure; the narcissistic satisfactions inherent in being alive and relating to real objects "persuade" the libido to sever its attachment to the object.

Why does the melancholic not also find greater pleasure in new objects? The nature of the original cathexis is different in the melancholic, Freud reasoned. This is not a relationship that was characterized by a simple exchange of pleasure, but a "narcissistic" cathexis characterized by a propensity toward regression to earlier psychosexual aims and intense unconscious ambivalence. Oral, cannibalistic components of the original relationship make the internalization of the object following its loss particularly pleasurable, and the abuse the patient heaps on the now-internalized object makes possible a highly pleasurable channel for the expression of the patient's sadism. Thus, in melancholia, in contrast to normal grief, the difference in the nature of the relationship, the prominence of oral and sadistic features, makes preserving the object through internalization more pleasurable than renouncing the lost object and finding new objects. This is a wholly consistent account based on *drive economics*—everything is explained in terms of the pursuit of drive gratification via the pleasure principle, the maximization of pleasure and the avoidance of pain.

Several years later, in *Group Psychology and the Analysis of the Ego* (1921), Freud made some further remarks about identifications which represent a distinct departure from the "Mourning and Melancholia" model and complicate the picture considerably. He speaks of very early identifications as "the earliest expression of an emotional tie with another person" (p. 105)—a dramatic and puzzling statement, for several reasons. First, Freud is broadening the concept of identification from a pathological mechanism to a general phenomenon of human development. Babies attach themselves to other people and identify with them in some sort of primary, irreducible way. Freud seems here to be stepping outside the borders of the explanatory framework of drive theory and venturing into the kind of perspective later developed by relational-model theorists.

Further, Freud seems to be separating identification from object loss, which he established in 1917 as the mechanism (wholly consistent with drive theory) through which identifications arise. If identification is the earliest expression of an emotional tie, what is the relationship between identifications and object cathexes? If early identifications are to be explained within the drive model, they have to be accounted for, in some fashion, as drive derivatives. But why would the child internalize an object that has not been lost? And how is it possible to cathect both a present external object and an identification? The broadening of the concept of identification in 1921 undermines the neatness of Freud's 1917 mechanism (identification as a consequence of object loss) and creates a crisis in theory construction. If Freud was to continue to give identifications such clinical prominence, he needed either to create a new metapsychological framework other than drive to house and derive them, or to find a way to account for them once again in terms of pure drive theory.

Freud might have made oral introjection a much more pervasive and fundamental process, leading to primary identifications (as Melanie Klein was later to do). Or he might have tried to tie identifications to inevitable momentary object losses within the context of a generally consistent relationship (as Mahler and Kohut were later to do). Both these strategies lead increasingly in the direction of a relational model. At this point Freud needed to find *some* theoretical construction which would enable him to carry the increasing clinical importance he was placing on early identifications.

He grappled with this basic problem of the psychodynamic origins and metapsychological status of identifications in 1923 in the third chapter of *The Ego and the Id*. Unlike the vast majority of Freud's writings, this chapter seems conceptually flawed, torn by an internal tension. By following his initial vacillations and ultimate solution, we get the impression that Freud was at first not sure which way he wanted to go; once having decided, however, there was no looking back. Does the clinical importance of early identifications merit assigning them a primary place in development and motivation? Or are identifications to remain under the explanatory sway of drive theory, to be understood as instinctual vicissitudes?

Freud opens the chapter by describing a "grade in the ego, a differentiation within the ego, which may be called the 'ego-ideal' or 'super-ego'" (1923, p. 28). He reminds us that in 1917 he had accounted for the painful self-accusations of the melancholic as the result of an identification with a lost, ambivalent object. He has discovered since that such identifications are not at all unique to melancholics, but are quite universal. The superego is the result of precisely this internalization process. The basic problem of this chapter becomes how to account for this fundamental, universal internal structure.

Freud notes, as he had in 1921, that some identifications seem to take place very early in life. "At the very beginning, in the individual's primitive oral phase, object cathexis and identification are no doubt indistinguishable from each other" (p. 29). This statement plunges us into metapsychological confusion, a blurring of motivational systems at their most basic level. If identifications and object cathexes are indistinguishable, the former cannot possibly be derivative of or a replacement for the latter. Freud seems to be toying with the possibility that identifications have an emotional primacy in their own right and are not, as he thought in 1917, simply a compensation for lost objects. He seems to be considering some sort of primary object relatedness as a basic motivational factor.

Yet in the next paragraph Freud returns to the mechanism he established in 1917. "The character of the ego is a precipitate of abandoned object-cathexes" (p. 29). Identifications *follow* the loss of objects; they remain an instinctual vicissitude. By the end of the same paragraph Freud shifts back again. There are cases, he notes, of "simultaneous object cathexis and identification," once again suggesting that identifications can occur independently of drive gratification and defense, a phenomenon which then needs to be metapsychologically grounded in some fashion. Yet in the next paragraph Freud shifts back again, suggesting that identificatory alterations in the ego are perhaps the mechanism underlying the transformation of object libido into narcissistic libido, making possible the process of sublimation. Identifications are a mechanism whereby the ego captures the id's love and, therefore, once again, identifications derive from and substitute for drive cathexes.

How does Freud resolve this vacillating contradiction? There seem to be early identifications whose metapsychological status remains ambiguous. "This is apparently not in the first instance the consequence or outcome of an object-cathexis; it is a direct and immediate identification and takes place earlier than any object-cathexis" (p. 31). Here we have a relational-model premise positing some sort of primary object relatedness. The most important character-building identifications, however, are those which result from the resolution of the Oedipus complex, and here Freud applies the 1917 drive-model mechanism—identifications as the consequence of abandoned object cathexes. The child in the throes of the Oedipus complex has powerful cathexes directed toward his parents as objects. These cathexes are renounced, and in their place the superego is established internally. Object cathexes have been replaced by identifications. The motive for the establishment of the superego is clearly within the interpretive range of drive theory. The superego provides a compensation for the object loss involved in renouncing oedipal wishes, and the superego operates as an ally of the ego for the purpose of defense against oedipal wishes. Thus, Freud concludes, the superego is "the heir of the Oedipus complex" (p. 36). It is both a compensatory substitute for oedipal object love and a defense against those desires.

Freud concludes the chapter by broadening his observations to consider religion, morality, and "social sense," and his observations here are highly relevant to the question we are pursuing. How is Freud going to derive social cohesion and attachment? This is another way of posing the question raised at the beginning of this chapter—what is the relationship between the drive concept and the relational matrix?

Social phenomena all reflect superego functions, Freud argues, and are therefore all based on compensations for, or reaction formations against, the expression of more basic drives. "The social feelings arise in the individual as a superstructure built upon impulses of jealous rivalry" (p. 37). Phylogenetically as well as ontogenetically, the superego and its attendant social bonds originated from the early historical events that led to totemism—the killing of the primal father for his sexual monopoly of women and the consequent longing and guilt over his loss.

Thus, for purposes of theory construction, Freud chooses to go solely with a model of mind based on drive as his foundation. He obviously does not believe that it is possible to grant weight-bearing significance to both drive and relational premises; he also does not believe "primary identifications" are simply accountable within the drive-model framework. So, he notes them as possibilities, but denies them central importance in his account of character formation. He does not go back and derive "primary identifications" from the drive model, nor does he retract his depiction of them. He simply derives all important later identifications from the drive-based mechanisms of superego formation. Thus, Freud drops totally the interactive, relational-model premise of a primary object relatedness which is implicit in his description of early identifications and derives all object relations within the drive-model framework.

What is so striking about the conclusion of this third chapter is how compelling it is for Freud to return to the explanation of identifications as abandoned object cathexes. In accounting for social feelings as reaction formations, he seems to have completely left behind his earlier suggestion that there are primary identifications prior to or simultaneous with object cathexes. Would not such identifications be a much more conceptually economical foundation for object attachments and social feelings? But it is clear that Freud has chosen not to follow that metapsychological option, nor to try to integrate it with drive theory. He leaves dangling the loose end of metapsychologically obscure primary identifications, and ends up accounting for later identifications as consequent to abandoned object cathexes. The clinical salience of identifications has been accounted for by drive-theory principles. Identifications are central psychodynamically, because they replace and defend against the powerful cathexes of the Oedipus complex.

By 1926 Fenichel, the codifier of classical theory and technique, removes all of the ambiguity with which Freud was struggling in 1923, leaving no room for doubt.

> The motive force of identifications is always supplied by the *drives* (or instincts). These, originating in somatic sources and imposing demands upon the ego, which controls motility, strive for *gratification*, that is, for an adequate alteration of the external world by means of which the tension at the source of the drive can finally be eliminated . . . It is thus plausible to describe identification too as an instinctual vicissitude. A change is made both in the *object* and the *aim* of the original objectual instinct which leads to the identificatory process . . . In the final analysis every identification is motivated by an economic factor, namely, the striving to find a substitute for lost gratification. (1927, pp. 97–101)

Thus, for Fenichel, there are no longer any loose ends; all identifications are derivable in terms of drive economics, and all evidence of Freud's flirtation with some sort of concept of primary object relatedness has vanished.

The Ego and the Id was a watershed in the development of psychoanalytic ideas, in that Freud found a way to stretch the drive model to encompass the growing clinical focus on object relations and identifications. His enthusiasm at the end of the third chapter for his derivation of all social relations from the drive-based Oedipus complex suggests his relief at being able to retain a coherent, consistent theory of mind, despite the stranded, abortive concept of primary attachments prior to or simultaneous with object cathexes.

If he had chosen to grant identifications a more fundamental role, instead of deriving them from the properties of drive regulation and defense, Freud's later theory would have looked quite different. He might very well have moved in the direction of subsequent authors in the British school of object relations, granting object attachment and object seeking a primary motivational status (as did Fairbairn and Bowlby), or viewing the boundary between external and internal objects much more fluidly (as did Klein). He very likely would have granted object relations a determining role in the origination and shaping of the drives themselves (as did Loewald and Kernberg). Freud chose the other fork, however, and in his subsequent writings ingeniously held together a theory virtually bursting at its conceptual seams; the other routes in theory building were left to later theorists.

Much of the complex and multifaceted history of psychoanalytic ideas can be understood as a series of alternative strategies for dealing with the central conceptual dilemma with which Freud was grappling in 1923—the clash between clinical data saturated with relations with others and a conceptual framework which relegates personal relations to a mediating, secondary role. Each of the major contemporary psychoanalytic schools of thought represents a tradition based on a particular strategy for dealing with this dilemma (Greenberg and Mitchell, 1983).

The Fate of the Drive Concept

Let us return to the question with which we began. Is it possible or useful to find a place for Freud's notion of drive within the context of the relational matrix? Do we want to do what Freud chose not to do—blend these two different models?

Since we are speaking here of interpretive systems, not "facts," answers to these questions can be neither "right" nor "wrong." "Drives" and "relational matrix" are organizational principles; they make possible certain ways of thinking, or arranging the infinitely complex tapestry of human experience into distinctive, consistent interpretive patterns. Integrated perspectives establish a claim that bringing together different preexisting lines of theorizing works conceptually and enhances our options. Any attempt to synthesize different theoretical systems succeeds or founders on the question of what it looks like when the different systems are made to stand side by side and are used together. Do they seem to work together in a smooth, consistent fashion that is mutually enhancing? Does the synthesis establish a coherent frame of reference, or a sense of being jolted back and forth between fundamentally different and mutually inconsistent vantage points? What happens when one tries to integrate drive theory with accounts generated from a relational-matrix perspective?

There are three possible answers to this question of model mixing, the same three options Freud faced in 1923. Each has distinct advantages and disadvantages, and each has found a substantial place in the psychoanalytic literature.

The first strategy is to claim that the relational matrix is tautological with respect to drive theory, that it is and always has been implicit in the drive model. According to this view, the very notion of a "drive" is impossible without some sort of relational field within which the drive seeks discharge or expression. Therefore, considerations of self-organization, object relations, or transactional patterns are largely redundant with the concept of drive; theories which explore these areas are merely filling out the world in which drives operate. Freud was always concerned with these dimensions, the argument runs, but to consider them without the concept of drive results in a shallow, eviscerated perspective, a world without a compelling theory of motive or meaning. Freud would have been adopting this tactic if he had derived primary identifications from drive economics, as Fenichel was later to do. Thus, the first solution to the problem of model mixing is to dismiss the question by claiming that the relational model is implicit *within* the concept of drive.

A second strategy is to claim that the kinds of theorizing which explore the relational matrix *do* represent a distinctive point of view not at all implicit in the drive model, but nevertheless highly compatible with it. According to this way of thinking (which has been the central strategy of Freudian ego psychology from Hartmann through Kernberg and Pine), relational-model accounts are best regarded as natural extensions of drive-theory accounts. Considerations of self-organization, object relations, and interpersonal transactions can be smoothly and seamlessly juxtaposed, and mixed together with considerations of drive; it is enriching to our thinking and clinical options to do so. Freud would have been adopting this model-mixing route if he had retained both primary identifications and drive economics as a dual basis for subsequent object relations.

A third strategy is to claim that the relational matrix and the drive-model perspective are fundamentally alternative, and in fact conceptually incompatible. This is not to say that they *cannot* be put together—any array of disparate concepts can be joined if one is clever enough. The question is whether it is conceptually and clinically economical—whether it is *useful* to do so. According to this way of thinking, juxtaposing and blending drive and relational-model accounts is cumbersome and confusing, and results in a hybrid which, despite its breadth, is in no way an improvement over either of its ancestors, a kind of monstrosity of inclusiveness that cannot move very much at all.

This position, in which model mixing is declined, is the route Freud chose to go, eschewing any role for primary relatedness in his theory and relying instead solely on drive economics. This third position on mixing drives with the relational is also the basis for this book; but here I am selecting the alternative fork—a purely *relational* mode perspective, unmixed with drive-model premises.

Let us consider more fully some of the implications of the three different options.

Loose Constructionism

The internecine struggles within the psychoanalytic world with regard to drive theory exemplify the universal human dilemma of relating present thinking to past ideas, relating current innovations to tradition. In *Object Relations in Psychoanalytic Theory,* Greenberg and I applied Kuhn's theory of scientific revolutions to the history of psychoanalytic ideas; old paradigms are stretched and accommodated to discordant observations until replaced by a radically different and novel vision. But this is not a process unique to science. Commitments to various psychoanalytic movements and schools have had, from their inception, powerful religious and political overtones, and the debate about what to do with Freud's legacy, particularly the drive theory, often sounds less like science than like religious debates over holy books such as the Bible, or political and legal debates over the function of the Constitution. Is the meaning of the seminal text fixed at the time of its writing, or is it subject to interpretation, changing over time? Can one add later books or amendments? How are these to be integrated with the original work? Can one disclaim the divine or unalterable status of the original document and still remain a true believer?

The first of the psychoanalytic strategies with regard to drive theory, based on the premise that object relations are merely vicissitudes of drives and therefore that object-relations theory is implicit in drive theory, is very much like the concept of loose constructionism in constitutional law.

So-called loose constructionists regard the Constitution as a document with no fixed meaning; the Founding Fathers could not have foreseen the enormous social and economic changes that have occurred over the course of American history, and the Constitution is therefore best used as a text whose interpretation is contingent upon changing circumstances. Its interpretation in later years might be totally different from anything the Founding Fathers had in mind or could have predicted. (The strict constructionist, by contrast, regards the meaning of the Constitution as limited by the specific intent of the Founding Fathers; if we are to use the Constitution as a meaningful basis for law, we ought to abide by that intent or else explicitly change the Constitution.)

If the central issue in constitutional law (generally a rationale for more political motives) is how we are to use the Constitution, the central issue in the history of psychoanalytic traditions (also often a rationale for more political motives) has been how we are to use Freud's legacy. The claim that what *seems* different in relational-model theories really is implicit in and derivable from Freud's text is a form of loose constructionism that is very appealing in a number of respects. It keeps Freud alive by continually updating and reworking his ideas and creates a sense of complete continuity with the past. Why not create a different text, less burdened by anachronistic meanings? Because Freud's language, in Loewald's view, is the archaic language of our discipline, with primordial resonances, evoking "primitive" forms of organization, bodily experiences, passionate desires—resonances that are lost in psychoanalytic discourse which omits "drives."

This is fine when the looseness of the construction is conscious and acknowledged. Loewald, for example, whose rich contributions have had a profound impact on contemporary psychoanalytic thought, explicitly acknowledges that his interpretation of Freud is what he calls imaginative—not a literal reading of what Freud had in mind, but a creative use of Freud's text to generate new meanings. "What psychoanalysis needs might not be a 'new language,' but a less inhibited, less pedantic and narrow understanding and interpretation of its current language, leading to elaborations and transformations of the meanings of concepts, theoretical formulations, or definitions that may or may not have been envisaged by Freud" (1976, p. 193). Loewald is essentially uninterested in how Freud *actually* understood things and how his (Loewald's) understanding differs; he is concerned with using Freud as a text and assigning new meanings as a vehicle for grounding, presenting, and developing his own thought.

What is troublesome, however, is when the looseness of the construction is unacknowledged, and Freud is made to read as if he actually *meant* to say what the current author now proclaims. This creates great confusion; basic differences in premises and conceptions are blurred, and an accurate exploration of the implications of these differences becomes impossible. This strategy depends ultimately on the illusion that using the original words *does* retain something of the original meanings.

Thus, modern adherents of the drive model frequently claim to be merely updating the concept of "drive" while changing it fundamentally and still claiming the authority and interpretive power of the original formulation. Brenner, for example, disconnects "drive" from any organic substrate or energic flow, treating it as a self-evident, purely psychological concept, yet he feels no need to derive the power of drive, which Freud based on organic tensions, from other sources. On the one hand, the original concept is radically redefined; on the other hand, all the connotations and attributes of the original concepts are still claimed.

Seldom do practitioners of this loose constructionist strategy clearly or explicitly redefine all the terms, because to make the redefinition clear or explicit is to break the spell, to make it apparent that one is no longer in the embrace of the prior vision but out on one's own. So new meanings are introduced under a soft focus, and the danger is a sacrifice of clarity.

Model Mixing

The second strategy, generally known as model mixing, is based on the claim that although contemporary theories do constitute a distinct paradigm or model quite different from the drive model, they are complementary and can fairly easily be integrated with the older theory. Even though the models often blur together, this approach is quite opposite in practice from the loose constructionism of the first strategy. While the latter expands the meaning of Freud's text beyond what Freud had in mind, model mixing involves a narrowing of Freud's concept of drive so that it can be set beneath or alongside other theories.

Model mixing tends to involve a juxtaposition of the models rather than a real integration of them. Some mixing strategies (those of Gedo and Kernberg, for instance) regard object relations and drives as constituting a sequence of different kinds of developmental phenomena, which emerge at different points in childhood, and interference with which generates fundamentally different kinds of psychopathology. According to this approach, issues concerning attachment and separation, the positioning of oneself in relation to others, are regarded as developmentally early problems, preceding later sexual and aggressive conflicts among id, ego, and superego, rather than as the fundamental psychodynamic issues throughout life that lend meaning to sexual and aggressive experiences.

Other mixing strategies (such as that of Pine) regard drives and object relations as different dimensions of human experience, the former pertaining to physical "urges," the latter to interpersonal attachments. Both these approaches involve a layering process. Rather than regard the drive model and the relational model as comprehensive interpretive systems, each accounting for all of human experience, each theory is condensed into an account of only part of human experience, either in horizontal layers involving particular developmental epochs or in vertical layers involving certain wishes and needs across developmental epochs (or as distinct sequential phases of treatment; see Modell, 1984).

The characterization of this sort of approach as model mixing is somewhat misleading in that it alters the models before mixing them and thereby diminishes the explanatory power of each system, at the same time obscuring the differences between them. Freud's concept of drive does not pertain solely to physical urges or solely to the oedipal phase. The power and utility of the drive model as a unified interpretive system lies in the way in which it illuminates *all* areas of experience, including attachment, by regarding them as derivative of the underlying drives. Similarly, an object-relations theory like Fairbairn's is not an account simply of discrete emotional needs for connection and attachment, or simply of the earliest relationship of the infant with the mother.

The power and utility of the relational model as an interpretive system stand or fall on their illumination of all areas of experience, including sexual and other physical urges, as taking their meanings from underlying ties to internal objects and patterns of interpersonal relations, as being shaped in an interactive, relational context.

Pine's work (1985) illustrates this problem. He wants to embrace object-relations theory, as well as self psychology and ego psychology, under a broad, flexible framework that will enrich Freud's drive theory, not supplant it. Having established each of these "psychologies" as a primary and initially independent motivational base, with distinctive developmental lines, he attempts to weave them together, relying heavily on an expansion of Waelder's principle of "multiple function" (1936)—every act has a meaning in terms of the psychologies of drive, ego function, object relations, and self.

The problem with Pine's mix is the assignment of priorities. The "essential unity" Pine decrees between object-relations theory and drive psychology (1985, p. 59) is possible only if their competing, underlying claims are radically reduced and their incompatibilities blurred. Having established the principle that everything means everything, Pine fails to provide coherent, consistent guidelines for ascertaining *how* different meanings or functions are ordered or arranged vis-à-vis each other, and how one selects among them clinically. Each of these theories layers motives in a different way; to hold all of them together in a single framework, they have to be flattened in terms of priorities.

Greenberg and I (1983) have argued that the drive and relational models are comprehensive interpretive systems which account for all dimensions of human experience, and that they are based on very different fundamental presuppositions about the generation of experience and meaning. Therefore, systems like Pine's, Kohut's (in 1977), and Sandler's, which try to keep these two interpretive systems delicately balanced, tend to topple in one direction or the other. Since the two models are inversions of each other, what is derivative in one model is fundamental in the other. They consume each other, and trying to combine them in the same framework is a little like trying to stand on one's feet and one's head at the same time. It can be done (if one is limber enough), but it is not very useful if one's intent is to go somewhere rather than demonstrate a capacity for balance. The most effective theory, while inclusive of the most data, is not necessarily inclusive of the most theories.

Kuhn (1962) has described different paradigms in science as different kinds of "thinking caps." Each model addresses the entire field of data, but engages those data differently. Consider the accompanying visual image, one of those used by standard psychology textbooks to illustrate reversals of figure and ground. If you look at the picture one way, you see two profiles; if you look another way, you see a goblet. What is figure in one view is background in the other, and vice versa. Each view uses the entire visual field, but different portions in different ways. The same principle applies to the drive and relational models. Each has interpretive power and breadth, but arranges the same data differently. What is figure in one model is background in the other, and vice versa.

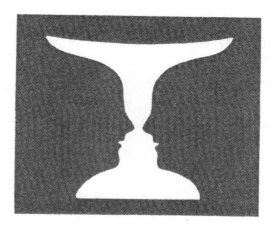

Reversal of figure and ground

From R. L. Atkinson, R. C. Atkinson, and E. R. Hilgard, *Introduction to Psychology*, 8th ed. New York: Harcourt Brace Jovanovich, 1983. Courtesy of Harcourt Brace Jovanovich, Inc.

Mixed-model approaches are like attempts to divide the visual field by trying to force attention to each area of the picture separately—there is a profile on the side, a goblet here, another profile here. Thinking caps have to be switched rapidly as one's gaze travels across the picture. One's vision is not enhanced thereby; it is fragmented, constrained, and narrowed. One loses the fullness which each single, complete vision provides. Similarly, each of the two theoretical systems is fundamentally altered when one tries to squeeze the drive and relational models into a common framework by collapsing them into specific developmental lines or needs.

To claim that model mixing is conceptually unstable and costly says nothing about how analysts use psychoanalytic theory in the consulting room, where one may frequently draw on one's reservoir of theoretical concepts in a fashion that is necessarily less than rigorous or systematic. Further, an analyst may use concepts from many different authors, but reset those concepts within an implicit, unarticulated, but generally consistent metapsychological framework of his own design. Similarly, the fact that some clinicians draw on different models for understanding and treating different kinds of patients, or the same patient at different times, says nothing about whether these various models fit meaningfully together in any logical sense. There are many interesting questions that one might ask regarding these issues: Do most analysts stay consistently within the framework of one particular model? How is the treatment affected by consistency within models as opposed to shifting from model to model? When analysts borrow concepts from various authors, do they remain true to the full original conceptualization of those notions, or do they translate and redesign those concepts to fit into their own fairly consistent model? To my knowledge, no one knows much about these questions; they have not been empirically tested, nor are they easy issues to tackle empirically.

An Integrational Relational Model

The strategy adopted in this volume has been to develop an integration of the major lines of relational-model psychoanalytic theorizing into a broad, integrative perspective—from which the concept of drive, as Freud intended it, has been omitted. Freud's concept of "drive" pervades the classical psychoanalytic understanding of all domains of psychoanalytic theory and technique. The major innovations in postclassical psychoanalytic thought have been shaped within a framework that regards mind as interactive, and this premise also pervades contemporary approaches to all realms of psychoanalytic theorizing. Rather than force an unnatural fit between two discordant visions, I have instead drawn together the major psychoanalytic schools which proceed from the interactive, relational-model vision. The "intrapsychic," the experience of the body, "one-person" psychology—all find a prominent role in this integration, not as separate from (and subsequently mixed with) relational considerations, but as derivative of the interactional field.

Gill has noted (in a personal communication) that to choose one model rather than another does not mean ignoring or minimizing any of the *data* which might lead some people to choose the other model. To choose one model rather than another entails giving up theoretical constructs, not clinical material or experience. (Strictly speaking, there *are* no clinical data totally separate from theoretical constructs.) The important clinical data which led Freud to develop the concept of drive—the *sense* of "drivenness," the phenomenology of pressure and urgency, fantasies of oneself as bestial, the recurrent use of metaphors referring to bodily parts and processes—these have often been deemphasized by theorists rejecting the metapsychological concept of drive. They must be accounted for in any persuasive psychoanalytic theory, and it is to these kinds of experiences that we turn in Part Two. Their inclusion and centrality is in no way contingent upon whether one retains or discards Freud's theory and language of drive. The richness and resonances of the classical tradition can be retained by radically recasting its clinical contributions within an interactive, relational theory of mind. In the long run, this seems a more economical and coherent basis for theory construction than retaining "drive" only semantically (loose constructionism) or limiting its interpretive range to one of only token significance by adding to it other, incompatible theories (model mixing).

The concept of drive places great emphasis on the "innate," that which is constitutional, a priori, in the construction of human experience. In relational-model theories deriving mind from the establishment and maintenance of connections and patterns of interaction with others, what happens to the innate? If we discard *Freud's* drive theory, is *some* concept of drive still necessary to account for that which is constitutional?

In a broad sense, trying to locate the innate in the relational model is impossible, because it takes a term which is central to one paradigm and tries to locate it within another, in which it necessarily has a very different meaning. This is a bit like trying to locate Ptolemy's epicycles within Copernicus' model of the solar system. For relational theorists, *all* meaning is generated in relation, and therefore nothing is innate in quite the same way as it is in the drive model. Even basic bodily events, like hunger, defecation, and orgasm are regarded as experienced through, interpreted in the context of, the symbolic textures of the relational matrix.

Thus, in a broader sense, the very establishment of the relational matrix is innate, and human development can perhaps be best characterized as a "continuous unfolding of an intrinsically determined social nature" (Stern, 1985, p. 234). How can we designate the processes which constitute that social nature, which lead to the construction of the relational matrix? Is it meaningful to speak of an innate drive toward relation?

Although I have no strong objection to such a concept, I am not sure it takes us very far. Either one depicts a relational "drive" in extremely broad terms, like "attachment," object seeking, bonding, which adds little in the way of specificity, or else one collapses the complexity of social and interpersonal relations to what are presumed to be more fundamental, underlying needs, such as dependency (Fairbairn), safety (Sandler), security (Sullivan), mirroring (Kohut), and so on. The latter reductions seem to me often arbitrary and lose something of the richness of the many forms of connection within the relational tapestry. (See Eagle, 1984, pp. 197–202, for a closely related argument against the "reductionism" of establishing "superordinate motives," whether drive, object relations, or self-psychological.) Further, as soon as one establishes a motive as innate, one ironically closes it off somewhat from analytic inquiry and thereby loses the opportunity to deepen an appreciation of its origins and resonances within the individual's particular relational matrix.

My preference is to use the notion of the relational matrix not in a narrow, discrete motivational sense, but in a broad, paradigmatic sense, as encompassing: innate wiring (like Bowlby's response patterns and the perceptual capacities and preferences of newborns), motivational intent (like Fairbairn's object seeking and Klein's drive toward reparation), and implicit interpersonal processes involved in self-definition (like Winnicott's "facilitating environment" and Kohut's self-object relations). Man's social nature leads him to seek many different forms of connection, familiarity, security, dependency, merger, safety, pleasure, validation, mutual knowing, and so on. What dimensions of the infinite variety of human connection become dynamically central and conflictual for any particular person depends strongly on the particularities of the cultural and familial context and the specific constellation of talents, sensitivities, and rhythms the individual discovers in himself within that context.

Part Two

Sexuality

THE EARLIEST and the most consistent clinical phenomenon Freud encountered was disturbance in the realm of sexuality. The seemingly bizarre symptoms of his patients, Freud soon became convinced, were not meaningless murmurings and sputterings of a nervous system gone awry, but were disguised aspects of the patient's sexuality, repressed and detached from the rest of life, forced to find expression only in circuitous and clandestine fashion. In fact, Freud came to feel, neurotic symptoms *constitute* the patient's sexuality; where sexuality is mature and well integrated with other aspects of personal relationships, neurosis is impossible. By 1910 Freud declared the splitting off of sexuality, which he now termed "psychical impotence," the inability to experience full sexual excitement in an intimate relationship, to be the most common mental disorder of our time, to be in fact universal. "Where they love they do not desire and where they desire they cannot love" (1910, p. 183).

How can "psychical impotence" be explained? The concept of instinctual "drive," Freud's basic metapsychological building block, was developed as a way of accounting for what, based on his clinical experience, he felt was the fundamental antagonism between sexuality and other dimensions of human experience. A powerful tendency toward debasement in sexuality is intrinsic to human nature, Freud argued, which makes a full integration of sexuality and love impossible. As he puts it in the retrospective gaze of the *New Introductory Lectures on Psychoanalysis*, "From the very first we have said that human beings fall ill of a conflict between the claims of instinctual life and the resistance which arises within them against it" (1933, p. 57).

Commitment to the drive model is often based on the clinical judgment that sexuality is central to and formative in human development, and that difficulties in the realm of sexuality underlie all psychopathology. Relational-model theories, in abandoning the drive framework, *do* often deemphasize the primary clinical importance of sexuality. This is an unfortunate historical artifact. Conceptually unnecessary, it detracts from the persuasiveness and comprehensiveness of relational-model theorizing.

In Chapter 3 I examine the close connection between Freud's grasp of the nature of sexuality and its psychopathology, and the concept of "drive" based on nineteenth-century biological principles and the scientific zeitgeist of Freud's day. I then consider in Chapter 4 what happens to our understanding of sexuality when the concept of drive is radically altered or translated into a relational-matrix framework. In the integrated relational model presented here, sexuality and relational issues are not seen as alternative foci. Rather, sexuality is regarded as a central realm in which relational conflicts are shaped and played out.

But the argument is, as our English friends say (and quite literally in this case), "arse about face." Humans are the most sexually active of primates, and humans have the largest sexual organs of our order. If we must pursue this dubious line of argument, a person with larger than average endowment is, if anything, more human.

—STEPHEN JAY GOULD

3   Drive Theory and the Metaphor of the Beast

Although Freud's clinical emphasis on sexuality and the metapsychological concept of drive became closely intertwined in the fabric of classical psychoanalytic theory, they did not emerge simultaneously in his thinking. Freud had argued for the sexual etiology of the neuroses (1894, 1896) for more than ten years before his introduction of the theory of infantile sexuality and the full development of drive theory (1905a). To grasp fully the relationship between sexuality and the metapsychological notion of drive in Freud's thought, we need to consider first the way Freud thought about sexuality prior to the development of drive theory.

Sex before Drive

The nineteenth century has been characterized as the "age of energy." The burgeoning technology of the industrial age had revealed ways of harnessing hydraulic, chemical, and electrical energy, making it possible to extend human resources and productive powers in proportions unimaginable just a short time earlier. Newton, the model for Enlightenment philosophers (Gay, 1969) and subsequent nineteenth-century natural and social scientists, had conceived of the universe as a vast, intricate machine, composed of mass in motion, all governed by common energic and physical principles. Most of Freud's contemporaries saw mind in the same framework, explainable in terms of matter and

67

energy, and Freud's metaphor of the psychic apparatus dramatically reflects this—mind as a hydraulic system of pressures, channels, dams, flows, backups, and diversions.

Consider further the context of the neurobiology within which Freud worked. Golgi's technique for staining a small proportion of brain cells at one time was developed in 1875, making possible the isolation and study of a select number of neurons within the otherwise tangled mass of brain cells. The very term "neurone" was not introduced until 1891; thus, Freud developed his model of mind in an era preoccupied with energy and alongside an explosion of research in brain physiology based on the dramatic discovery of the conduction of electrical impulses along nerve cells. This was a heady period for the study of brain and mind.

Freud's earliest efforts to explain psychopathology vividly reflect the excitement of this intellectual milieu. Neurosis is understood from the beginning to be a disorder of energy regulation. Freud maintained throughout that the essential function of the nervous system is the mastery of excitation. Neurotic illness represents an energic overload, a quantitative level which has exceeded the nervous system's capacity for regulation. Following Charcot and Breuer, Freud regarded traumas as the cause of neuroses, and trauma is understood in energic terms as an excess of stimulation. "A trauma would have to be defined as an *accretion of excitation* in the nervous system, *which the latter has been unable to dispose of adequately by motor reaction*" (1950, p. 137; italics in original). It is evident that Freud is speaking of excitation not as a metaphor, but quite literally and concretely. He speaks of "special chemical substances" that are "produced in the interstitial portion of the sex-glands" and compares neuroses to the condition of intoxication (1905a, p. 215). Too much of a stimulant creates a toxic state, flooding the system; the neurotic is addicted to excitations which, since they cannot find motoric outlet, become dammed up.

What is the source of these excitations? Prior to 1897 Freud understood the origins of pathogenic sexual excitations to be specific kinds of external "impressions, sexual seductions in early childhood." Based on the then-dominant "reflex arc" model of mental function, sexual seductions were seen as stimuli which led to blocked, "dammed-up" responses. The pathogenic impact, Freud reasoned, is not at the actual time of the seduction (at which point he felt the child is protected by naiveté and prepubertal lack of passion); only later, with the hormonal upsurge of puberty, does awakened sexuality impart to the memories of seduction a disturbing, overexciting, "traumatic" intensity. As Freud puts it in the "Project for a Scientific Psychology" of 1895, "a memory is repressed which has only become a trauma by *deferred action*" (p. 356; italics in original). Thus, the toxins in Freud's early theory of sexuality are products of contamination; infantile seductions, with their delayed effect, flood the nervous system with stimulants (memories and affects) which cannot be assimilated and processed by the child's immature psychological organization within which they were experienced. Hysterics, as Freud and Breuer put it in 1893, "suffer from reminiscences"— that is, disturbing memories.

The theory of infantile seduction provided an explanation for Freud's most consistent clinical problem—psychic impotence. In this account sexuality has split off from other aspects of experience and personal relations because it has been aroused too much and too soon. The energic capacities of the nervous system can contain intense sexual excitement when that excitement emerges in its proper time and context, at puberty. Precocious sexual experience, when joined later with the full physical force of puberty, overruns the capacities of the system (which begins to break down) and leaks out around the edges. The other person, it should be noted, plays the key pathogenic role in this version. In these early formulations Freud was thinking very strongly of sexuality in the context of early relations with significant others. Parental seducers had sown the seeds of neurosis by molesting their children, precociously arousing unacceptable feelings and establishing memories which would be impossible to assimilate.

Sexuality and Drive

The death of Freud's father, his self-analysis, his increasing clinical sophistication, all led in 1897 to a dramatic turn in his understanding of neurosis and sexuality. The memories of seduction reported by his patients, Freud decided, were not necessarily veridical. Further, many children are subjected to sexual experience without becoming neurotic. Mere memory by itself lacks the purpose, the force, to overrun the nervous system, to cause the dammed-up state and flooding which is the pathogenic source of neurosis. The contaminant model of infantile seduction was too simplistic—the excess of stimulation fueling neurotic symptomatology had to be accounted for some other way.

The drive theory was the solution. The pressure is generated from

Infantile Seduction (what) was replaced by drive (why)

within the organism. As Freud explained in a letter to Fliess as early as 1897, "the psychic structures which, in hysteria, are affected by repression are not in reality memories—since no one indulges in memory activity without a motive—but *impulses*" (1985, p. 239). The accretion of stimulation in neurosis is a product not of *im*pression from without but of *ex*pression from within. Thus, the concept of drive allowed Freud to see sexual motives as present at the very beginning, pushing for discharge, rather than aroused by external stimulation. A more interactive approach has been replaced by a theory of mental life as patterned a priori; the drives contain in themselves all the force and organizational principles through which the mind unfolds and structures itself.

The *Three Essays on the Theory of Sexuality* (1905a) represents Freud's formal presentation of this solution. His argument is directed against the then-current "popular" notion of the nature of human sexuality, which was understood as largely a response to the charms of a person of the opposite sex leading to the species-serving aim of reproduction. Freud uses the perversions and the neuroses to claim a much broader and more varied range of sexual phenomena, including many different kinds of objects, many different kinds of aims, and extends sexuality back into early infancy.

The pivotal feature of the position Freud stakes out here is that the "object" has been granted too much importance in our understanding of human sexuality. It is not the charms of the object which evoke a sexual response, Freud argues; sexuality appears as a powerful collection of internal pressures, in many forms, polymorphously perverse, which can become attached to many different kinds of objects. In fact, in its very beginnings the sexual instinct has no object, but stumbles across objects through self-preservative activities such as feeding. Thus, Freud wants to "loosen the bond" between the instinct and the object, which is no longer regarded as part and parcel of the instinct (1905a, p. 148).

From his current vantage point, Freud finds himself guilty of granting too much importance to the object in his earlier theory of infantile seduction, in which the object evokes the sexual response. Now Freud claims that the object is a minor factor, tacked on later, one among an infinite number of possibilities for the highly promiscuous, highly mobile, internally pressured sexual instinct to attach itself to. Freud has shifted the focus from the object to the internal pressure. He repeatedly compares libido to a kind of ravenous hunger, which in its natural form encompasses an enormous range of objects and aims. "Normal" sexuality is what is left after culture has inhibited infantile sexuality in its many forms. Rather than evoke sexuality, the object is simply the lucky survivor after all other possible forms of sexual pleasure have been excluded by social restrictions!

A comparison of the variations in wording between the 1905 and 1915 editions of the *Three Essays* reveals the gradual consolidation of Freud's view that spontaneously arising expression of internal pressures and not interaction with external objects is the key feature of human sexuality. In 1905 he defines the sexual instinct as "a contribution from an organ capable of receiving stimuli . . . an organ whose excitation lends the instinct a sexual character" (p. 168n). Note that here the sexual organs are still portrayed as directed outward, interacting with and receiving stimuli from the outside world, acted upon by the object. This wording was replaced in 1915, when the sexual instinct is defined as "the psychical representative of an endosomatic, continuously flowing source of stimulation, as contrasted with a 'stimulus,' which is set up by *single* excitations coming from *without*" (p. 168). Now the sexual organs are driven from within, receiving stimuli emerging from the soma and seeking external objects as vehicles for "organ pleasure" (p. 126).

Thus, Freud progressively consolidated the concept of drive as the motivational energy impowering the psychic apparatus, as a "demand made on the mind for work" (p. 168). Throughout his writings Freud stresses the energic quality of drives, as "a certain quota of energy which presses in a particular direction. It is from this pressure that it derives the name of 'Trieb' " (1933, p. 96). The energic imagery through which Freud envisions the workings of libido is perhaps nowhere more vivid than in the posthumously published *Outline of Psycho-analysis*. "There can be no question but that the libido has somatic sources, that it streams to the ego from various organs and parts of the body" (1940, p. 151). Sexuality is an expression of the sexual drives, and the drives arise out of, gain their peremptory power from, and always refer back to, the body. "The aim of an instinct is in every instance satisfaction, which can only be obtained by removing the state of stimulation at the source of the instinct" (1915a, p. 122). Although Freud's clinical analysis of the psychodynamic transformations and vicissitudes of libido is often extremely intricate, he continually emphasizes the specific organic underpinnings of libidinal satisfaction. "This can be attained only by an appropriate ('adequate') alteration of the internal source of stimulation" (1915a, p. 119).

What has happened to the role of experience, the "impressions" derived from objects? Freud is much too complex a thinker to leave out the input from experience, but it is obvious that the center of gravity of the theory has shifted from interactions with others to the unfolding of inborn pressures. The entire field of interpersonal relations has been collapsed around spontaneously arising impulses with encoded, a priori meanings. The reflex arc model of nervous system function still prevails; the stimulus which sets the process in motion has just been shifted from an external impression to an internal pressure, the drive. "An urgent state of tension, caused chemically and manifested through a sensory stimulus, is to be discharged" (Fenichel, 1945, p. 54). Objects are now facilitators for the expression of inherent needs. The object is "what is most variable about an instinct and is not originally connected with it, but becomes assigned to it only in consequence of being peculiarly suited to make satisfaction possible" (Freud, 1915a, p. 122).

Freud thus comes to understand the role of the object as operating much like the day residue of the dream, which provides the link to the preconscious, making it possible for the real motive force of the dream, the infantile wish, to find an outlet. "The constitutional factor must await experiences before it can make itself felt; the accidental factor must have a constitutional basis in order to come into operation" (1905a, p. 239). In Freud's drive theory the fundamental motivational thrust in human experience, powered by the drives, is toward the reduction of internal pressures, the pursuit of pleasure and the avoidance of pain. Sexuality in its varied forms is the manifestation of this impersonal force, employing interpersonal experiences to express a priori themes and fantasies.

"Loosening the bond" between the drive and the object is essential to the new solution for the clinical problem of psychic impotence. Although expressed in experiences with others, sexuality is universally problematic not because of anything its objects do or do not do, but because in its very nature sexuality is *antagonistic and offensive to the other*. The conflict-filled fragmentation of sexuality is not contingent on specific traumas, but is inherent in the rapacious nature of sexuality itself. It is the id, Freud explains in his last writings, that "expresses the true purpose of the individual organism's life. This consists in the satisfaction of its innate needs" (1940, p. 148). And for Freud the innate needs of the individual organism necessarily and inevitably clash with other features of social and interpersonal relations.

Freud and Darwin

Throughout the many centuries of Western civilization prior to Freud's day, human beings were understood to have originated in a fall from a higher state. Plato saw human experience, indeed all life in time, as a descent from an eternal world of ideal forms, and the Judeo-Christian tradition portrayed man as fallen from a paradisiacal harmony designed by a divine creator. The evolutionary perspective which Darwin introduced, and which dominated the scientific zeitgeist of Freud's day, was an abrupt reversal of prior centuries of Platonic-Christian thought. Man had not stumbled from above, Darwin argued, but had gradually evolved from below. Man was not a fallen angel, a chip off the divine block gone astray, but a more or less refined beast. This reversal provided a fresh and exciting perspective on human nature and experience, and Freud was very much a beneficiary. In fact, Sulloway has forcefully argued that Darwin "paved the way" for Freud's theories and was the most dominant influence on his thinking (1979, p. 238). (Earlier psychoanalytic authors had also noted, in much more limited fashion, Darwin's influence on Freud. See, for example, Jones, 1957, III, 302–333; Rapaport, 1960, pp. 22–23.)

In the broadest sense, Freud's clinical theory of sexuality, and the drive theory metapsychology which encases it, was a brilliant analogue of the structure of Darwin's theory of the evolution of the human species. Just as lower organisms evolve into higher forms of life, bestial sexual and aggressive impulses are transformed into the entire array of civilized human activities. "Primitive" impulses bubble up from the id, a "cauldron full of seething excitations" (Freud, 1933, p. 73), and are worked over by a "secondary" process concerned with adaptation to external reality, to fuel "higher" functions. Phylogeny is recapitulated not only in ontogeny, but in the very process of thought itself. And in Freud's system, sexuality (and after 1920, aggression) is the crucial link to our animal past.

The general strategy of finding meanings in the present by uncovering a *prehistory* of the individual in a remote ancestral past dominated the natural sciences in the second half of the nineteenth century, inspired not only by developments in biology but by advances in geology as well.

Preceding the development of Darwin's theory of bestial prehuman ancestors was the discovery of what McPhee (1980) has called deep time. Contrary to the biblical account, which dates mankind from the very beginning of things, geologists in the first half of the nineteenth century were beginning to grasp that only a small fragment of the vast age of the earth coincides with human history (see Gould, 1987a). The present, the surface, what is manifest, pales in significance before what has gone earlier. What Berlin refers to as the historicism of the nineteenth century reflects this tendency to look for answers in the remote past. "History alone—the sum of empirically discoverable data—held the key to the mystery of why what happened happened as it did and not otherwise" (1953, p. 11). And this historicism, combined with Darwin's dramatic discoveries, had a powerful influence on Freud and early psychoanalytic authors. Ferenczi pushed this approach to its limits in his call for a "depth biology, that would explain how phylogenetic memory-traces accumulated in the germ plasma, imprinting there 'all the catastrophes of phylogenetic development' " (quoted in Kermode, 1985, p. 5).

The traditional psychoanalytic preference for "genetic" explanations, arrived at through "developmental reasoning" (Pine, 1985, p. 19) derives partly from the enthusiasm of scientists of Freud's day concerning their discoveries about the early history of life on our planet and of the planet itself. The distant geological and phylogenetic past became a rich source of metaphor on which Freud drew to explain current difficulties in living (see the recently discovered manuscript of Freud's *Phylogenetic Fantasy*). "It was important to be able to map neurosis, genitally and so forth on to an indefinitely protracted past, or, as he himself put it, 'to fill a gap in individual truth with prehistoric truth' " (Kermode, 1985, p. 5).

The Darwinian-inspired theory of sexuality which became the basis for drive theory provided Freud with a powerful explanatory model for illuminating the conflicts involved in psychic impotence. Sexuality is difficult to integrate with other dimensions of interpersonal relations because it is a vestige of man's primitive origins, of his early days as a precivilized protohuman, as well as of the prehuman ancestors in his phylogenetic development as a species. Thus, Freud regards what is distinctively human and special in mankind as a tenuous overlay upon a rapacious, bestial core, which is only with great difficulty brought under the control of civilized motives.

Sulloway argues that Freud, because he wanted to portray psychoanalysis as a totally unique and autonomous discipline, tried to conceal the extent to which his theories were drawn from evolutionary biology, but there are many places where Freud makes quite explicit his belief that many specific features of sexuality have a prehuman or subhuman foundation. The pregenital organizations, for example, are actual residues of the sexual morphology of subhuman species, "vestiges of conditions which have been permanently retained in several classes of animals" (1918, p. 108). (For a similar comparison, see 1905a, p. 198.) Orality and anality are linked, as Gould puts it, to a "quadrupedal ancestry before vision became a dominant sense and eclipsed a previous reliance upon smells and tastes" (1977, p. 157). The genitals, Freud argues in a dramatic combination of Victorian prudery and species chauvinism, are a concrete holdover from bestial days. "The genitals themselves have not taken part in the development of the human body in the direction of beauty: they have remained animal, thus love, too, has remained in essence just as animal as it ever was" (1912a, p. 189).

Freud frequently speaks of the sexual instincts as being hard to educate, like a dull and stubborn dog, the last to be wrested from the dominance of the pleasure principle (1911), and his portrayal of civilization is always as a secondary counterfoil to man's bestial nature. "For society must undertake as one of its most important educative tasks to tame and restrict the sexual instinct . . . for with the complete irruption of the sexual instinct, educability is for practical purposes at an end. Otherwise the instinct would break down every dam and wash away the laboriously erected work of civilization" (1916–17, p. 311–312).

Freud inevitably viewed human history through the ethnocentric eyes of nineteenth-century anthropology and its overly simplistic "cardboard Darwinism" (to adapt a term from Gould, 1987b), as a grand and prolonged struggle to attain the acme of human development, nineteenth-century Western European culture. From this vantage point, non-Western, so-called primitive peoples are seen as expressing raw animality in a pure form, less camouflaged and transformed by culture (Freud, 1940, p. 200). In "savages" we find "a well-preserved picture of an early stage of our own development" (1912–13, p. 1), and earlier periods in Western European history likewise were times of greater sexual gratification and less culture (1915a, p. 131). Whereas *physical* ontogenetic recapitulations in the human fetus are fleeting stages on the way to irreversible higher structures, in Freud's model of mind *psychic* recapitulations never fade, but continue to exist beneath higher mental processes. As Freud puts it in *Civilization and Its Discontents,* "Only in the mind is such a preservation of all the earlier stages alongside of the final form possible" (1930, p. 71).

Thus, Freud's id became the repository of man's phylogenetic and historical evolution. (Jung's theories of archetypes and a racial unconscious draw on similar early Darwinian and Lamarckian premises.) The "id, with its inherited trends, represents the organic past" (1940, p. 206). And the past which Freud believes, quite literally, to be encased within the id is an array of bestial desires. Civilized man lives always in the tension between his social existence and his primitive past, which is alive in him as a powerful motivational core. Freud uses the metaphor of the Zuider Zee to characterize the analytic process: "Where id was, there ego shall be" (1933, p. 80). But in a larger sense, all of social existence represents a reclamation project, operating on borrowed territory, with the continual threat of being overrun once again by primeval, instinctual forces. This is why in Freud's view psychic impotence is such a pervasive condition. Sexuality is a vestige of our bestial ancestry, always a threat to our superimposed civilized demeanor. At heart, argues Freud, everyone regards the sexual act "basically as something degrading" (1912a, p. 186). At heart, each of us is literally a wolf in sheep's clothing. The loved object is shielded, protected from bestial desires. Self-fragmentation is the inevitable price of intimacy.

THE INTERPRETIVE power of Freud's understanding of the nature of human sexuality has been extremely compelling and has pervaded the way in which we have come to experience and understand sexual phenomena. Thus, from a literary point of view, Bloom (1986) has argued that Freud's "conceptions . . . have begun to merge with our culture, and indeed now form the only Western mythology that contemporary intellectuals have in common." Sociologists Simon and Gagnon (1973) argue that Freud's vision of sexuality, in its "natural state," as bestial, has pervaded our culture and shaped the very way in which we experience ourselves.

Central to the experience of sexual desire in its innumerable forms is a sense of its deep power, a "drivenness," of engorgement and climax, tension and release. Sexuality is often experienced as if it were something more fundamental, more primitive, more peremptory, than other motives. Sexual desire seems to break through, disrupt, overpower, more mundane, tamer, more civilized aspects of experience. Freud's postulation of an atavistic, polymorphously perverse array of bestial sexual tensions as the primary source of psychic energy provides a powerful explanatory framework for understanding why we experience ourselves the way we do. Yet, from the very beginning, Freud's account of the sexual instincts was not without serious contradictions.

The Problem of Adhesiveness — *i.e. what explains attachment to unsatisfying objects*

By loosening the bond between the sexual instinct and its object, Freud developed an elegant and powerful model of mind and a compelling account of psychic impotence. It is not the objects or the discordant experiences which necessitate repression and self-fragmentation; the child brings to his objects and experiences an array of rapacious desires *and rageful/sadistic* which make social living and loving, by definition, a process of self-restraint and concealment.

Nevertheless, if the unconscious operates on the basis of the pleasure principle, using objects as vehicles for its hedonistic aims, why do we so regularly get stuck in pursuit of early objects which bring so little satisfaction and such enormous pain? Freud portrays libido as "polymorphously perverse," capable of continually shifting its aims and objects, characterized by an enormous "plasticity" (1933, p. 97). Based on this hedonistic vision, people should turn out differently than they do, resisting the demands of civilization or finding devious ways to reap clandestine pleasures out of the necessities of civilized life. Yet Freud's patients were miserable. True, they were seeking pleasure through the various libidinal aims concealed within their symptoms, but they did it poorly. The pleasures they sought were from inaccessible, impossible others, substitutes for original incestuous objects; hence, their pursuit of pleasure was always doomed. If pleasure seeking is so powerful and plastic, why is it so systematically and universally derailed? If we are beasts at heart, why are we such ineffectual beasts?

Freud's stress on unconscious conflict and original incestuous objects makes some contribution to solving this riddle. It is only the libido that is pleasure seeking, not the reality-oriented ego, and the original pleasure-seeking aims of the libido cathect dangerous oedipal objects, with aims that make retaliation likely. Yet unconscious conflict between pleasure-seeking oedipal cathexes and regulatory and punitive controls does not fully account for the repetitive restructuring of

attachment

neurotic misery. Why are the original cathexes not more easily renounced in favor of less troublesome, less conflictual pleasure-seeking aims? Why is the beast so easily tamed? The problem, as Freud saw it, was what he termed the adhesiveness of the libido, its tendency to get stuck on, fixated to, its first objects, and thus to maintain a lifelong dedication to unsatisfiable desires (1905a, pp. 242–243 ; 1916–17, p. 348; 1918, pp. 115–116).

The drive model thus led Freud to a difficult paradox. We are driven by a powerful, urgent pursuit of pleasure; yet psychopathology in all its multitude of forms is characterized by the systematic reproduction of pain and misery. Freud's description of the libido as "adhesive" is an elegant metaphor which highlights the problem; it does not resolve it. He called the "pertinacity of early impressions" a provisional psychological concept, a factor of unknown origin (1905a, p. 242) and was clearly puzzled by it. Freud's integrity as a clinician often led him to describe areas he had trouble accounting for within the model he was using at the time. Having established the pleasure principle as the modus operandi of drive theory, he kept bumping again and again into the systematic pursuit and reproduction of pain within human experience.

Why was Freud so uneasy with libidinal adhesiveness? Sulloway points out that the "exclusive attachment of an instinct to its first-eliciting object" was actually a common biological principle of Freud's day (1979, p. 266). Why not simply think of libido as operating on the basis of a kind of imprinting? Like ducks and their mothers, the libido simply fastens onto whoever is around. But as we have seen in our discussion of primary identifications, Freud could not have embraced as primary an imprinting sort of concept without fundamentally altering his theory. If the salient feature of libido is its attachment to early objects, the pleasure principle is seriously jeopardized. The ducklings follow their mother around not because she provides sensual gratification, but because *she is there;* they are not so much pleasure seekers as object seekers. To put primary motivational emphasis on attachment to early objects would have moved Freud's model in the direction of a more purely relational model, like Fairbairn's object-relations theory or Bowlby's theory of attachment. This is not the route Freud chose. He wanted to loosen, not tighten, the link between libido and its objects, to put explanatory emphasis on the Darwinian-inspired notion of sexuality as an inherent, rapacious drive. So the pleasure principle is retained as the reigning motivational concept, and adhesiveness is acknowledged as a puzzling mystery. The mind is shaped by powerful forces pressing for expression, but these somehow become entangled and thwarted by the first targets they encounter. Bestial sexuality is retained as the motivational bedrock, and civilized, nonsexual relatedness is the secondary veneer. Yet somehow the sheep's clothing seems to be controlling the wolf; or, to shift metaphors, the tail ends up wagging the dog.

It should be noted that with the introduction of the death instinct (1920a), Freud finally found an explanation for painful adhesive attachment to early objects as a simple characteristic of mental life—a tendency to repeat earlier states, deriving from the death instinct, operating "beyond the pleasure principle." Freud certainly never felt that he could adequately account for masochism, attachments to early painful experiences, within the framework of libido theory, and the theory of the death instinct appealed to him partly for this reason. Masochism presents "a truly puzzling problem to the libido theory; and it is only proper if what was a stumbling-block for the one theory should become the cornerstone of the theory replacing it [the death instinct]" (1933, p. 104). In explaining the phenomenon of psychic impotence in terms of a phylogenic primitivism in the very nature of sexuality, Freud reduced the importance of the object metapsychologically. All the same, it returned to haunt him clinically, and his subsequent explanation for adhesive attachments to early objects, the death instinct, has not been a compelling solution for most theorists and clinicians.

Sexuality and Contemporary Freudian Theory

Throughout the history of psychoanalytic ideas there has been a persistent linkage between sex as a clinical focus and drive as a metapsychological concept, as if they were bound together by necessity. To lose either, subsequent authors seemed to agree, meant the other was diminished. Theorists and clinicians for whom it was important to maintain the clinical focus on sexuality tend to preserve also the concept of drive. In their view, those who abandon the drive concept are closing their eyes to the body and the bestial core, backing away from unseemly and disturbing truths about the central place of sexuality in human experience. The decision to identify oneself as a specifically "Freudian" psychoanalyst is often adhered to on this basis.

On the other hand, theorists and clinicians who find it difficult to preserve drive theory as the basic metapsychological framework, such as those within the interpersonal, British object-relations, existential, and (more recently) self psychology schools, tend also, relatively speaking, to deemphasize the clinical importance of sexuality per se. George Klein points to the implicit agreement of both camps on the link between drive and sexuality:

> So ingrained and unquestioned is the assumed identity of drive theory with the clinical theory of sexuality . . . [that the rejection of drive] is automatically considered a denial of the motivational primacy of sexuality. Neo-Freudians have agreed on this equation. Expressing their dissatisfaction with the drive model, they usually conclude by disputing the importance of sexuality in the structuring of personality. (1976, p. 17)

Authors who have broken with drive theory completely tend to see sexuality as a developmentally later phenomenon which becomes conflictual only when drawn into the problems of earlier stages. Thus, Sullivan reverts to a pre-Freudian understanding of sexuality, terming it "lust" and dating its emergence at the hormonal surges of puberty, thereby minimizing the importance of the deeply sensual nature of experience in infancy and early childhood. Fairbairn and Kohut both locate sexuality in the oedipal phase of childhood, but regard any oedipal and sexual conflicts as *derivative* of earlier, preoedipal conflicts, the vehicle of infantile dependence for Fairbairn and of underlying disorders of the self for Kohut.* For many relational-model theorists, sexual experiences and fantasies tend to be viewed as "sexualizations" of other motives, an acting-out of needs and feelings more appropriately and constructively experienced in other ways.

Thus, moving away from the drive concept seems to imply a deemphasis on sexuality as motivationally central and problematic in its own right. Sexuality is only experienced as conflictual and bestial when more fundamental problems are operative; under normal circumstances, sexuality is integrated smoothly into nonsexual aspects of emotional life. The phenomenological experience of sexuality as pressured, conflictual, and not easily integrated with other aspects of life is an artifact, a derivative of earlier, more fundamental difficulties.

---

* In Kohut's posthumously published *How Does Analysis Cure?* he speaks of specifically "oedipal self-object" functions, disturbance in which may generate specifically oedipal disorders; but he indicates that parents failing in these functions would most likely also have had difficulty with earlier self-object functions.

In my view, both of these theoretical traditions have suffered because of the implicit linkage of sexuality and drive—the "Freudians" because preserving Freud's clinical theory of sexuality necessitates the preservation at all costs of the scientifically anachronistic concept of drive (Schafer, 1976; Eagle, 1984); and the neo-Freudians and post-Freudians because the linkage has led to minimization of the motivational and structural role of sexuality.

How can the frequent phenomenological accuracy and clinical utility of Freud's theory of sexuality be retained without yoking it to outmoded and implausible notions of drives as phylogenetic vestiges? This has been the central challenge for contemporary "Freudian" authors, and the most important contributions have emerged in the work of George Klein, Holt, and Schafer.

The essential strategy of this group of authors, whose work extends beyond considerations of sexuality to all areas of psychoanalytic theory, has been to argue that Freud's work is more or less divisible into two realms, two very different types of concepts and theories, a clinical or psychological theory, on the one hand, and a more abstract, philosophical, metapsychological theory on the other. The latter is seen as deriving from the mechanistic, physicalistic philosophy of science of Freud's day, borrowing concepts from now-outmoded nineteenth-century biology and neurophysiology. Each of these authors, in his own distinctive fashion, has attempted to discard the anachronistic metapsychological dimension of the drive concept while at the same time preserving what he regards as the significant clinical dimension of Freud's theories. Klein (1976) and Schafer (1976) have been most ambitious with respect to various areas of clinical theory, the former recasting Freudian concepts into a theory of relational meanings, and the latter translating Freudian concepts in an "action language" framework heavily influenced by British analytic philosophy.

Klein claims that the drive concept is not at all essential to Freud's understanding of the nature and function of sexuality, but instead was superimposed on his clinical grasp of sexual phenomena. Klein argues that sexuality is not driven from within, but evoked from without, by others. He develops a model which stresses the interactional, relational meanings of experience, what he calls the "superego" dimension of Freud's vision, arguing that social factors not only determine what will be done with sexual arousal, but govern the actual arousal itself. Klein redefines instincts not in terms of drives, but in terms of a kind of inherent responsivity. "Instincts" can refer to "capacity, to potential activity" (1976, p. 49).

Similarly, Holt (1976) presents a powerful critique of the concept of sexual arousal as a product of buildup of tension. (The only appetite for which this is the mechanism, Holt argues, is urination.) Sexuality depends for arousal, Holt suggests, not on deprivation but on external stimulation. He goes on to imply that Freud and his contemporaries greatly misunderstood the nature of both human and animal sexuality as well. "Recent careful observational and experimental studies of nonhuman animals, which were the classical embodiments of 'animal instinct,' do *not* support the notion of sex as an internally arising drive or tension that causes the organism to seek out need-satisfying objects" (1976, pp. 175–176). Animal sexuality is evoked by specific external stimuli; if the stimuli are not present, there is no sexual behavior, no buildup of tension—in effect, no sexuality. Holt quotes Frank Beach, the distinguished authority on sexuality in animals:

> To a much greater extent than is true of hunger or thirst, the sexual tendencies depend for their arousal upon external stimuli. The quasi-romantic concept of the rutting stag actively seeking a mate is quite misleading. When he encounters a receptive female, the male animal may or may not become sexually excited, but it is most unlikely that in the absence of erotic stimuli he exists in a constant state of undischarged sexual tensions. This would be equally true for the human male, were it not for the potent effects of symbolic stimuli which he tends to carry with him wherever he goes. (in Holt, 1976, p. 173)

Beach's phrase "symbolic stimuli" might easily be translated into the psychoanalytic concept of internalized object relations.

It is ironic that contemporary studies of animal behavior suggest that sexuality in nonhuman species depends for arousal, even more than in humans, not on spontaneously arising internal pressures but on the sensory awareness and experience of the other. The "driven" beast in Freud's instinct theory seems to bear little resemblance to behavior in nonhuman species. The experience of bestiality in human sexuality seems to have little to do with phylogeny; it is, somehow, a uniquely human phenomenon and must be accounted for in other ways.

The history of human representation of other animals is complex and fascinating. Historians of the menagerie have noted that "the appearance of early menageries was concurrent with the rise of urbanization" (Veltre, 1987, p. 2) and concepts of and interest in "wild" animals have been closely tied to cultural developments and social structure (see Loisel, 1912). Anthropomorphization is probably a universal phenomenon in all cultures. The experience of the self and one's sexuality as bestial is the product of an unconscious projection of human sexual experience onto an image of animals romanticized as being free of social constraint, then a subsequent identification with these semidetached, projected aspects of experience. I shall consider this process in more detail in the next chapter.

FOR FREUD, sexuality is powerful motivationally because the drives provide the energy which runs the mind, and the pressured expression of the array of sexual desires shapes experience according to the predesigned configurations of those desires. Early sexual experiences and memories are structurally formative because they are linked with primitive wishes which are still seeking discharge. Sexuality is difficult to integrate with tenderness and intimacy because of its primitive, prehuman features, encased like atavistic remnants in our pregenital organizations. The deletion of the drive concept from Freud's theory of sexuality, as in the work of G. Klein, Holt, and Schafer, removes the ground for those explanations. Sexuality becomes a response or an action rather than an internal pressure, and we are thrown back on the kinds of questions Freud's drive theory so neatly solved: *Why does sexuality become central, motivationally and structurally? Why does sexuality become so problematic?*

Contemporary Freudians tend to answer the first question by centering on the concept of pleasure. Sexuality is motivationally and structurally central because of the intensity and engrossing nature of early pleasurable experiences. Thus, George Klein defines sexuality as a "capacity for a primary, distinctively poignant, enveloping experience of pleasure" (1976, p. 19) and suggests that the centrality of sexual motives derives from the durability of early sensual experiences in memory. "Once experienced it continues to be savored; the record of its occurrence is hard to relinquish" (p. 26). Klein feels it is possible to retain Freud's clinical theory of sexuality while dropping the metapsychological notion of drive; the peremptory power of sexual motives simply derives from the vast pleasure they provide. Does this revision remain true to the central thrust of Freud's vision, *his* understanding of the nature of sexuality?

For Freud, the pleasure principle operates on the basis of somatic tension (the source of the drives). It is more accurately an unpleasure principle: "psychical rest was originally disturbed by the peremptory demands of internal needs" (1911, p. 219). For him the drive is a somatopsychic process, originating and ending in a bodily organ; the conscious or unconscious wish and its derivatives and the pleasure they seek are intervening processes generated by organ tension and aimed at relieving organ tension. By eliminating the drive concept one also lops off the beginning and the end of Freud's understanding of the nature of the sexual impulse (in eliminating the source and aim) and thereby strands (one is tempted to say, castrates) the libidinal impulse. The concept of pleasure no longer has any precise somatic referents, which makes it much less specifiable and truncates its explanatory power.

Klein is not unmindful of this problem and brings other explanatory concepts, relational in nature, to bear on the question of what sorts of experiences become pleasurable and why they are retained. He suggests that sensual pleasure does not operate autonomously in human motivation; it is not "sought after simply for its own sake" (1976, p. 38). Sensual experience does not "drive" a person, but "he seeks sensual experience because of meanings that have become associated with it in the course of his development" (p. 28).

The removal of the somatic drive concept from our understanding of psychological pleasure seems to *necessitate* the introduction of relational and social factors to take up the explanatory weight. Freud's "beast" is no longer an phylogenetic residue, but a piece of phenomenology, a metaphor for organizing and describing experience. The thrust of this approach is quite different from Freud's own, and Klein seems to generate more confusion than illumination in claiming that it is fundamentally the same as Freud's, or a part of Freud's. (For a similar argument see Eagle, 1984, p. 89.) For Freud, the meaning and power of sexual motives are endogenous and a priori; for Klein, the meaning and power of sexual motives derive from the relational context, which he characterizes as a "system and schema conception" (1976, p. 63). He has not merely deleted the drive concept from Freud's theory of sexuality; he has introduced an alternative explanatory framework into which he has reset Freud's theory.

The position proposed by Brenner (1982) is representative of current mainstream efforts to deal with this problem and makes an interesting comparison to Klein's approach. Brenner does not want to drop the term "drive"; yet he agrees that the notion of drives' having a specific organic "source" is no longer feasible. So Brenner declares "drive" to be a purely psychological construct, dropping the anachronistic tension-discharge elements in Freud's theory of sexuality and ending up with the full explanatory weight resting on the pleasure principle. Unlike Klein, however, Brenner does not introduce other explanatory concepts but limits himself to Freud's now-truncated drive theory, and in so doing, demonstrates how impoverished Freud's explanations become when they are simply separated from their original somatic underpinnings. Freud could explain *why* sex was a primary motivational force—it results from specific organic tensions that demand discharge. Brenner can only arbitrarily claim that libidinal drives are empirical facts.

If one deletes the somatic source and aim of drives, as Brenner has, and still insists that pleasure is the single motive of mental life, the very definition of pleasure, the nature of pleasure seeking, grows impossibly obscure. In Brenner's system, unlike Freud's, it is not at all obvious why sexual pleasures are any more central motivationally than any other forms of pleasure, or in what sense sexual and aggressive activities, many of which generate anxiety and pain, are to be construed as "pleasurable" at all. Brenner is driven to defend the pleasure principle as a single motivational criterion by insisting post hoc that whatever the person does, no matter how painful it feels and seems, *must* be pleasurable in terms of some unconscious wish. This is a strategy reminiscent of Skinner's invulnerable yet tautological defense of his concept of operant conditioning as the sole basis of learning on the grounds that whatever the subject eventually does was chosen because it must have been positively reinforced.

Brenner also claims that any wish, once activated, follows its pleasure-seeking path until it succeeds (p. 32). This becomes a very peculiar pleasure principle indeed. Brenner starts out with the proposition that the sole governing principle of mental life is the search for pleasure; libidinal and aggressive wishes are pursued on this basis. Once experienced, pleasure-seeking wishes are active forever, and the rest of life is thus dominated by the earliest libidinal and aggressive wishes. Brenner portrays the mind, instead of being pleasure seeking, as being fatefully committed to whatever early wishes happen to emerge within it. Why is there such fixation on first wishes despite their generation of a lifetime of unpleasure and frustration? While Freud himself had trouble explaining attachments to first objects, he could at least account for the persistence of early aims as necessitated by continuous stimulation at somatic sources. With the notion of somatic sources eliminated and drives reduced to pleasure-seeking wishes, Brenner's drives seem to appear arbitrarily and persist, with no convincing explanation of why they operate in the way Brenner claims they do. The comparison of Brenner's position with Klein's suggests that efforts to delete the anachronistic features of the drive concept greatly impoverish the explanatory power of Freud's theory of sexuality. It is only by relocating Freud's clinical insights in a relational framework (as does Klein, implicitly) that compelling explanations for the motivational and structural centrality of sexuality can be generated.

The second question answered by the drive concept and reopened by its deletion is, Why does sex become so problematic? As a manifestation of drive, sexuality is problematic because of its very nature as a collection of atavistic, bestial remnants. Without the drive concept, sexuality is a general capacity for sensual pleasure. Why does it then become so fraught with conflict? Contemporary Freudian revisionists who have abandoned the drive concept also necessarily lose the explanatory power which that concept provides; they tend to place full explanatory weight on the *incestuous* nature of infantile desires. Our early sexual responses, so compelling in their intensity (although not necessarily bestial), are all directed toward parental caretakers; because of the incest taboo, these desires become forbidden, inevitably conflictual. It is the clash between the poignancy of infantile sensual experience and its inevitably doomed and tragic fate which generates the sexual conflicts that underlie psychopathology.

Why is infantile love doomed? Society forbids it. But this does not explain the problem; to invoke incest merely displaces the taboo from an individual to a cultural plane. Freud's understanding of the incest taboo rested on the drive concept. Culture *must* oppose early incestuous love precisely because its bestial qualities, its prehuman nature, threatens the very basis on which civilization rests. For Freud, civilization is constructed upon borrowed territory, siphoning off energy from archaic desires ontogenetically as it did phylogenetically (in the guilt generated by the murder of the father in the primal horde). Without the drive concept, the incest taboo needs to be explained in some other way; we are left once again with the question, Why does sexuality—via social restrictions—become so difficult for the individual?

Some authors, particularly those drawing on Freudian ego psychology, attribute the problematic nature of sexuality and the taboo associated with incestuous love to the universal dangers and conflicts of early primary relationships; they thereby locate the problem within the inevitably conflictual interactive domain of the relational field. The mother who becomes the first sexual object is also the symbiotic matrix from which the child emerges in developing a rudimentary sense of self and early tentative boundaries. From this viewpoint, very similar to various relational-model theories to be considered in the next chapter, the incest taboo is fundamentally a bulwark against dedifferentiating regression. Thus, Schafer regards the fear of dedifferentiation from what is experienced as the "devouring mother" as an underlying cause of much sexual dysfunction, and he points to both the universality of these fears and their persistence throughout life. He describes

> the difficult, stressful, and unstable differentiation of oneself as an active figure—a person—in relation to the caretaking and terribly powerful maternal figure . . . The young child imagines loss of individuation to be a kind of devouring engulfment or annihilation that is perpetrated either by the mother or on the mother—a fantasy that, paradoxically, and like the castration fantasy, is experienced both excitedly and with shuddering horror. This archaically conceived struggle for and against individuation seems to remain a lifelong project. (1978, p. 157)

Loewald similarly depicts oedipal love as containing in its very core, features of primary identification and symbiosis. The function of the incest taboo thus becomes the strengthening of the separation from early undifferentiated objects, barring the confusion of identification and object cathexis, reinforcing the child's separation and freedom from the enveloping environment. Both oedipal wishes and oedipal guilt are universal for Loewald, not so much as a direct expression or derivative of drives, but because of the unavoidably conflictual struggle for self-definition within a relational matrix. "The self, in its autonomy, is an atonement structure, a structure of reconciliation" (1978, p. 394).*

Freud puts strong emphasis on the fear of castration in accounting for the universal, conflictual nature of sexuality. But *Freud's* castration com-

---

* Fromm too regards the regressive pull and danger of dedifferentiation as the basis for oedipal conflicts and the universality of the incest taboo. "Incestuous wishes are not primarily a result of sexual desires, but constitute one of the most fundamental in man: the wish to remain tied to where he came from, the fear of being free, and the fear of being destroyed by the very figure toward whom he has made himself helpless, renouncing any independence" (1964, p. 134).

plex is, once again, tied closely to his understanding of the function and power of drive. The child's incestuous wishes are overpowering in their intensity—nothing can stand in their way—and the idea of eliminating or castrating all rivals is a natural and inevitable solution. This then becomes the basis from which the child fears his own castration by the retaliatory father as punishment for his sexual strivings.

If one removes the metapsychological notion of drive, the clinical understanding of castration fears necessarily changes. If sexuality is aspired to because of a diffuse pleasure seeking, *would* the child begin to plot murder and castration to actualize his desires? *Would* the simple projection of these impulses onto the parents be able to generate intense castration anxiety? Without drive theory, castration anxiety as a clinical phenomenon seems to require (and is in fact now generally discussed in terms of) a shifting of explanatory weight onto interactional factors such as parental seductions; double binding; actual threats; fears of maternal engulfment and demasculinization; deeply divided, exclusive loyalties; intense paternal competitiveness and sadism; and so on.

Whether oedipal conflicts are attributed to universal struggles in the development of the self or to specific family dynamics, these contemporary versions of Freud's theory of sexuality are markedly different from Freud's own. The problem of sexuality is located not in its a priori nature, but in an interactive, relational field—the vicissitudes of object relations—from which it takes its meanings. The literal beast of nineteenth-century Darwinism, residing in the id and driving the psychic apparatus, has been replaced by the beast as metaphor in the struggle to establish and maintain the self within a relational matrix.

KLEIN, HOLT, and Schafer have made rich contributions to our clinical understanding of sexuality and its relation to nonsexual dimensions of human experience. Their common political strategy rests on the premise that the drive concept can be dropped without fundamentally altering Freud's clinical theory of sexuality. This position seems to me unconvincing. We have seen that the concept of drive in its cardboard Darwinian implications was designed to solve specific clinical problems, foremost among them psychic impotence. It is the nineteenth-century Darwinian connection and the image of the beast which it generated that provided Freud's theory of sexuality with its explanatory "bite." For Freud, the image of the beast is not at all metaphorical. We retain bestial impulses in the very tissues of our bodies, and they are the source of both the power and the problematic nature of sexuality. Sexuality without drive is a very different phenomenon: bestiality becomes a metaphor, generated as a way of symbolizing one's relationships to and feelings about oneself and others. Whether or not to designate these reformulations as "Freudian" is a political question that involves the role of semantics in preserving and altering theoretical traditions. Much more important is recognition of the changes in understanding which are inevitably linked with eliminating the drive concept.

In my view, removing a component of Freud's vision as essential as the drive concept does alter the theory fundamentally, creating an explanatory vacuum which needs to be filled in some fashion. If sexuality is not a powerful, dangerous, preconstituted push from within but a response or action within an interactive context, sexuality becomes a function, an expression of the relational matrix. While Freud "loosened" the bond between the instinct and the object, the logic of a position that eliminates drive seems to demand a *strengthening* of that connection. Indeed, Holt and Klein definitely point in this direction. There is in this tradition what might be characterized as a drift toward relational-model theorizing. Holt suggests that "the phenomena that psychoanalysts have long conceptualized in purely intrapsychic (or intraorganismic) terms must be accounted for in a way that takes serious account of the person's environment, especially the threats and opportunities it presents" (1976, p. 191). And Klein understands the psychodynamic significance of sexuality in terms of what he calls self-world values. "It is this relation to selfhood and to attitudes toward other people as objects that distinguishes sexuality in man from that of animals" (pp. 39–40).

These authors stop short of granting the pursuit and maintenance of object relations a primary motivational status in its own right. Having removed drive as the metapsychological framework and motivational prime mover, there seems to be a reluctance, perhaps partly because of continued loyalty to tradition, to replace it with another principle—for example, Fairbairn's notion of object seeking. We are left with the clinical centrality of sexuality within a larger theoretical framework composed of broad, abstract categories such as wishes (Holt), actions (Schafer), imbalances and mismatches (Klein), a framework that in my view fails to provide sufficient explanatory specificity and interpretive power.

It is possible to employ the relational matrix as a basic framework in a way that does not detract from the clinical importance of sexuality, but rather provides it with a more meaningful theoretical context, illuminating *why* sexuality becomes and remains so central in human motivation and *why* psychic impotence is such a pervasive problem.

Shifting Models

What does it mean to say that a particular understanding of the nature and function of sexuality operates from within a relational model rather than a model based on the motivational primacy of drive?

Theoretical models arrange phenomena with respect to surface and depth, figure and ground. No matter how much we try to listen to the patient's experiences from within the context of his or her own phenomenology, no matter how scrupulous we are to not superimpose our own theoretical presuppositions on clinical data, to listen is to arrange. As Spence (1982), Schafer (1983), and others have argued, there is no unstructured listening, unmediated by theory. The patient's associations become organized in the analyst's listening, and the principles of that organization are theoretical postulates which assign greater depth to some elements, stronger motivational and structural priority. The analytic process does not and could not operate on a flattened plane of meaning: "There's this and this and this and this." The analytic process entails a collaborative, slowly emerging, and painfully won three-dimensional understanding of the patient's experience: "There's this, which underlies that, which leads to that, which infuses that with meaning." Surface and depth are slowly differentiated, their intricate counterpoint delineated and charted.

Different theoretical models orient the analyst to different kinds of deep structures which are felt to underlie the fabric of human experience. The drive model regards rhythmic, endogenous pressures, their channelization and control, as the deep structure of experience. Relational models regard the establishment and maintenance of relational patterns as the deep structure of experience. These two models do not refer to different areas of experience—one model to physical urges, the other to interpersonal transactions. They are inversions of each other; both models account for the totality of clinical data, but they arrange that totality differently. For the relational theorist, it is not, as Freud believed, prewired "organ pleasure" itself that gives sexuality its mean-

and the insane complexity that entails (see p. 88)

ing and power, but the meanings that have become attached to those physiological sensations in the context of an idiosyncratically structured exchange with a particular other.

Compare the difference in interpretive strategies based on the two models. The drive model presumes that the fundamental motives and meanings of all human experience are provided by, derived from, the component instincts. Elements of the patient's life and free associations are broken down and grouped according to the categories provided by the drives. In essence, the variety of life is seen as an array of metaphors for sexual and aggressive wishes. Abraham's (1921) classic paper, "Contributions to the Theory of the Anal Character," provides a dazzling example of the application of this model. Different facets of anality are delineated and then applied to every imaginable aspect of life. Anal wishes or defenses against anal wishes are seen as structurally underlying and generating concerns with cleanliness, messiness, order, power, hoarding, control, sadism, envy, pleasure in one's creations and creativity, avarice, extravagance, ambivalence, balance, symmetry, reversals, oppositionalism, interest in looking at the other side of issues, separations of all kinds, giving and getting, submission and dominance, all regularization, mastery, and all conflict. The use of the drive model entails the discovery, in every imaginable feature of experience, of metaphoric representations of bodily, sexual, and aggressive themes.

The relational model provides different categories, different underlying structures into which experience can be organized. Here the establishment of strong connections to others, in reality or in fantasy, is presumed to be primary. Forms of relationship are seen as fundamental, and life is understood largely as an array of metaphors for expressing and playing out relational patterns: discovery, penetration, domination, surrender, control, longing, evasion, revelation, envelopment, merger, differentiation, and so on. The body is still centrally important. Sexuality and bodily experiences are viewed as particularly apt arenas for this activity, since sexuality is enormously multiform and plastic. The number of different body parts, the variability of interactions, the poignancy of the sensations, the immense number of combinations—the almost infinite variety of human sexual possibilities makes this an enormously fertile reservoir of metaphors for expressing different types of relationships, different configurations of connections, between self and others. Thus, the way in which the relational model construes the relationship between sexuality and object relations is the precise inverse of the way in which it is construed in the drive model. For Freud, object relations are the realm in which drive impulses are expressed, gratified, or defended against. For the relational-model theorist, sexuality and other bodily processes are the realm in which relational configurations are expressed or defended against. Both theories contain all the data, but they are organized very differently. It is precisely because of this reversal of means and ends that Freud's drive theory and object-relations theories such as Fairbairn's cannot be juxtaposed or mixed without radically changing one or both of them.

WHAT OF infantile sexuality? Does a relational-model perspective inevitably minimize the significance of infantile sexuality, which is so central a feature of the drive model? While it is true that infantile sexuality, like sexuality in general, has been underplayed by most major relational-model theorists, this is more a historical artifact than a necessity dictated by the premises of the model. Infantile sexuality, like adult sexuality, surely exists; the question is—what is it? Is the child driven toward certain predetermined experiences and fantasies, or do the exquisite sensations provided through bodily experiences with others take on passionate significance and meaning from the relational context in which they occur? In Chapter 4 we shall see how a relational-model perspective can provide a different way of understanding the motivational and structural centrality of both infantile and adult sexuality.

Freud's solution to the problem of psychic impotence was to loosen the tie between sexuality and its objects. The problem does not concern the object per se, but lies in the constitutional nature of sexuality as a prehuman and protohuman vestige of our animal past. Relational-model approaches take the opposite tack. Rather than loosen the tie between sexuality and its objects, they broaden it. Surely Freud was correct in challenging the popular notion of sexuality as evoked at puberty by the charms of the object. Yet perverse sexuality can be understood not as minimizing the importance of the object itself, but as reflecting different types of object ties—not less connection to the object, but *alternate routes*. Sexuality provides pathways through which relational configurations are established and maintained. From this perspective, "adhesiveness" is not an anomaly but reflects the very nature of early interpersonal relations, and sexuality in all its polymorphous variations is seen as an array of different kinds of self-organizations and object ties. Thus, psychic impotence is a result not of the fallen, bestial nature of sexuality, but of splitting, anxiety, and fragmentation in the search for and maintenance of connections with others.

and individuation

All we are able to imagine is what makes everyone like everyone else, what people have in common. The individual "I" is what differs from the common stock, that is, what cannot be guessed at or calculated, what must be unveiled, uncovered, conquered . . . So it was a desire not for pleasure (the pleasure came as an extra, a bonus) but for possession of the world . . . that sent him in pursuit of women.

—MILAN KUNDERA

4   Sex without Drive (Theory)

In the previous chapter we considered contributions to an understanding of sexuality apart from drive by theorists who attempted to disentangle drive theory metapsychology from Freud's clinical theory of sexuality. The centrality of sexuality as a motivational prime mover is maintained, but its *nature* as a mover, the justification for its centrality, seems to grow obscure. Without the drive concept and without any other similar alternative motivational framework, the motivational and structural centrality of sexuality seems to float in metapsychological space. If sexuality is not mandated by a pressured expression of inner necessity, *why* does it become so essential in personality development and psychopathology?

There have been various attempts to answer this question by developing a theory of sexuality within an explicitly relational perspective. These contributions can be roughly divided into two groups, those that focus on the *object* dimension of the relational matrix and those that focus on the *self.* Both depict the same relational matrix within which the self becomes structuralized through its interactions with others. One group of theories stresses the tie to the other, how it is established and how it is preserved; the other group of theories stresses self-continuity and the preservation of identity. Although in the rhetoric of psychoanalytic literature much is made of such differences, I believe that these strategies are more complementary than mutually exclusive and both are extremely rich clinically. Let us first consider theories stressing the role of the tie to others in sexual experience.

Sexuality and the Object

It is ironic that Melanie Klein, despite her devoted allegiance to drive theory, laid much of the groundwork for a very different understanding of the nature of sexuality and its place in human relations. For Freud, as well as for traditional Freudian ego psychology, genitality appears only at the end of the period of infantile sexuality, after much emotional development and psychic structuralization has already taken place. The fundamental distinction between oedipal and preoedipal psychopathology rests on this late dating of genitality. Klein, on the other hand, locates the entire complex array of object relations (including genitality, oedipal difficulties, and superego development) in the first year of life (1945, 1957). Whatever questions might be raised about this controversial dating, it has had enormous and very constructive implications for understanding the nature of sexuality, because it places sexuality squarely in the middle of the emergence and structuralization of the self in its relation to others. For Klein, sexuality is not a developmentally later phenomenon which will be untroubled as long as earlier, more basic issues are worked through; sexuality is the major vehicle for playing out and working through the powerful struggles between hate and love, between destructiveness and reparation, which constitute the core of early object relations. In my own view (elaborated in Chapters 5 and 6), it is not necessary to date sexuality so early to explain why oedipal issues are central to early object relations; rather, so-called preoedipal issues (or issues of object relations) are central throughout the life cycle, and sexuality is a major arena in which they are developed and worked through.

For Klein, the depressive position provides the context for the meanings which the child assigns to his or her sexuality. There is a powerful struggle between love and gratitude toward the mother for the nurturance, caring, and pleasure she provides, and hatred and envy toward the mother for disappointments, frustrations, and resistance to omnipotent control by the child. Destructive fantasies are extremely powerful and very real. The child fears he has destroyed the mother and her insides, where all good things are to be found, and also fears retaliation in which the mother strikes back in kind. Powerful reparative longings arise, involving a deep sense of regret and a poignant need to make up with the mother, to put her back together again, to heal her and give her pleasure instead of pain.

It is in this context that the giving and receiving of sexual pleasure takes on such significance. For both men and women, giving sexual pleasure to another has meaning in terms of repairing the mother, overcoming depressive anxiety by generating more joy than misery, more pleasure than pain. Providing a satisfying sexual experience for oneself and another is a testimony to the triumph of one's reparative capacities over one's destructiveness, to one's ability to keep alive and nurture both one's internal and one's external objects. Similarly, receiving and experiencing sexual pleasure from and with another has meaning in terms of identification with one's internal objects, now experientially alive and happy rather than depleted and destroyed. The capacity for sexual pleasure is a testament to the integrity of one's body, not destroyed by the mother (as had been feared) in retaliation for fantasies of destroying her insides. "The desire to give and receive libidinal gratification is thus enhanced by the drive for reparation. For the infant feels that in this way the injured object can be restored, and also that the power of his aggressive impulses is diminished, that his impulses of love are given free rein, and guilt is assuaged" (Klein, 1945, p. 381).

From this perspective reproduction also takes on very powerful significance. In Freud's theory, the deepest psychological meanings of sexual reproduction are in terms of substitutions or symbolizations of body parts and organ pleasure. For the man, impregnating a woman represents sexual possession over the mother and triumph over castration fears; for the woman, pregnancy and babies are compensations for the missing penis and a salve to penis envy. In Klein's formulation, the psychological meanings of sexual reproduction are more primary and fundamental; they concern a person's basic sense of self in relation to others. For the man, impregnating a woman carries meanings involving restoration of the mother, a healing of her insides previously destroyed in fantasy; for the woman, pregnancy signifies a healing of the mother, via identification with her as an internal object, and also proof that her own insides have not been destroyed by the mother's retaliation, that she is whole and can generate life. "The sexual development of the child is inextricably bound up with his object relations and with all the emotions which from the beginning mould his attitude to mother and father" (p. 390). For Klein, sexual pleasure and impregnation have strong significance in terms of our deepest anxieties and longings, which are never fully resolved but remain open and often raw in each interpersonal encounter.

Although many features of Klein's larger vision are highly controversial, her placing of genital sexuality in the middle of issues involving basic object relations rather than subsequent to them has had an enormous impact on many authors who do not identify themselves as "Kleinian." Khan and Kernberg have been two of the most creative cultivators of the path Klein opened in our understanding of the nature and function of sexuality.

Khan blends some of Klein's basic concepts into a Winnicottian perspective, with particular emphasis on the notion of "transitional" experience. Winnicott depicts development as passage from an original state of "subjective omnipotence" to an eventual appreciation of "objective reality." In the former, the child believes, with considerable help from the mother, that he is omnipotent, that his wishes and gestures create the objects of his desires. In the eventual world of "objective reality," we come to appreciate the limits of our power over others and their own subjective reality. Between these two states of being lie transitional experiencing and transitional objects, whose status in relation to the self is ambiguous and paradoxical. We have not exactly created these others (for example, the traditional teddy bear), but all the same we feel them as extensions of ourselves and experience a special relationship to and control over them.

Khan locates sexual perversions within this transitional realm. The mother of the pervert-to-be has lavished intense nurturance and body care on the infant, but in a distant, impersonal way. The child internalizes this "thing-creation" of the mother's, and because of the mother's failure to relate in a more personal, differentiated way, the child becomes addicted to the early physical sensations, constantly trying to repair the damage, to reanimate this aborted self. Thus, the "reparative drive [is directed] towards the self as an idolized internal object" (1979, p. 16).

In Khan's view, the other person for the pervert is never really an "other," but a transitional object whom the pervert manipulates and arranges in order to re-create the tie with the mother and thus feel whole. The perversion operates as a "technique of intimacy which is profoundly solitary in nature . . . even though two persons are involved in a heightened instinctual modality essentially it is all the invention of one person . . . There is no object relatedness; hence no nourishment"

(p. 23). Khan depicts the mental state of the pervert as akin to that of a creative artist or as similar to a dream. A kind of illusory, omnipotent control has been established over the object (with the other's complicity) and is essential; any resistance breaks the spell. Thus, for Khan as for Klein (and unlike Freud), sexuality does not itself trigger action endogenously, driving the person into relations with others; rather, the physical and physiological features of sexuality are employed to establish and express prior relational patterns and needs. "It is all engineered from the head and then instinctual apparatuses and functions are zealously exploited in the service of programmed sexuality" (p. 15).

Khan focuses almost exclusively on pathological sexuality, but a few of his remarks suggest the possibility of expanding his analysis to the entire realm of sexual phenomena. For example, the use of the other as a transitional object, to be arranged and controlled for one's own pleasure, may be an essential ingredient not just in perverse sexuality but in the most mature sexual relationships as well, where the partners shift back and forth between the roles of subject and object, actor and acted upon. In this view, the common experience of loss of sexual interest in intimacy over time has less to do with boredom than with inhibition. "In ordinary so-called normal genital sexuality, many disturbances accrue from the incapacity to relate to the object in this dual fashion: distantly and impersonally as a body-thing-person, and affectively as a cherished being" (p. 178).

The experience of "romance" seems to entail precisely the tone that Khan ascribes to perversions, where an alternative realm is created outside the usual objective reality, where the playful mutual surrender to the illusions of the other creates a kind of spell which makes passion possible—and which can easily be broken through noncompliance. For many people, drugs or alcohol are used to create this altered state which, because of constrictions, they cannot take full responsibility for creating themselves.

Kernberg also has employed Kleinian concepts in his explorations of the varieties of sexual experience and the capacity to love across the range of different types of psychopathology. One fundamental feature of Kernberg's approach has been his persuasive challenge of the basic, classical Freud-Abraham characterology which derives personality types from the point of libidinal fixation. Within classical drive theory one's sexuality is the centerpiece of personality; the other dimensions merely reflect or express underlying sexual development. If "genital primacy" is achieved, psychological health is assured. In Kernberg's blend of Kleinian theory with Mahlerian ego psychology, personality structure centers on different organizations of object relations, and sexual functioning is a manifestation and expression of those object relations. Thus, Kernberg argues, in some types of severe characterological disorders, sexual functioning is quite intact and serves to reinforce a deep splitting of object relations. Ironically, as the analysand improves and various dimensions of relatedness become more integrated, sexual functioning often becomes more conflictual and inhibited. Similarly, in higher-functioning neurotics, Kernberg regards sexual experience as contingent upon and derivative of underlying relational configurations rather than vice versa. "Clinical study of couples indicates the significant effect of the nature of their total relationship on their sexual experiences: the frequency of intercourse, the intensity of its erotic quality, the excitement related to the enactment and sharing of sexual fantasies—all depend on the quality of the couple's object relationship" (1980, p. 297).

Kernberg, like Klein, regards sexuality as reflective of—in fact, as constituted by—configurations of object relations and therefore portrays sexual experience as inevitably carrying meanings pertaining to various relational needs and issues. He extends Klein's focus on early oral aggression by emphasizing the crucial and often problematic integration of feelings of envy and rage into sexual excitement. He also extends Mahler's concepts of symbiosis and separation-individuation by emphasizing the importance and inevitable dangers involved in the experience of crossing boundaries in sexual intimacy.

Sexuality and Self-Organization

A second and closely related approach to understanding the prominence and power of sexuality without the metapsychological concept of drive has focused on the role of sexual experience in shaping and maintaining a sense of self or identity. In classical drive theory psychosexual urges and wishes propel experience and behavior, and one's sense of self is derivative of the expression of these underlying motives. Various authors from different traditions have turned this causal sequence around, arguing that the maintenance of a sense of identity and continuity is the most pressing human concern and that sexual experiences often derive their meaning and intensity by lending themselves to this project.

For Fromm, sexuality is a vehicle for expressing and maintaining underlying character orientation. Whereas Freud regarded libidinal fixations as determining character type, Fromm regards character type as more fundamental and as manifesting itself in particular libidinal styles; he relocates Freud's psychodynamic descriptions of libidinal organizations into a framework which stresses character in a broader cultural and historical context. Sexuality becomes "the expression of an attitude toward the world in the language of the body" (1941, p. 320). Fromm believes that the structure of the character and the position of the self in relation to the world of others is always the predominant psychodynamic concern; sexual experience and sensations provide materials out of which this structure is assembled.

Lichtenstein, in "Identity and Sexuality," approaches the meanings of sexuality in remarkably similar fashion. In contrast to lower species, Lichtenstein argues, man lacks a biologically given identity, and must construct his own. Precisely because of the lack of biological mandate, "the maintenance of identity in man has priority over any other principle determining human behavior, not only the reality principle but also the pleasure principle" (1961, p. 189). The core of individual identity, Lichtenstein suggests, is created in the early sensual interactions between the infant and the mother, a "partnership of sensual involvement," which "imprints" on the infant an "irreversible identity theme" (p. 208). The specific content of that theme derives from the mother's unconscious wishes, which the infant inevitably is drawn into gratifying. "While the mother satisfies the infant's needs, in fact creates certain specific needs, which she delights in satisfying, the infant is transformed into an organ or an instrument for the satisfaction of the mother's unconscious needs" (p. 207).

More recent contributions approaching sexuality from the point of view of identity have focused specifically on gender identity and point to the establishment and maintenance of a sense of oneself *as a man,* or *as a woman,* as the motive underlying much sexual behavior and fantasy. These authors have drawn heavily from the influential sociological study of human sexuality undertaken by Simon and Gagnon, who developed an elaborate and persuasive critique of Freud's concept of sexuality as an innate and dangerous instinct.

Simon and Gagnon argue that all aspects of sexual experience, including arousal and satiation, derive from social contexts and carry social meanings, which they call scripts. "Scripts are involved in learning the meaning of internal states, organizing the sequences of specifically sexual acts, decoding novel situations, setting the limits on sexual responses, and linking meanings from nonsexual aspects of life to specifically sexual experience" (1973, p. 19). Although scripts draw their meaning from the interpersonal social field, they become intrapsychic phenomena which generate motivation, arousal, and commitment. From this vantage point, Freud's understanding of the means-end relationship between sexual motives and social behavior is the reverse of the way it actually operates. "Social roles are not vehicles for the expression of sexual impulse but . . . sexuality becomes a vehicle for expressing the needs of social roles" (p. 45).

Stoller (whose early contributions predate and whose later contributions draw upon the work of Simon and Gagnon) also understands sexual behaviors, particularly perversions, in terms of the enactment of scripts. In Stoller's view, the scripts embedded within sexual passion always have to do with an intent to humiliate another, as a reversal of and triumph over childhood traumas and humiliations. These childhood events were so traumatic, Stoller argues, because they represented threats to one's "core gender identity." "I see castration anxiety as a mild misnomer for a threat that is best put in identity terms; for humiliation is about 'existence anxiety' " (1985, p. 20n). Once again, there is a reversal of Freud's understanding of the relationship between sexual factors and social role. "Identity stands behind anatomy. Men, that is, do not fear loss of genitals per se (castration anxiety) as much as they fear to lose their masculinity and—still more fundamental—their sense of maleness" (p. 35).

Similarly, Person has traced the role of sexuality in terms of what she calls "the mediating structures of gender and sex print" (1980, p. 630). Sexual experience and behavior sustain gender identity. In men, Person argues, where gender identity is much more fragile and easily threatened than in women, sexuality seems more compulsive and appears "driven." (Classical drive theory institutionalizes this male "hypersexuality" through what Simon and Gagnon call the myth of naturalness, which conceals its derivation and significance in maintaining gender identity.) Thus, Person argues, "the meaning of sexuality will always be linked to nonsexual meaning because of the infantile intertwining of sensuality and object relations . . . Sex qua sex, without these other meanings, is an impossibility. Sex will always be permeated with meanings that attach to individual and social parameters" (p. 627).

Kohut initially distinguished more differentiated or nonnarcissistic sexuality (object libido) from sexuality which carries narcissistic meanings (narcissistic libido). But, as he eventually came to see *all* psychopathology as deriving from disorders of the self, sexuality in general, or any sexuality that is impassioned enough to be interesting, is seen more and more in terms of its meanings vis-à-vis the self. Stolorow and Lachmann deftly trace the developmental sequence of various sorts of sensual, psychosexual experiences and their role as "psychic organizers" in the building of stable images of self and other. "Nature, in her evolutionary wisdom, has harnessed the exquisiteness of sensual pleasure to serve the ontogenesis of subjectivity" (1980, p. 148).

Various self-psychology formulations regarding the motivational underpinnings of sexual experiences highlight the close connection between the need to preserve a sense of continuity and coherence of the self and ties to experiences with early significant others. Some perversions, for example, are understood as a search for healthy self-object functions such as mirroring. Other perversions (for instance, Mr. Z's masochism in Kohut, 1979) are understood in terms of a preservation of pathological self-object integrations as the only basis on which self-cohesion can be maintained. Still others are understood in terms of the reproduction of physical sensation as proof of one's own existence, given the lack of vitalizing connections with others.

Although different relational-model strategies for understanding sexuality can be separated into those focusing on connection and attachment and those focusing on identity, this is a difference more of emphasis and tradition than of basic conception. Taken together, these currents demonstrate how embeddedness within and loyalty to an interactional, relational matrix can be employed as an alternative to classical drive theory in accounting for the enormous variations, power, and range of human sexual experience.

WHY SEX? Why does sexuality become the arena in which fundamental relational issues and struggles are played out? Four factors seem crucial.

First, bodily sensations, processes, and events dominate the child's early experience. The mind develops initially, as Winnicott (1988) puts it, in "the imaginative elaboration of body functioning." The child draws on and generalizes from the major patterns of bodily experience in constructing and representing a view of the world and other people. Thus, the world and other people are regarded variously as potential nutriment or potential excrement, as soothers or invaders, as harbingers of sexual pleasure or harbingers of pain. Early bodily experiences become basic organizational signifiers for more complex later experiences; they become, as Schafer (1978) has suggested, paradigms for all subsequent psychological events.

Second, the fact that sexuality entails an interpenetration of bodies and needs makes its endless variations ideally suited to represent longings, conflicts, and negotiations in the relations between self and others. Sex is a powerful organizer of experience. Bodily sensations and sensual pleasures define one's skin, one's outline, one's boundaries; and the dialectics of bodily and sexual intimacies position one in relation to the other: over, under, inside, against, surrounding, controlling, yielding, adored, enraptured, and so on.

Third, the powerful biological surges in the phenomenology of sexual excitement, the sense of being "driven," provide a natural vocabulary for dramatic expression of dynamics involving conflict, anxiety, compulsion, escape, passion, and rapture.

Critics of classical drive theory often mistakenly underplay the relevance of physiology and temperament in the phenomenology and dynamics of sexuality. It is vitally necessary to distinguish between what Person (1980, p. 611n) calls the "initiating event for arousal," the original trigger, and various pressures brought into play as mechanisms or consequences of arousal. Freud thought of spontaneously arising, endogenous physiological pressures demanding discharge as the trigger. Holt, Person, and others cite considerable evidence that sexual physiology in both animals and humans does not *generate* its own energy; rather, it is a system of response to *external* cues, social triggers. Hormones, for example, do not generate internal pressure, but control *arousability,* responses within an interactive, relational field of interpersonal relations and internalized object relations. Thus, the biology of sexuality is extremely important in an interactional perspective, providing the medium—often the central medium—within which relational struggles are played out.

Fourth, the very privacy, secrecy, and exclusion in one's experience of one's parents' sexuality make it perfectly designed to take on meanings concerning a division of interpersonal realms, the accessible vs. the inaccessible, the visible vs. the shadowy, surface vs. depth. Sexuality takes on all the intensity of passionate struggles to make contact, to engage, to overcome isolation and exclusion.

Thus, one does not require a metapsychological notion of drive to account for the universality of sexual conflict and the peremptory experience of sexual desire. To view the subjective experience of conflict and "drivenness" as a product of an accretion of physical tensions obscures the meaning of sexual desire as a powerful, physiologically mediated response within a particular interplay of self and other, within a larger, subjectively structured, inevitably conflictual, relational design. Let us now consider some of the ways by which sexuality becomes the vehicle for experiencing and representing universal relational themes.

Search, Surrender, and Escape

Libido, Fairbairn argues, is object seeking. What does this mean? The child is seeking not pleasure per se, but contact, emotional exchange. Because he tends to focus on the earliest relationship between infant and mother, Fairbairn often writes as if availability for contact, receptivity to the child's object seeking, is a cut-and-dried business. There are good objects and bad objects, mothers who are available and mothers who abandon. But relationships between children and parents are much more complex and subtle. Parents are highly variable emotional presences, whose experience of the child is entangled with their own security needs and therefore embodies narcissistic meanings. The parents' capacity to be reached and moved by the child is necessarily obscured by and hostage to the vulnerabilities and conflicts of the character structure of the individual parent. Human beings are deceptively elusive creatures, which makes object seeking, the search for access to and connection with others an engrossing and intricate process. The palpable visibility of the human face belies the complex privacy of experience. (Winnicott, 1963, for one, believed that the core of the true self is always incommunicado, inaccessible to others.)

There has been frequent reference in the psychoanalytic literature to the sense of mystery which the child attributes to the parents' secret sexual life with each other. But parents are mysterious to children in more pervasive and encompassing ways. The intense and highly personal curiosity toward the analyst which each analysand eventually develops is always partially a re-creation of the child's generally thwarted and repressed curiosity about and search for the inner, personal experience of the parents. Thus, if attachment and object relatedness are taken beyond a simple, literal physical presence, the object seeking Fairbairn speaks of is a very complex, subtle process. Each parent is accessible in some situations, inaccessible in others; in some ways reachable, in some ways always out of reach. If object seeking is to be regarded as a fundamental human motivation, we are referring not to literal presence or absence, but to a complex array of desires, identifications, and behaviors which reflect efforts to reach others. Khan (1979, p. 22) points out that the word "intimacy" is best understood by considering its verb form, "intimate," defined by the *Oxford English Dictionary* as "to put into, drive or press into, to make known." The language reflects a sense of interiority—a gap or space between oneself and the other which one strives or longs to overcome.

Winnicott presents a view of early relatedness that is quite different from Fairbairn's. Fairbairn emphasizes the child's search for the parent; the problem is the parent's unavailability. Winnicott portrays the child as happily self-absorbed, generating spontaneous wishes and gestures which become actualized by the "good-enough mother," who provides the belief that he has in fact created all he desires. Ideally, the mother is invisible. The problem in Winnicott's account is not unavailability, but "impingement"; the caretaker responds to the infant in a way which takes little notice of the infant's own spontaneous needs and gestures, breaking in on the child's subjectively experienced, blissful self-sufficiency. Whereas in healthy development the mothering one is exquisitely sensitive to the child's wishes and actualizes them, in mothering which generates a false self, the caretaker misses the child's wishes more or less completely and sees only her own image of the child, her own agenda.

What happens to the child in such circumstances? Winnicott argues that the child cannot maintain genuine wishes and needs in an unreceptive environment—it is too painful. The true self is unattended to, either kept secret or repressed. Further, the caretaker's agenda must be dealt with; relatedness is essential to physical and emotional survival. So the child learns to shape himself or herself according to the contours of the mother's vision, becoming the "mother's son," or the "mother's daughter," a "false self on a compliant basis" (Winnicott, 1954a).

Winnicott introduced this description in connection with more severe character pathology; a close reading of his later work, however, suggests that he came to consider it as operating not only in cases of severe disturbance but across the entire range of psychopathology. All patients, all of us, are cared for by parents who only imperfectly grasp our wishes and experience. In addition, the amount of connection and attention desired by most children generally exceeds the parents' physical and emotional resources. The child learns to become more visible to the parent by becoming more like the parents' image of him or her. Thus, there are elements of falseness and compliance in all personalities.

Farber characterizes this process as "promiscuity," in its original meaning an "indiscriminate mingling," a tendency for one to feel "driven to scatter their overtures, as though they would be everything to everyone" (1976, pp. 195–196). Freud's concept of the superego is predicated on a similar assumption that the child finds it necessary to bend himself out of shape to accommodate himself to the social environment; but for Freud, accommodation is necessary because of more fundamental asocial drives. Relational-model theorists like Winnicott, Sullivan, and Farber assume a powerful primary need for interpersonal connection, which makes it necessary for the child, to one degree or another, to shape himself to the parents' vision of him; to present himself in a way that is both visible and palatable; to become, in Sullivan's terms, the parent's definition of "good me." Thus, the child inevitably becomes captive to the parents' world of meanings and values.

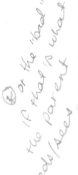

or the "bad" me if that is what the parent needs/sees

The pressure to comply with the images and values of the other often creates a counterpressure, to escape from the strictures of compliant relatedness. The surrender to the tyranny of the impinging object generates an anxiety in which the child, and later the adult, feels there is nothing about him that is real or genuine, nothing apart from his socially styled, acceptable appearances. So counteridentifications are established, unconscious (or conscious and secret) realms which are anathema to the primary object, which sabotage the surrender to "goodness" and acceptability. Identifications with parents are often counterbalanced against each other in this manner. Sometimes there is a secret and forbidden identification with a parent or other significant figure who is largely absent or cast in a malevolent or degraded role. The central identification with the primary, more powerful parent is preserved, with its elements of compliance, while a clandestine pact with the prohibited object provides a surreptitious excitement and vitality.

Fairbairn, and Bowlby as well, portray the child as seeking after unavailable objects; Winnicott portrays the child as submitting to and secretly evading intrusive objects. What is the relationship between these two processes? Guntrip (1971) sees them as pertaining to two different kinds of mothers, resulting in two different kinds of psychopathology. I think they are more universal, that every parent is in some sense unavailable and in some sense impinging; this is why relational conflict plays such a ubiquitous psychodynamic role. The child's relationship with each significant caretaker, all later intense relationships between adults, are a blend of self-protective molding to the other's vision and values, counterpressure to escape those unavoidable accommodations, and, at the same time, a search for the other's deeper, more private experience. One or the other of these processes may be more prominent in any relationship, but I believe they are generally all present.

The predominant meanings of sexuality in the lives of analysands often derive from these basic relational patterns of search, surrender, and escape. Fairbairn speaks of pleasure or pain as a "channel" to the object. Relationship is mediated through activities and sensations. If the other offers pleasurable activities, Fairbairn suggests, these are sought as a mode of contact. But the function of pleasure within intimacy is more subtle than this. If the emotional access to the object is as complex as I have suggested, intensely pleasurable mutual experiences have multiple meanings. Because sexual excitement entails such a powerful physiological response, and because the full emotional responsiveness of the other, in contrast to the physical presence of that other, can never be taken for granted, sexual encounters always contain elements of risk and implicit drama. Will the other be there, and in what way? When sexuality approaches true intimacy, an unritualized search for open emotional exchange, one places oneself in the other's hands (the double meaning is intended). Thus, sexuality plays a central role in most intimate relationships. This is not because pleasure regulation itself is the fundamental human aim, and therefore, as Freud understood it, loving is "the relation of the ego to its sources of pleasure" (1915a, p. 135). Rather, it is establishment and maintenance of relatedness that is fundamental, and the mutual exchange of intense pleasure and emotional responsiveness is perhaps the most powerful medium in which emotional connection and intimacy is sought, established, lost, and regained.

When sexuality is operating in the service of intimacy, it is the fact that it is the particular other who is responding to the vulnerability inherent in sustaining desire that generates intensity and meaning. It is precisely the physiological intensity of the sexual response that lends the sexual encounter its dramatic interpersonal significance. This suggests that it is a mistake to regard the role of sexuality in relation to needs for relatedness and attachment as a "sexualization," which implies that sex is

⊛ my ♡ was only emotionally
available to me through the
drama of projected shame

carrying something that can and somehow should be attended to in other ways. (Although this is sometimes the case.) The distinction between preoedipal and oedipal developmental levels often implies such an artificial and misleading separation between sexual experience and issues of attachment and connection. There is perhaps nothing better suited for experiencing and deepening the drama of search and discovery than the mutual arousal, sustaining, and quenching of sexual desire. (See Stern, 1977, for a discussion of the importance of "attunement" in relation to what he calls vitality affects between mother and infant.)

The inability to sustain desire in relation to another is a common thread which runs across the entire continuum of psychopathology from neurosis to the more severe character disorders. The obsessional, in particular, often deals with the vulnerability inherent in sexual desire through elaborate, ritualized power operations (Schimel, 1972). In the capacity to provide or withhold sexual availability and satisfaction, the other is experienced as very powerful, and thus very dangerous. The sense of being at the mercy of the other is countered by assigning imperious claims to one's own sexual desire. Sex is demanded in the name of love, and its absence is experienced as betrayal and humiliation. Lack of sex is experienced in terms of mounting sexual pressure, which has more to do with anxiety than with arousal. Sexual release is experienced not just in terms of tension reduction, but as desperately sought reassurance against abandonment and betrayal. Who does what to whom, and how often? These are crucial issues in the obsessional's approach to sexuality, often elaborated into a complex arrangement characterized by Sullivan as "double-entry bookkeeping." Sex becomes the arena in which the same questions are played out over and over: If I need you, will you be there? Will you gratify or deplete and exploit me? If I sustain my desire for you without diverting or depleting it, will the satisfactions outweigh the pain and disappointments?

Masturbation often provides an escape from these dilemmas, a form of self-arousal and self-gratification in which the physiological drama has implications for sustaining and soothing the self, as well as the interpersonal message, Who needs you anyway? I can both arouse and gratify myself, regulate my own desire, independent of your availability and accessibility. The pressure driving compulsive masturbation is not an endogenously arising tension, but anxiety about and solution to a sense of intense interpersonal vulnerability experienced in physical terms. Thus, some obsessionals will masturbate as soon as possible following a satisfying sexual experience with another, as if reclaiming their own autonomy, using the physiology of sexual arousal and satiation as the vehicle for establishing their self-sufficiency with regard to the other, whom they long for and whose importance to them they therefore dread.

In more severe disorders, the threat connected with experiencing desire in relation to another is often so great that it precludes ever allowing oneself to really want anything from anyone. Kernberg (1980) describes borderline patients whose desire is wholly self-referential, where any possibility of the other's presenting an occasion for arousal or a source of satisfaction is eliminated. Higher-functioning borderlines may allow themselves sexual gratification with others, who are eventually and inevitably experienced as degraded or worthless. The degradation is not, as Freud thought, in the a priori meaning of the sexual activity itself; the degradation is assigned to the sexual activity as a way of minimizing the significance of the other. Sullivan's concept of the "malevolent transformation" and M. Klein's concept of "envy" are both accounts of the systematic destruction of hope and desire, massive spoiling efforts to avoid being in the position of *needing something important from someone important,* which is experienced as equivalent to placing oneself at that person's mercy.*

Perversions in a Relational Perspective

Freud regarded the variety of so-called perversions as evidence for the heterogeneous nature of sexuality; libido is not a unitary drive, but a collection of component drives, each emanating from a tension in a different body part. From a relational-model perspective perversions, like all forms of sexuality, attain their meaning from the manner in which they lend themselves to the vast array of relational motifs.

Anality often takes on meanings related to a sense of the other as

---

* Eating disorders such as anorexia nervosa and bulimia dramatically illustrate the manner in which bodily states and desires can be manipulated to preserve illusions of self-sufficiency and total omnipotence over relations with others, complete control over desire and interpersonal exchange. In these states hunger as an endogenous physiological stimulus has become insignificant; the acts of eating, burning calories, and excreting often are transformed into symbolic statements of complete freedom from desire and vulnerability to others. The bodily preoccupations and self-scrutiny of the anorexic are dramatically reminiscent of the careful gaze of the mother of the newborn, watching for problems of feeding or elimination and measuring ounces.

elusive, to be reached only through hidden entrances or back doors, enabling one to reach behind the mask, under the surface, to secret recesses where, in fantasy, the other actually resides. Anal eroticism can represent for both parties a kind of access to mysteries and intrigues not accessible to others, not reachable in other ways. Analysands with these dynamics have often had parents who kept secrets from them regarding their own inner worlds, and sometimes crucial facts about their own early history. As adults, genital sexuality often seems shallow, something easily granted to everyone; being allowed anal penetration carries meanings of deeper, more meaningful disclosure and intimacy, access to secrets otherwise forbidden.

Sadism often takes on meanings related to a sense of the other as hidden or holding back, to be reached only by overcoming some resistance, causing some pain, wresting something away, making a dramatic impact. Sadists often regard the masochistic surrender of their partner as a kind of second deflowering and an exclusive intimacy, feeling no jealousy about the partner's having intercourse with another, but feeling betrayed if masochistic surrender is also then involved.

Similarly, masochism often takes on meanings related to a sense of contact with and impact on the other, to be attained only through exposure and surrender. Enduring pain at the hands of the other becomes a sign of devotion, evoking a fantasied response from the other not reachable in any other way. Passive fantasies (in both men and women) of being raped, for example, are often employed by analysands to represent a disguised passionate surrender to an overpowering parent, whose intrusiveness is guarded against in all other ways.

One female analysand, an only child of a widowed father, had been turned to by her father with emotional pleas and nearly explicit sexual gestures which she found overwhelming. Her subsequent character was a finely balanced composition of surrender to and resistance against his protection and intrusion. Efforts to control all aspects of living and, ultimately, her own passive longings dominated her experience. Her life seemed designed to preclude the possibility of anything spontaneous or organic; she had difficulty, for instance, in growing plants because she would be unable to restrain herself from opening the new shoots rather than allowing them to unfold at their own pace. Sex was unpleasant to her, and intercourse was actually painful; yet her erotic life centered around a fantasy of being overcome, tied down, and raped by a dashing stranger. Her father's lack of control had made it necessary for her to isolate herself from him both behaviorally and internally, and it was dangerous for her to allow herself to recognize her longings for contact with him. Yet the sexual fantasy, and the masturbatory experiences accompanying it, made possible a secret, passionate, cataclysmic engagement with her father, terrifying to allow or even desire in any other way.

Voyeurism and exhibitionism most vividly express the quality which is central to all perversions, as well as to sexuality in general—a dialectic between surface and depth, between the visible and the secret, between the available and the withheld. Voyeurs are often found to have had depressed parents, for whom the emotional surface of things was experienced as dead and meaningless. Life is inside, hidden, under wraps; what is exciting is seeing into hidden recesses, watching others in realms and actions otherwise inaccessible. Similarly, exhibitionism often becomes prominent in analysands from families where it was difficult to make an impact or be noticed. There is a sense that the normal interchange among people is shallow, meaningless, self-absorbed. Nothing happens; no one is really touched or moved. Passion and true contact come from shock, seizing attention, taking someone by surprise.

The privacy of the body, one's own and that of others, makes sexuality perfectly suited for the experience and the symbolization of object seeking, longings for contact with and access to others. Sexual passion, whether concretized into repetitive compulsive scenarios or allowed free rein in a more spontaneous and authentic interpersonal context, draws its excitement and vitality not from simple pressure on erogenous zones, but from the dramatic play between the visible and the hidden, the available and the withheld, the longing and the revelation. As anyone knows who has spent time on a nude beach, nothing kills eroticism as effectively as total visibility; guaranteed access, in any form, strips the physiology of sexual pleasure of the relational meanings which are the underpinnings of passion and desire. When developmental vicissitudes allow object seeking to be pursued with verve, sexuality becomes a compelling and enriching realm; when developmental vicissitudes make object seeking a dangerous and desperate project, sexuality becomes a search for symbolic reassurances and illusory guarantees. Thus, in compulsive promiscuity the elusiveness of the person is replaced by the concreteness of the genitals, in an endless and futile search to get behind or underneath the intricate latticework of accessible and inaccessible regions which constitute human character.

*   *   *

A SECOND major set of relational meanings which are often expressed in sexual fantasies and behaviors concerns not a longing for the object, but a flight from the object. Here sexuality takes on meaning as the one realm in which independence from the impinging other is possible. The primary object is surrendered to, and sexuality with this object has the deadened, ritualized, artificial quality which characterizes all dimensions of the surrender. Impotence or frigidity with the legal spouse often has this quality, where all interactions are clothed in respectability and conformity to social norms. Each feels he or she has surrendered so much to the other already that the withholding of sexual excitement becomes a secret point of pride, a way of holding back some vestige of selfhood. Genuine sexual excitement, in contrast to false sexual compliance, becomes buried in what Winnicott calls the true self, whose very existence must never become known to the tyrannous, impinging other.

For others, genuine sexual responsiveness remains available, but only in counteridentifications. Here sexuality becomes designated a secret realm, beyond the purview and control of the primary object, in which defiance of the primary object is played out, either in fantasy or in actuality. In this looking-glass realm, relationships are often built upon *inversions* of the structure of primary relationships. Thus, patients whose actual intimate relationships are characterized by submissiveness to others will develop sexual fantasies or sexual liaisons characterized by dominance and aggression. Patients whose compulsive role in primary relationships is one of domination will often play out sexual fantasies of passivity and surrender. McDougall provides a moving description of a sexual sadist whose nonsexual relationships were marked by a pervasive compliance to others:

> His world was split into two: an outer one, where all was treachery and deception and where he had to control his every word and movement to achieve his "superadaptation" to it, and an inner world, the "real" one, where he was alone with his body and his fantasies. I attempted to put into words the two worlds he had so carefully delineated for me in the last few sessions: one valueless, colorless, controlled, and kept at a distance, and the other, intimate and sensual, the kingdom of sexual desire in which he was the sole sovereign. (1980, p. 39)

Stoller argues that the primary motive in perversions is to humiliate, and that sexual passion in general always has a predominantly aggressive component. In my view, the frequent aggressive element in sexual passion represents neither a discharge of some elemental drive, nor only a reversal, as Stoller argues, of childhood traumas and humiliations, but a defiance of the primary mode of object relatedness. This applies to the almost universal link between sexuality and dirtiness, naughtiness, evil. Freud placed great emphasis on the anatomical proximity and overlap of sexual and eliminative functions in this linkage as well as the phylogenetic achievement of repression of olfactory sensuality in the transition to walking on two legs. In my view, an important aspect of the link between sexuality and dirtiness is its function in escaping from what are presumed to be the primary object's demands (as the socializing agent) for cleanliness, goodness, compliance, an escape precisely into what Sullivan calls "bad me." In this view, the "dirty," kinky meanings of sexuality are not inherent in anatomy or physiology, but are assigned to it in the creation of a defiant, counterobject realm, in which one's pleasure is not hostage to the wishes and values of the other. Woody Allen, in his film *All You Ever Wanted to Know about Sex,* captures this dimension of sexual passion when he asks, "Is sex dirty? Only if it's done right."

In more extreme versions of this dynamic, objects and activities may be chosen precisely because they are alien, repulsive to the primary object. The fascination with prostitutes and the separation of the opposite sex into two categories of saints and sinners often reflects this phenomenon. Freud understood it as deriving from the premise that sexuality is inevitably experienced as degrading: one cannot with ease imagine performing such acts with parents whom one loves, and therefore sexual objects are chosen on the grounds of their differences from oedipal choices.

From a relational-conflict perspective, this phenomenon originates not with the experience of the sexual impulse as degrading, but with the elevation of the parental object as ideal, saintly. One finds in these cases parents who were extremely demanding, virtuously tyrannous; to remain connected with a person of such high standards requires total devotion and self-improvement. Prostitutes or women declared inferior and devalued are appealing precisely because one need not worry about pleasing them, meeting their standards, gaining their approval for one's own impulses and desires. A variation is seen in the person who requires an explicit display of sexuality from the other, which he or she experiences as both exciting and wanton, or who requires an overt sexual invitation by the other person in order to feel that his or her own sexual interest is acceptable. It is the compulsive preoccupation with the judgments of the other, not the initial experience of sexuality as degrading, which underlies these kinds of splits in categorizing members of the opposite gender.

Similarly, perversions involving excretion, in which urination and defecation on the other's body becomes the central erotic experience, often tend to develop in people who have been tyrannized as children into regimes of cleanliness and control. There is a self-perpetuating cycle in the tension between the inverse realms of compulsive conventionality and excessive constraint on the one hand and the fantasy or experience of total (sphincter) release, dirty naughtiness, an orgy (often rageful) of self-absorbed indulgence on the other.

FREUD REGARDED fetishes as symbolizing the mother's missing phallus, and therefore as operating in the service of a denial of castration anxiety. The fetish represents a refusal to acknowledge the anatomical differentiation between the sexes and the castration threat implied by that differentiation. From a relational-model perspective, the fetish is seen as expressing relational themes not capable of being integrated into the main channels of integrations with others. The fetish becomes a crucial element in a subtly balanced composition of relational configurations. This is best illustrated by an example.

A young philosophy student in his twenties—like the hero of Jensen's *Gradiva* (Freud, 1907)—had a secret obsession with a certain curve of ankle in women, which became the centerpiece of his sexuality. He would maintain a relationship with a woman toward whom he was extremely tender and devoted but who lacked this anatomical trait, arranging things so that these relationships were largely asexual. He would then use his state of sexual deprivation as a rationale for pursuing the obsession; eventually, invoking the visual image of the ankle line became a necessary prerequisite to orgasm.

This analysand had been the cherished object of his mother's devotion, an extremely depressed and frightened woman who used her only child as a confidant and substitute for the massive sense of deprivation she felt in relation to her husband, and before that, to her parents. The mother had hobbled him with her solicitousness and overprotectiveness, and would literally use him as a clotheshorse while she tailored her garments. His emotional life, and later his sexual life as well, was arranged as a carefully counterbalanced blend of surrender to the mother's ministrations, becoming the mother's son, and a defiance of the mother's claims (interwoven with identifications with his hypermasculine father).

The fetish was an exquisitely constructed weave of these themes. On the one hand, worshiping at the woman's feet revived, through role reversal, his mother's early devotion and attention to him. He would fantasize and occasionally act out an elaborate process of arranging the ankles, now this way, now that way, re-creating the mother's physical ministrations toward him as an infant and her later manipulation of him as an extension of herself beneath her clothes. The transformation from passive to active made possible the re-creation of this fusion with and surrender to the mother, otherwise dreaded as devouring and crippling. On the other hand, the obsession itself created a private world in which he was free of the mother or whatever other woman was momentarily the object of his devotion. He would arrange his life to make possible hours of search in pursuit of his rare game, identifying with his father who had maintained an elaborate clandestine life of which his fearful wife was ignorant. Midway through the analysis, the analysand dreamed of himself as a centaur, with a hidden pair of hind legs which folded up for concealment beneath a waistcoat, but on which he galloped alone during the night. Thus, the dichotomy between his nonsexual devotion to women and the fetish as an erotic obsession corresponded with an inner sense of himself as bifurcated between a formal and constricted person and a surreptitiously powerful, passionate creature.

When sexuality takes on this kind of relational meaning, passionate intensity is often extreme. The passion comes not from a buildup of sexual need per se, but from a kind of suffocation anxiety. In the primary surrender to the object, there is a sense of giving away too much, of one's distinct selfhood being smothered; the counterobject defiance, whether in fantasy, masturbation, or secret liaisons, becomes desperately sought. Often what is experienced as great sexual need reflects a mounting anxiety concerning a loss of self, and a need for the escape and defiance which the sexuality can provide. The real meaning of certain sexual infidelities is often obscured precisely because of this confusion between the need for defiance and the physiological tensions which become the vehicles for this need. Thus, sexual betrayals are often experienced as necessitated or "driven" by deprivation, by incompatibilities in levels of desire, and so on, as if the betrayal is an unfortunate consequence of the intensity of the physical need. Often it is the betrayal itself that is the point, while the sense of inexorable need reflects not peremptory sexual drive but the imperative force of anxiety.

An analysand who found her sexual life with her husband to be unsatisfying felt driven to flirtations with other men, which her husband invariably discovered—either through direct observation or through her guilty, often unintended (consciously) self-disclosures. Analytic inquiry revealed that the flirtations, although pleasant in their own right, were largely the vehicle for what was much more emotionally salient—revenge and atonement. She was extraordinarily solicitous of the husband, whose relative sexual indifference was experienced as a betrayal of what she felt was an implicit contract between them; devotion and attention ought to earn reciprocal devotion and sexual availability. (Her relationship with her mother had been structured around such a contract, her devotion earning her mother's love.) The flirtations served as a protest against her feeling that he had violated their unstated contract, and the self-disclosures served as confessions in which she pleaded for atonement, establishing her "goodness" and virtuous devotion once again. In this neurotic cycle she believed that her resistance of the temptation to engage in actual adultery, and the sincerity of her confession and plea for forgiveness, would surely earn her husband's reward in terms of increased attention and sexual interest. When this expectation was disappointed, she felt once again the pressure to seek revenge and an occasion for demonstrating her virtuous devotion.

Another analysand portrayed himself to himself as a "greedy baby." He felt himself to be riddled with powerful, primitive impulses of an oral and sexual nature, constantly fighting the temptation to eat chocolate and to initiate adulterous liaisons with women. He experienced himself as a hungry baby who had been severely deprived by an extremely depressed mother, who herself had been greatly deprived as a child. Analytic inquiry revealed that he arranged his life in such a way that he was always tormented by the impulses he barely managed to resist. He would eat just enough chocolate to keep himself physiologically slightly addicted, and would involve himself in flirtations with women which left things just ambiguous enough to be constantly tempting to him. The purpose of this self-designed teasing, we discovered, was to establish the possibility for heroic restraint. His mother had social pretensions and felt she had married beneath herself. She viewed her husband as crude and animalistic, greedy in fact, and what little she was able to value in her son involved his "goodness," that is, his restraint. In his experience of himself as a greedy, sexual baby, he was able to maintain a secret, forbidden identification with his father, and at the same time consolidate his tie to his mother through virtue and renunciation. Like Odysseus tying himself to the mast so as to fully experience yet resist the sirens' call, he designed his life so as to continually stimulate yet resist his own "greedy," "infantile" impulses.

The physiology of sexual arousal makes sex ideally suited for embodying protests against accommodation to "goodness," precisely because sexual arousal cannot be willed or controlled. Autobiographical and novelistic accounts of the tortured struggles of adolescents in highly religious, sexually repressive cultures (such as Joyce's *Portrait of the Artist as a Young Man* and Davies' *What's Bred in the Bones*) capture the agony of efforts to squeeze one's experience into acceptable molds and the perpetual protest of the "unruly member." In such an interpersonal matrix, it is precisely the "bad," demonic features of sexual responsiveness that embody what remains of personal spontaneity and authenticity.

An element of the relief often experienced in connection with sexuality in the context of these dynamics is the manic triumph over the object which much counterobject sexuality enacts. In fantasies and activities involving anonymous, exchangeable others, casually picked up and discarded, the depressive anxiety inherent in the needful primary relationship is overturned. Thus, promiscuity is often the end product of a dedifferentiation, in which the particularity of the primary object is challenged in a flight from dependence and depressive anxiety. One might describe this process, which underlies much sexual experience and perversion, in Freud's original terms of a loosening of the link between sexuality and its object. Whereas Freud saw this loosening as an inherent feature of human sexuality, it can be understood instead as a universal escape from the inevitable anxieties and pressures of human relatedness.*

SINCE INDIVIDUAL human consciousness is a distinctly temporal phenomenon, personal relationships are never static. In the best of relation-

---

* There seem to be consistent differences between men and women in terms of the ease with which sexuality can be separated and abstracted from intimacy. Culturally defined gender differences seem crucial here, but differences in physiology and early male-female differences in the origins and qualities of object relations may also play a part (see Gilligan, 1982; Stoller, 1985; Silverman, 1987).

ships, there is a recurring conflictual drama of involvement and detachment, accommodation and defiance, search and discovery. "The tragedy of sexual intercourse," Yeats once noted, "is the perpetual virginity of the soul." I prefer to think of it not as a perpetual virginity, never penetrated, but, in the continual flux and privacy of experience, a perpetually regenerated virginity, never permanently deflowered, accessibility never presumed. The richest and most integrated sexual experience is one characterized by an openness to this interpersonal drama and an inclusion of various relational themes characterized by both mutual discovery and mutual defiance, where meanings pertaining to search, accommodation, and rebellion (both against each other and, jointly, against social norms) find a place within the same sequence of actions. The psychopathology of sexuality might be measured against this ideal; in psychopathology a single relational motif predominates, and search, surrender, or escape is enacted through a stereotyped, compulsive, and concrete iconography of body parts rather than in the delicate emotional dialectics of intimacy.

I do not mean to imply in all of this discussion that sexual desire is always a tremendously solemn business, involving ponderous passions of one sort or another. As with cigars, sometimes sex is just sex. The centrality of sexual experience for most people, however, and its key role in psychopathology derive not from its inherent properties, but from its interactive, relational meanings.

The Metaphor of the Beast

Adherents of the drive model believe that it is "drives" that empower and impassion sexuality; the abandonment of drive theory is often regarded as resistance to the acknowledgment of one's own bestial nature, resulting in a theory that is shallow, a cowardly retreat from unpleasant truths. Certainly the disavowal of drive theory *can* be used in the minimizing of the sexual meanings of clinical material. Any theory offers opportunities for self-deception and what is probably a universal longing to disguise the ambivalences and ambiguities of the human experience; if one presupposes drives, the abandonment of drive theory is obviously a form of denial and self-deception.

But if one begins with the relational matrix as the basic premise, the idea that sexuality is a product of phylogenetically vestigial "drives," still vibrating and pulsating in the very tissues of our bodies, whether proclaimed by an analysand or by a theorist, appears in a different light. This reified bestial metaphor is often proclaimed with a chest-thumping pride, which effectively conceals the manner in which the drive theory itself can be regarded as a retreat from a fuller and more meaningful responsibility for sexual passion and the central role it plays in experience and behavior. Viewing sexuality from within a relational-matrix perspective does not detract at all from the centrality of sexuality, but it accounts for that centrality and the whole experience of sexuality as driven and bestial in a different way.

Schafer (1976) has argued that the concept of an aggressive drive, building up, seeking discharge, and boiling over, represents what might be considered an anal theory of anger. The analysand's angry actions are disclaimed, separated from himself as agent, and assigned anal meanings, serving various purposes—central among them, disavowal. It is not that the analysand does angry things, but that the analysand has a substance inside which builds up, seeks cathartic release, and so on.

Understanding sexuality as a manifestation of bestial drives can be seen as serving a similar function. It is not the analysand who wants to gain access, penetrate, surrender, capture, defy, vilify—it is the libidinal drives, phylogenetic remnants encased within bodily tissues, originating outside the mind and making claims upon it. Rather than impassioning sexuality, the concept of drive actually places it at one remove from the person.

The experience of oneself as bestial is probably universal. The question is, Why is experiencing oneself as if one were a beast so compelling? And why does it emerge as a common metaphor for self-organization? To be bestial suggests a disregard for the other person, a pure, animalistic (that is, in our romanticization of animals) seizure of pleasure and the use of the other for that end. To be bestial is to throw off the constraints of object relatedness, to *depersonalize* the other—sometimes as a way of reaching them more fundamentally, sometimes as a way to escape their claims. To be bestial together can entail a mutual usage of each other, thereby providing a clarity and immediacy which may not be available in the subtle choreography of other dimensions of emotional intimacy.

But what happens when this experience of bestiality is reified into a theoretical entity, when the experiential metaphor is taken as a verity, reflecting an *inherently* loosened bond between sexuality and its objects? Just as the theory of anger as a contaminating substance can be employed to disavow angry actions, the bestial theory of sexuality, whether attached to drives or not, can be used to depersonalize and disclaim the conflictual relational meanings inherent in sexual experiences, particularly those that serve motives of counterobject defiance and escape.

Many analysands, both male and female, experience their own bodies as something to be put at the service of their lover, for the lover's pleasure, rather than as an instrument for their own pleasure. Thus, sexual inhibitions often involve the inability to feel free to "use" the other in the service of one's own passion. Careful solicitousness and wariness of the other cannot be suspended long enough to become lost in one's own sensation, movement, and rhythm. Often in such cases one's own sexuality is experienced as bestial, dangerous to and unable to be integrated within, intimacy with another. Consider an example.

A middle-aged lawyer avoided sex with women, which he found almost totally uninteresting, and instead cultivated rather elaborate masturbatory fantasies. He was the son of an erratic, often assaultive mother and a self-absorbed, narcissistic father and was seen by both of them as the bad kid, selfish and greedy. He had himself elaborated that role, and although quite talented and socially adept, had come to regard other people as basically not offering him anything, not likely to enjoy him or want to provide him with pleasure. Analytic inquiry revealed his experience of sex with another person as an act of his servicing them; he could not imagine their being interested in or able to provide him with any pleasure, certainly nothing that approached the pleasure he could provide for himself.

This analysand had a passing acquaintance with psychoanalytic theory and considered himself to be wholly understandable in terms of Freud's theory of instinctual drive and the structural model. He was filled with bad, bestial drives and therefore had to keep himself always on a short leash. It was crucial to be solicitous always of other people, providing what they seemed to expect, as a way to keep his badness concealed. He felt he had a harsh superego, a projective extension of the primitivity of his own bestial impulses.

Analytic inquiry within the framework of the relational model suggested a different sequence. Involvement with his parents, particularly his scapegoating and abusive mother, necessitated the internalization of her image of him as bad and animalistic, and the fashioning of a false-self personality, extremely attentive to the expectations of the other, hiding any spontaneous needs or wishes. This compulsive compliance with others regularly generated considerable rage and a longing to escape this interpersonal pressure, to be free of the need to be good—to be, in fact, the bestial bad boy his parents had felt him to be. Thus, the superego introjects came first, and the bestial wishes and impulses were a defiant reaction to them, a protest in which he asserted his right to his own existence and pleasure in the only form available to him, the image of himself as greedy and animalistic. These experiences redoubled his need for the harsh parental introjects, providing him with critical judgments he felt necessary to keep himself under control and out of trouble.

The phenomenology of bestiality thus is often part of a neurotic loop (see Wachtel, 1982) within the relational matrix. It is generated as a defiant reaction to compliance and a compulsion to elevate. The metaphor of the beast serves to conceal the personal and interpersonal, relational-conflict significance of that defiance, which in turn consolidates the need for further compliance, which generated the wish to be bestial in the first place. For some analysands it is extremely important to maintain the image of themselves as bestial and captive in order to be able to experience themselves as truly heroic in their renunciation and protection of the beloved from their dangerous nature. The metaphor of the self as beast provides an essential, dramaturgical ingredient for the analysand to portray himself to himself and others as extraordinarily devoted and self-sacrificing.

The historian Peter Gay points out that for Enlightenment philosophers, who provided the basis for so many of Freud's basic values and attitudes, the fascination with "primitivism" was a reaction to and a kind of mythical solution for what were regarded as the "artifices of urban culture."

> Montaigne's wry praise of cannibals, and Dryden's felicitous term "the noble savage," retained their popularity in the age of the Enlightenment. While most philosophers, and most philosophes, celebrated cultivation, a minority of cultural critics eloquently voiced their disgust with civilization and exploited the paradox that the very acquirements polite men valued most were most baneful. (1969, p. 94)

Freud brought these currents together: an enormous dedication to and love of civilization, particularly science, with a romanticization of animals and early man as somehow closer to pleasure. Thus, Freud established sexuality as a realm of unfettered pleasure, free of the tyranny of the object and social necessities, a "nature preserve," like a zoo in the middle of an urban setting.

Seen from this perspective, the metaphor of the beast institutionalized in drive theory has enormous appeal. A part of us, that which is most fundamental, has escaped the tyranny of the object, has been loosened from its objects and exists apart from and prior to the necessary accommodations of interpersonal relations. Sexuality is a realm which has escaped the encroachment of socialization. In this way the concept of drive and the reification of the metaphor of the beast can be used as a device for obscuring the structure and quality of one's own relational patterns, the manner in which one's sexuality expresses or defies relational configurations. Ironically, the linking of sexuality with drives can serve to conceal the meanings and true appeal of experiencing sexuality as an atavistic holdover from our bestial ancestry. Like other metaphors which serve important functions in terms of self-organization, the experience of the self as beast arises within the complex pressures and conflicts of the relational matrix. The importance of sexuality is not minimized by viewing it in an interactive, relational context; rather, its importance is more accurately understood.

Part Three

Infantilism

I N HIS 1906 essay entitled "My Views on the Part Played by Sexuality in the Aetiology of the Neuroses," Freud went public for the first time with the dramatic turn in his understanding of the neuroses, which had taken place nearly a decade earlier. What had appeared to be simple "memories" were more complex constructions, greatly transformed and sometimes even created by the child's own fantasies. The theory of infantile seduction had been replaced by the theory of infantile sexuality. Freud notes that despite the changes in his theory, "there are two positions which I have never repudiated or abandoned—the importance of sexuality and of infantilism" (pp. 277–278).

At later points in his development, Freud established various other criteria as constituting the *essential* psychoanalytic principles. Nevertheless, infantilism, along with sexuality, has remained a traditional pillar of psychoanalytic belief, and those who would exclude as "unpsychoanalytic" opposing points of view are often charged with its neglect.

Infantilism—the central role of concepts of early development in psychoanalytic theory and practice—is the subject matter of Part Three. In Chapter 5 I consider the importance of infantilism in classical drive theory and its very different although equally central function in developmental-arrest formulations. The transition from the drive model to the developmental-arrest model in fact might best be described as a shift in the way in which infantilism is understood. I then develop a third, quite different view of these issues, derived from a relational-conflict perspective. In Chapter 6 I look at the considerable clinical implications of these differences.

Nostalgia runs deep in the human psyche . . . it converts healthy dissatisfactions into an atavistic longing for a simpler condition, for a childhood of innocence and happiness remembered in all its crystalline purity precisely because it never existed. —PETER GAY

5　The Metaphor of the Baby

What does Freud mean by infantilism? The analysand presents himself for treatment as an adult, with an enormous complexity of experience, the meanings and interrelations of which are by no means apparent. Some areas of experience (neurotic symptoms) are ego dystonic and may be wholly opaque to the analysand himself. Other areas are only dimly noticed or reflected on. Many features of his life are "understood" in a fashion which, under the scrutiny of analytic inquiry, is revealed to serve the purpose of rationalization and distraction, deflecting attention from other more salient and more distressing meanings.

Psychoanalytic experience has shown that the scattered and complex fragments of the analysand's background are often powerfully integrated and illuminated by viewing them in terms of infantile experiences. (Freud customarily uses the term "infantile" to refer to the entire span of childhood from birth through resolution of the Oedipus complex at six years or so, although his specific clinical focus was most often on the older, "oedipal" years.) Whereas the *analysand as adult* appears to be operating in obscure and puzzling fashion, viewing the *analysand as child* often helps us to organize the pieces and fragments of the analysand's experience into coherent, understandable patterns. The analysand is motivated by some infantile longing, or hoping to escape some infantile terror, or struggling to obtain some parental ministration or function. It becomes possible to see the fragments of the analysand's experience and associations as related to underlying patterns of early life, a process which often dramatically orders and illuminates the analytic data, like the organizing impact of a magnet beneath a paper of scattered iron filings. In employing infantilism as a basis for interpretation, we are using our image of the baby as a metaphor. The analysand is not literally a baby, but if we think of him in those terms, as wishing, fearing, and experiencing like a baby—we find meaning and patterns in otherwise inchoate fragments of experience.

Metaphors can suggest varying degrees of similarity. To say that A is like B may not imply at all that A *really* has anything to do with B, but merely that A resembles B in a way that can be useful to our understanding and appreciating A. To say that A is like B may also suggest that in some underlying, deeper sense, A and B are closely related, or even are transformations of the same phenomenon.

The kind of comprehension generated by employing infantilism and the metaphor of the baby depends greatly on how one understands the nature of *development* and the relation of the present to the past. In much of the psychoanalytic literature, the present has been regarded as a direct derivative of the past, as a thin veneer behind which the more causally potent past steers psychic life. In this usage, according to so-called psychic reality there is no distinction between past and present; the present *is* the past, played out over and over again. Although *memories* of past events may not be literally accurate, infantile motives and experiences operate beneath the appearance of maturity, guiding and shaping feelings and behaviors. The reification of the experiential metaphor of the beast in drive theory was noted in the last chapter; in the same way infantilism often ceases to be a metaphor and becomes a psychic reality. Psychodynamically speaking, the analysand *is* the baby.

We examined earlier what Berlin has termed the historicism of Freud's era. Freud's sense of what it means to "explain" something was clearly influenced by the Copernican discovery of deep space, the geological discovery of deep time, and the Darwinian discovery of man's remote, prehuman ancestry. Explanation for Freud means going beneath the present, the surface, the manifest, into the past. His technique of dream interpretation, in which the seeming coherence of the narrative is regarded as a diverting disguise to be broken into pieces (Aron, 1988), reflects Freud's conviction that meaning is to be found not by magnifying the surface (Levenson, 1985), but by chopping it up and tracing the latent, invisible paths of its fragments to their remote origins.

Thus, Freud's stress on infantilism, the salience of the most distant, personal past, is closely linked to his basic sense of what it means to explain something analytically, to what has been termed his archaeological metaphor (Spence, 1982). Freud often seems to take the "baby" seemingly revealed through the analytic method as having had (and in fragments, still having) as literal an existence as ancient Rome. And the bestial desires of the baby who still exists carry the powerful, inherent forces that shape experience. Developmental-arrest theories, which minimize or drop completely the concept of drives, thereby change the bestial nature of Freud's baby; nevertheless, they often maintain a reified baby of a different nature.

From Freud's Baby to the Modern Baby

What is the metaphorical psychoanalytic baby like? There is no uniform answer to this question. Different theorists and different clinicians invoke vastly different kinds of babies as organizing metaphors for psychoanalytic data. Freud's pre-1897 baby was a passive victim of adult molestation, registering and later suffering from "impressions" from the external world. The baby of Freud's later drive theory, on the other hand, is essentially bestial in nature; driven by powerful instinctual urges, fantasies, and terrors; dominated by the pursuit of pleasure in all its polymorphously perverse variety; and fearful of retaliatory mutilation. After Freud's shift away from the seduction theory, his baby is much more active, with constitutionally given, somatically based drives and primary, universal fantasies and fears providing the basic categories of mind.

Freud's baby is necessarily riddled with conflict. There is a fundamental antagonism between his nature as a reflexive pleasure seeker and the surrounding physical and social environment. Life run by the pleasure principle does not work well; reality soon intrudes, often very painfully. In Freud's model of mind, the very emergence of mental life as we know it is born of conflict—the clash between the baby's reflexive primary process and the exigencies and realities of life. As Fenichel succinctly puts it, "The noninstinctual part of the human mind becomes understandable as a derivative of the struggle for and against discharge, created by the influence of the external world" (1945, pp. 11–12).

The nature of Freud's baby determines the manner in which it is employed as the organizing metaphor for clinical data. The fragments of the analysand's experience are organized along selected dramatic lines. The analysand is understood and portrayed as rent by powerful conflicts; he desires a great deal, and his desires are experienced as forbidden and frightening, in conflict with one another and likely to precipitate overwhelming, life-threatening "danger situations" because of their impact on the social environment. Freud's baby, and the analysand who is understood via Freud's baby as metaphor, are inevitably tormented.

In the last several decades a different sort of baby, a relational baby, has emerged as an organizing metaphor within the psychoanalytic literature, largely in the traditions of American ego psychology, British object-relations theory, and self psychology. This baby is of crucial significance in developmental-arrest theories; he has a different face, a very different sort of nature, from Freud's baby. This baby is seen as requiring certain basic environmental conditions and parental functions for his growth and development, variously characterized as holding, containment, mirroring, the provision of opportunities for symbiotic merger, separateness, idealization, and so on. In this view the provision of appropriate environmental conditions is felicitous and calming, allowing uninterrupted development. It is only in the absence of necessary parental provisions that tensions and difficulties arise. Growth is aborted, and the child is driven to aggressive responses and the compulsive seeking of inferior substitutes, as he tries to wrest from the interpersonal environment what he desperately needs to survive and continue to grow. While Freud's baby is inevitably a conflicted troublemaker, his instinctual wishes continually bumping against the external world, the modern baby sometimes seems almost more botanical than zoological, preconflictual, innocent. The modern baby is portrayed, under normal circumstances, as fitting in smoothly with his interpersonal environment, as unabrasively seeking, like a plant bending toward the light, the conditions necessary for his development.

The nature of the modern baby too determines the manner in which it is employed as an organizing metaphor for clinical data, selecting and highlighting certain issues, minimizing the importance of others. Here the analysand is understood and portrayed as a victim of what Winnicott has characterized as a "deficiency disease." As it would be in a plant without the right mineral nutriments, growth has been aborted. The analysand's psychopathology is viewed as a necessary arrangement in the face of deprivation, the product of an effort to make do, to find compensatory substitutes, to protect himself.

Thus, the developmental-arrest model combines monadic and inter-active assumptions about psychological life. The early experience of the child is regarded as significantly interactive; psychic structure is shaped in dyadic exchanges within an interpersonal field made up of the baby and the caregivers. Once early emotional growth has been arrested, mental processes become largely monadic. Infantile needs become fro-zen and static; the deepest, most significant psychological recesses of the personality become isolated, buffered from new elements in the inter-personal field. The child within the adult transfers infantile longings onto each new interaction in an ongoing search for what was missed. Relational configurations established through interaction become in-variant, with inherent forces shaping all subsequent experience.

The analytic situation and process as well are viewed differently within the developmental-arrest model. Whereas Freud's baby requires analytic abstinence to highlight and eventually to renounce, in the light of secondary process, early wishes and fears, the modern baby requires, in addition to insightful understanding, actual experiences with the analyst to replace the missing parental functions—or at least enough like the missing parental functions to stimulate the aborted developmental pro-cess to proceed once again. Without these experiences, Winnicott (1954a) argues, nothing else can happen. Although this has not been spoken about openly because of the political specter of being accused of advocating anything like Alexander's "corrective emotional experience," the modern baby as metaphor is generally associated with an emphasis on the noninterpretive aspects of the analytic relationship, that is, the experiences provided rather than the information conveyed.

What are we to make of this shift? Why has the metaphorical psy-choanalytic baby changed, and what are the implications of this pro-gression? Probably the most common understanding is that this change in babies is a direct product of scientific advance, that the burgeoning field of infancy research, as well as data emerging from psychoanalytic experience, has simply led to a revision of Freud's baby in the direction of the modern baby. Certainly this is partially correct. The major figures in the shift, Winnicott and Mahler, spent a great deal of time observing babies, and (as we saw in Chapter 1) many of the theoretical concepts emerging from the British school of object relations, ego psychology, and self psychology find ample support in the data of infancy research (see Lichtenberg, 1983). To regard the shift in psychoanalytic babies as merely a scientific advance is misleading and overly simplistic, however. It presumes, first of all, that there is general consensus within the scientific community about what babies are like, about the most important and lasting influences in their development. This is not the case.

There are probably few phenomena which lend themselves to more multiple interpretations than psychoanalytic patients, but babies are among them. Babies are extremely complex, often inconsistent, and very obscure—they make perfect "blank screens" on which all of us in general and child psychologists more formally, project their fantasies. Schafer (1983, pp. 237–238) has noted that theories about infancy are often presented as mere fact finding, when it is evident that infancy researchers, like all researchers, are prepared ahead of time for what they find. And Kagan (1984) has pointed out how much our image of the nature of the child changes according to different fashions, fashions that are very much influenced by factors other than data or observation.

We have seen that Freud's image of the baby as bestial was colored by the scientific and intellectual milieu in which he lived and worked, particularly by the prominence of Darwin's theory of evolution. Darwinism was new, exciting, and controversial. To approach man as essentially animalistic opened many breathtaking conceptual angles on human experience never before possible in the same scientifically compelling way. The baby as beast became a direct link between adult humans and our animal ancestors. As "ontogeny recapitulates phylogeny" became a rallying cry, the devotion to Darwinism made Freud's baby very persuasive. Similarly, Kagan argues, the image of the baby introduced by Erikson (1950) was also informed by larger intellectual and social forces. Erikson, himself a refugee from wartorn Europe, was writing in this country at a time when there was considerable debate among biologists and psychologists concerning the economic and social difficulties of European immigrant groups. Political interest was growing in the view of social experience rather than inherited instincts as formative and as the basis for differences among peoples.

These intellectual, social, and political meanings and uses, Kagan argues, lend a "ring of truth" to whatever image of the baby is in vogue at any particular time; Freud's comparison of the baby's satisfaction at the breast to postcoital glow becomes compelling to his contemporaries, as does Erikson's comparison of the same phenomenon to adult trust. One might extend this analysis to the meaning of concepts like symbiotic "oneness," a "holding environment," and "empathic mirroring" to those of us living in an increasingly depleted environment threatened with contamination and extinction.

Does this discussion imply that theories about babies are fictional, that like the philosopher's "thing-in-itself" the "baby-in-itself" is either nonexistent or unknowable? Not at all. It implies only that our images and understandings of babies are theory saturated, serving *themselves* as metaphors laden with meanings and assumptions. It cautions against overly concrete use of developmental concepts and metaphors as explanations for clinical data, against overeagerness to make the leap, as Lachmann (1985, p. 17) has put it, "from the crib to the couch." It suggests further that, as with our psychoanalytic theories in general, it behooves us not to take our theories about babies too seriously, certainly not to assume that they have any universal consensual validity among people who do not already tend to think like-mindedly. (There are many child psychologists, for example, who question virtually every aspect of the modern baby of psychoanalysis, regarding many of the developmental stages which we see as products of emotional processes and achievements as, instead, reflecting cognitive and physiological maturational advances.)

There is a second reason for caution in our use of the baby as metaphor, a reason that has to do with the key political role which theories concerning the nature of the baby have played in the history of psychoanalytic theorizing over the past several decades.

Theory Change and the Developmental Tilt

Melanie Klein evolved an elaborate account of human experience as a passionate struggle between murderousness, malevolence, and envy toward significant others, and a deep sense of love and gratitude and the desire to save and restore them. Balint depicts human relations as a search for a perfect unconditional love, offering the possibility of passive surrender to a trusted and caring nurturance. Winnicott came to see psychopathology as centering on the struggle between an authentic and spontaneous expression of impulses and wishes and the need to shape oneself around the way others see one, according to the image others provide and seem to require. Mahler locates the experience of self in a pervasive dialectic between the need for autonomy and self-definition and the desperate longing to surrender to and fuse with another. Kohut characterizes the self as a bipolar structure generated from the tension between the need for warm and embracing recognition, and the need to identify with admired others.

Each of these contributions (obviously noted here in collapsed, schematic form) constitutes a relational-model theory applicable to human experience at all points in the life cycle. Each offers an account of life's central passions, an account at considerable variance with that provided by classical metapsychology, in which human experience is portrayed as a struggle to negotiate between the claims of body-based, asocial psychic tensions and the demands of social reality. In each relational-model account the human organism is seen as inherently social, embedded in a matrix of relationships, establishing connections with others in a primary and fundamental fashion. In each relational-model account the passions depicted characterize human longings and fears at all ages. The struggle between destructiveness and hopeful benevolence, the search for all-embracing love, the tension between self-expression and pandering, between autonomy and a longing to fuse, the need for supportive recognition and admired heroes—these are fundamental dimensions of human relations, from infancy through senescence. These various theories all draw on the relational model, whose basic premises are at variance with the classical drive model. They all depict the relational matrix as the fundamental motivational framework for psychodynamic inquiry, with different theories stressing different facets of that matrix.

The most essential feature of what are generally considered "object-relations" theories is exactly this broad and pervasive departure in fundamental paradigm. Yet the dynamic issues the theories depict tend to get characterized as infantile, preoedipal, or immature; their persistence in later life is often regarded as a residue of infantilism, rather than as an expression of basic human relational needs. Why this tendency to collapse relational needs into the earliest years?

DEVELOPING A psychoanalytic theory is a process not dissimilar to designing a house, to constructing spaces within which people live and act. Various kinds of spaces can be envisioned; the problem in design is to arrange those spaces so that they fit together, so that the more microscopic and circumscribed clinical insights and emphases rest comfortably on the fundamental metapsychological premises of the theory.

In classical Freudian theory (prior to ego psychology) the conceptual foundation is provided by the concept of drive. All motivational, developmental, and structural phenomena, both in life in general and in the psychoanalytic situation, are understood in terms of drive derivatives and defenses against drive derivatives. Classical theory encompasses an account of relations with others, but these relations, like all other phenomena, are understood to consist in transformations of underlying drive pressures and defenses, serving either as vehicles for drive gratification or as bulwarks in the ego's defense against drive pressures. In this sense classical drive theory is internally consistent, a well-designed and amply supported conceptual edifice.

Drive theory was intellectually satisfying to early analysts partially because, in addition to its Darwinian flavor and internal consistency, it was perfectly congruent with the philosophy of science of its day, as well as with what was known of brain physiology and neuroanatomy. This is no longer the case. The principles of tension reduction, the reflex arc model, the closed energy system—these have all been superseded in our understanding of how the brain operates. Consequently, even zealous defenders of the drive concept have struggled to update it, Brenner by stripping it of particular somatic sources, Rothstein by separating it from energic considerations, Kernberg by viewing drives as derivatives of early object relations, and so on. It can fairly safely be said that for most contemporary theorists and clinicians, drive theory (at least as Freud conceived and developed it) is no longer by itself a serviceable metapsychological system (Greenberg, in preparation).

Further, in the more recent history of psychoanalytic ideas (since the late 1940s), increasingly greater emphasis has been placed on relations with others, past and present, real and imaginary, in the collection of theories which operate within the relational matrix. Some have emphasized self-organization, some attachment, some interpersonal transactions. In general, most psychoanalytic clinicians and theorists have begun to grant relations with others a more central and more pervasive role than before, and this has created a crisis of design. The increasing clinical and theoretical emphasis on object relations has placed an enormous strain on the classical model, like a group of cantilevered beams which are called upon to bear more and more ornamentation until they threaten to collapse under the increased weight.

Greenberg and I (1983) argued that the various strategies within the complex array of object-relations theories can be grouped around two basic positions, which we termed the strategy of radical alternative and the strategy of accommodation. Strategists of radical alternative have abandoned the drive model completely and substituted an alternative conceptual framework to replace the weight-bearing function of the original foundation. Sullivan, Fairbairn, and Bowlby are the purest practitioners of this approach. Strategists of accommodation have remained loyal to drive theory and have developed various, often ingenious devices (including loose constructionism and model mixing) for bracing and buttressing the drive model, for stretching and altering it, to enable it to contain an ever-greater emphasis on object relations.

How does one both preserve a theory and introduce into it new concepts at variance with its basic thrust and underlying assumptions? More specifically, how can one both grant that Freud was correct in his characterization of psychopathology as entailing conflicts over drives and defenses centered on the Oedipus complex, and at the same time grant a primary role to the development and patterning of relations with others?

One device has been to alter one or more component parts of the original model to encompass relational processes and issues. Hartmann, for instance (1939), transforms the concept "ego" from an agency whose sole purpose is the control and regulation of the drives into an agency encompassing complex and primary relations with the environment (including the interpersonal environment), relations which are relatively independent of the drives. Other theorists have transformed the concept "id" so that the repository of the drives themselves is subject to the impact of early object relations (Jacobson) or actually composed of relational configurations (Kernberg). Another device has been the strategic use of diagnosis (Kernberg, Kohut, and Stolorow and Lachmann): classical theory and the structural conflict it depicts is correct for neurosis; however, for more severe disorders (borderlines, narcissistic personality disorders, developmental arrests, and so forth) a new model focused on object relations is required.

One of the primary devices through which accommodation has been accomplished, leading to pervasive implications for the way object-relations concepts have been shaped, is what may be termed the developmental tilt, which postulates that Freud was correct in understanding the mind in terms of conflicts among drives *and* that object relations are also important, but *earlier*.

The pillar of classical metapsychology, the structural model, is understood by strategists of accommodation to provide an adequate framework for an account of human experience, both normal and pathological.

That account depicts the conflicts among various drive derivatives, and between drive derivatives and the defensive functions of the ego and the superego. When theorists following this strategy want to introduce various relational needs and processes as *primary in their own right*, as irreducible, as neither merely gratifiers nor defenders against drives, they often introduce them as operative *before* the tripartite structures of id, ego, and superego have become separated and articulated. Theorists concerned with linear continuity necessarily preserve the classical theory of neurosis as centered around sexual and aggressive conflicts at the oedipal phase. They set object-relations formulations into preexisting theory by arguing that they pertain to a developmental epoch prior to the differentiation of psychic structures, in the earliest relationship of the mother and the infant. The traditional model is jacked up, and new relational concepts are slid underneath. In terms of our architectural metaphor, it is as if a complex and roomy foundation level has been set beneath an older edifice; the upper stories remain just as they were, but the center of gravity shifts downward. The original structure is intact but unoccupied; the scene of the action has moved to the lower levels.

Such a strategy in theory construction entails the introduction of the modern baby *beneath* Freud's baby, or, in the language in which this is usually couched, "preoedipal" issues developmentally precede "oedipal" issues. Since analysis of preoedipal issues is generally presented as simply an advance since Freud's time in the understanding of early childhood, it is easy to overlook the profound shift in theoretical framework which is implied, the enormous difference in the kind of "past" which is viewed as underlying and controlling the analysand's current experience. As we have seen, the preoedipal (modern) baby is quite a different creature from the historically earlier (presumably developmentally later) oedipal baby.

Although conceptually cumbersome, the use of the developmental tilt to position the modern baby beneath Freud's baby has very compelling political advantages. The new features of the modern baby serve as a banner in connection with which theoretical innovation can be politically palatable. Whereas it has been difficult for loyalists to challenge classical concepts simply on clinical, logical, or aesthetic grounds, the developmental research which has produced the modern baby makes possible a challenge on empirical grounds. Because we are talking about direct observation and experimental manipulation of infants and children, developmental theory can seem (in my view erroneously) less subject to interpretation than clinical data drawn from the analytic setting. Thus, use of the modern baby (via the developmental tilt) as apparent fact instead of as metaphor lends a scientific credibility to theory change.

The fear of charges of disloyalty or cowardly revisionism has haunted psychoanalysis from early on. The appeal to empirical data serves as a preemptive defense. Sex and aggression are still central, but facts, after all, are facts. Pine has provided an unusually frank and extraordinary catalogue of the hazards of theory change:

> The awesome power of Freud as mentor and of one's own analyst similarly; the need for referrals, which lead to caution in what one presents about one's work to the world; the ease with which the motives of revisionists can be interpreted in this field (i.e., the resort to ad hominem argument) and the "timelessness of teaching," that is, the tendency to teach what we were taught rather than what we ourselves have come to think or do. But the advent of child analysis and then of early developmental research, providing a new data base and anchored in the data-gathering frame of reference of the larger science outside the analytic community, helped to change this in some ways. (1985, pp. 26–27)

Thus, the research credentials of the modern baby make seemingly disloyal theory change thinkable, by allowing theoretical innovations to be wrapped in a mantle of empiricism.

The modern baby has also made possible innovations in long-cherished principles of traditional psychoanalytic technique. The classical rule of abstinence was fashioned in the context of drive theory and fits seamlessly with the drive concept. Neurosis is caused by regression and the failure of repression, by wishful impulses seeking alternative routes to gratification through symptom formation. As resistances to the analytic process develop, the same impulses seek satisfaction in the transference. The analyst's refusal to gratify is a sine qua non of analytic change, because it intensifies and highlights the impulses, forcing their reconsideration in the light of secondary process and their eventual renunciation. Transference gratifications, while tempting to both analyst and analysand, mask the underlying drive derivatives and thereby rob the analysand of the opportunity to experience fully and work through the residues of infantile life. Within the drive-theory framework, therefore, the rule of abstinence is essential, virtually unchallengeable.

The modern baby, however, opens things up. If some psychopathology, or some dimensions of all psychopathology, derive from deprivations, certain kinds of gratifications in the transference become thinkable. "Needs" for necessary developmental provisions become distinguishable from "wishes" for drive gratification. New diagnostic concepts like "borderline" and "narcissistic personality disorder," to which structural conflict and abstinence do not apply, are strategically introduced. The analysand feels better not because some infantile longing is satisfied, but because the self is reached (Winnicott, 1954a). The patient needs something special (Silverman, Lachmann, and Milich, 1982), and it now becomes feasible to want to give it to him. One is not satisfying old infantile wishes, but providing something new that was missing the first time around.

Goldberg, for example, credits Kohut's concept of the child's need for self-objects with the freedom to respond to patients outside of what Goldberg clearly experienced as the confining structures of classical technique.

> Whether or not one is committed . . . to the self psychologist's position of permitting various non-interpretive responses to the patient, ranging all the way from a greeting on the street to a measure of sympathy at the death of a loved one, there is now a rationale for alternative forms of behavior. (1983, p. xvi)

Thus, part of the appeal of the modern baby is the solutions it provides for those who want to move beyond psychoanalytic classicism in theory and technique, but who do not wish to challenge directly classical drive theory and the rule of abstinence which derives from it.

AUTHORS WHO preserve drive theory, but introduce relational dynamics as earlier, end up with a bifurcated view of the life cycle. To regard relational issues as prior to drive issues separates human development into two kinds of concerns: young infants have relational needs; older children and adults (those who are healthy or suffer only from neurotic difficulties) struggle with conflicts between instinctual impulses and defenses. Winnicott therefore distinguishes between early needs and later instinctual wishes; Stolorow and Lachmann distinguish between developmental arrests and later structural conflicts; Kohut distinguishes between disorders of the self and later structural neuroses; and Mahler distinguishes between disorders involving the separation-individuation process and later oedipal conflicts.

Is it accurate or feasible to limit relational issues to the earliest developmental phases? Do relational issues emerge sequentially over the course of early infancy, becoming progressively resolved and allowing the child to move on? The latest thinking of some of the more prominent infant researchers suggests that they do not.

Stern (1985), for example, challenges the notion that the separation-individuation issue as depicted by Mahler is accurately assigned to an early phase of development. Developmental theorists such as Mahler, as well as Erikson and Spitz, have tended to regard one early phase of life as bringing to a head and essentially resolving a particular life-crisis issue, relational in nature, such as the establishment of basic trust, autonomy, separation-individuation, and the like. Stern argues, by contrast, that these issues are most accurately viewed as lifelong struggles. The dialectic between union-fusion and differentiation-autonomy experiences, for example, is a lasting facet of human existence, manifesting itself in the infant through visual gaze behavior, in the toddler through motility, and in the older child and adult through various symbolic processes. These are differences not in meaning or dynamic issues, but in the equipment, motoric and cognitive, through which the child is able to experience the same issue. Thus, collapsing lifelong relational issues to early, circumscribed phases via the developmental tilt distorts the very nature of those issues and the ways they manifest themselves at different points throughout the life cycle.

The developmental tilt has generated what at times seems to be an infinite regress in claims to developmental priority. A psychodynamic account which each author regards as more basic, more primary, than structural conflict, is presented as earlier, as leading to attribution to the newborn of extraordinarily complex affective and cognitive capacities (M. Klein), to assignment of great weight to prenatal and birth experiences (Winnicott, 1949b), and even speculation on the effects on the embryo of parental attitudes at the point of conception (Laing, 1976). "Deeper" is translated into "earlier," rather than into "more fundamental," as if dynamics attributable to the first months of life or to prenatal existence still occupy the most basic layers of experience, underlying and governing psychic events and processes of later chronological origin. This mode of introducing theoretical innovation strains credulity; it also skews these innovations in a peculiar way, by collapsing relational issues into the interaction between mother and infant during the earliest months of life.

Let us consider as representative several key concepts from the work of Michael Balint, who introduced rich object-relations concepts, while attempting to maintain also the basic principles of drive theory. Balint developed the concepts of "primary love" and "basic fault" in an innovative and clinically useful effort to account for transference-counter-transference impasses with certain kinds of difficult patients. The principle of abstinence central to classical technique, Balint points out, was developed in the context of drive theory. The patient's impulses and wishes must not be gratified, lest they become further entrenched rather than transformed into memory and renounced. Nevertheless, certain patients become stuck in analysis, demanding a responsiveness from the analyst without which they seem unable to progress. Balint characterizes these longings and the patient's efforts to gratify them as a need for "primary love."

> In my view, all these processes happen within a very primitive and peculiar object-relationship, fundamentally different from those commonly observed between adults. It is definitely a two person relationship in which, however, only one of the partners matters; his wishes and needs are the only ones that count and must be attended to; the other partner, though felt to be immensely powerful, matters only in so far as he is willing to gratify the first partner's needs and desires or decides to frustrate them; beyond this his personal interests, needs, desires, wishes, etc., simply do not exist. (1968, p. 23)

Balint has provided an account of the analytic encounter which is based on relational concepts and is alternative to that generated by the drive model. It is not gratification of specific impulses that the patient is seeking, but establishment of a certain kind of relationship—a state of unconditional love. What is puzzling is Balint's restriction of such longings to the earliest and most "primitive" object relationships.

It appears that Balint's depiction of the longing for primary love has wide applicability. Surely we might define "mature love" as a relationship characterized by mutuality. "When the satisfaction or the security of another person becomes as significant to one as is one's own satisfaction or security, then the state of love exists" (Sullivan, 1940, pp. 42–43). Such mutuality, though, seems an ideal, not a normative practice. No matter how mature and healthy, all love relationships are characterized by periodic retreats from mutuality to self-absorption and demands for unconditional sensitivity and acceptance. Many patients (not at all as "regressed" as those Balint sees as suffering from a "basic fault") take years before their relationships are weighted in the direction of mutuality rather than self-absorption. Sullivan argued that *most* of us are chronically juvenile, integrating relationships on the basis of our own egocentric concerns and lacking the capacity for intimacy, for seeing things from the other's perspective as well. It seems particularly odd to depict as "primitive" the emergence in the analytic situation of a preoccupation by the patient with his own needs and an experience of the analyst as existing only in relation to those needs. One might argue that the analytic situation is *defined* precisely in this way. Most patients experience, or struggle to resist experiencing, the analyst only in relation to themselves; in fact, the absence of such feelings is often understood to reflect a resistance to the transference. Balint's concept of primary love provides an illuminating account of relational longings and conflicts throughout the life cycle; but, as with many object-relations formulations, these accounts have been collapsed into earliest infancy, "a very primitive and peculiar object-relationship."

It might be argued that the impact upon object-relations concepts produced by the developmental tilt is insignificant. The basic relational-matrix concepts are there anyway. What difference does it make if relational issues are understood as operating essentially prior to the differentiation of psychic structure and the inception of instinctual conflict?

Such a view would necessarily minimize considerations of economy in theory construction, for theories employing the developmental tilt tend to be exceedingly (often unnecessarily) complex and contrived. Relational issues are granted temporal priority, but the theory must move inexorably toward the establishment of instinctual conflict as the core of neurosis. Bridging this conceptual gap is not easy and often requires the kind of ingenuity for which Rube Goldberg was famous. Kohut's postulation of two separate libidinal energies and developmental lines (narcissistic libido and object libido) and his "principle of complementarity" and Kernberg's use of "general systems theory" are the best examples of shifting terminology and strained arguments which serve as bridging concepts, allowing the theorist to start with the relational matrix and arrive at the traditional version of the Oedipus complex. (Mitchell, 1981, gives an extended analysis of these strategies.) The resultant theories have an oddly unsettling, implausible quality, reminiscent of the architecturally notorious residential college built at Yale whose exterior facade, facing earlier buildings, is done in traditional Gothic style, while the interior facade opens onto a colonial courtyard. One enters the building (or theory) in one century and exits in another! External continuity is preserved at the price of internal contradiction and tension. The most important impact of the developmental tilt on object-relations concepts, however, is in terms of its clinical implications. I shall examine these in the next chapter.

Developmental Reasoning

First, let us consider some other features of infantilism by looking more broadly at the traditional psychoanalytic tendency to think about adult clinical data in infantile terms, or, as Kohut puts it, "the firmly established thinking patterns of the analyst [that] lead me immediately to the childhood situation" (1984, p. 128). The conceptual power and clinical utility of this kind of thinking is part of what makes the modern-baby metaphor so compelling. What we observe in the present, this line of reasoning goes, proceeds from, grows organically out of, that which has gone before. Earlier is more fundamental, foundational. That which is earlier still exists, is still operating beneath later events and processes. The past underlies the present. "The child is father of the man," or, rather, children of various ages and developmental levels in some sense coexist *within* the man.

This way of thinking about development and structuralization is basic to understanding psychopathology in both the drive and the developmental-arrest models. The various components and organizations of the sexual instinct unfold sequentially over time, argued both Freud and Abraham, and culminate, under conditions of health, in genital primacy as the centerpiece of adult maturity. In psychopathological conditions the earlier the fixation, the more severe and distorting the personality warp.

Freud and Abraham viewed development in terms of component instincts. This kind of reasoning was extended, however, to the very different view of development, in the context of a relational matrix, provided by more contemporary ego-psychology and object-relations theories. Development traverses different relational stages, variously described: from autism, through symbiosis, to separation-individuation (Mahler); from the paranoid-schizoid position to the depressive position (M. Klein); from infantile dependence to mature dependence (Fairbairn); and so on. The earlier the difficulty, the earlier the fixation and the more severe the psychopathology. Pine summarizes this approach, which he terms developmental reasoning, as based on

> two modes of thinking characteristic of psychoanalytic thinking in general: (1) to look for early normal periods of development that provide the *anlage* for, that give shape to, later forms of pathology, based on the assumption that these later forms must have had an earlier edition; and (2) to reason that the severer the pathology the earlier the "earlier edition"—that is, the point of "fixation." (1985, p. 47)

According to the assumptions underlying developmental reasoning, we would expect that later psychopathology is fairly predictable from the vicissitudes of childhood experience, and especially that extreme trauma early in life should itself cause distinct later emotional damage. Yet neither of these expectations seems well supported by the evidence.

> In spite of the fact that these views [of sequential sensitive phases of development] have been prevalent for many decades, there have as yet been no prospective longitudinal studies that support the very clear predictions of these theories. Psychological insults and trauma at a specific age or phase should result in predictably specific types of clinical problems later on. No such evidence exists. (Stern, 1985, p. 23)

In a broad survey of research data on the long-term effects of maternal deprivation on intellectual, social, and behavioral functioning, Rutter similarly questions the utility of the concept of discrete "critical periods" during the early years. He notes that (contrary to developmental reasoning) environments which improve only in middle and later childhood *do* lead to major gains, and that good experiences in early years *do not* protect children from the ill effects of later deprivation. He concludes

> that single isolated stresses in early life only rarely lead to long-term disorder, that multiple acute stresses more often do so, and that long-term damage is most likely when multiple acute stresses arise against a background of chronic disadvantage. (1979, p. 293)

Freud noted early how much easier it is to reconstruct what he took to be causal sequences than to predict future effects from current presumed causes.

> So long as we trace the development from its final outcome backwards, the chain of events appears continuous, and we feel we have gained an insight

which is completely satisfactory or even exhaustive. But if we proceed the reverse way, if we start from the premises inferred from the analysis and try to follow these up to the final result, then we no longer get the impression of an inevitable sequence of events which could not have been otherwise determined. We notice at once that there might have been another result, and that we might have been just as well able to understand and explain the latter . . . in other words, from a knowledge of the premises we could not have foretold the nature of the result. (1920b, p. 167)

Freud's subsequent explanation for this dilemma is a perfect piece of Newtonian thought. Newtonian physics, which dominated thinking in the natural and social sciences well into the twentieth century, claims that if all the mass of the universe were known, along with its location, velocity, and direction, it would be possible to predict all future events in the universe from now until the end of time. Freud extends this metaphor of universe as mechanism to the development of mind over time.

> It is very easy to account for this disturbing state of affairs. Even supposing that we have a complete knowledge of the etiological factors that decide a given result, nevertheless what we know about them is only their quality, and not their relative strength. Some of them are suppressed by others because they are too weak, and they therefore do not affect the final result. But we never know beforehand which of the determining factors will prove the weaker or the stronger. We only say at the end that those which succeeded must have been the stronger. Hence the chain of causation can always be recognized with certainty if we follow the line of analysis, whereas to predict it along the line of synthesis is impossible. (1920b, p. 168)

Like Newton, Freud is confident that if only one knew the pieces and forces, all subsequent events could be predicted.

Another way to explain why the so-called chain of causation is easy to reconstruct and impossible to predict is that there is no chain of causation. It may be that later difficulties in living are often *not* direct causal products of earlier deprivation and problems, but a complex combination of the impact of early experience and reactions to later stresses and conflicts. From this perspective, prediction is impossible because no simple cause and effect is operative; reconstruction *is* possible because a good reconstruction can always find earlier versions of later phenomena and attribute causal significance to them.

Certain kinds of issues (such as fusion and separation, love and hate, dependence and independence) are basic to human experience throughout the life cycle. Thus, the developmental reasoner—whether drive theorist or developmental-arrest theorist—can always find infantile experiences which are similar or structurally parallel to adult issues. What makes genetic reconstruction so compelling (and so dangerous) is the ease with which one can attribute causation to structural parallels, can claim that the earlier phenomenon somehow underlies or causes the later one.

Consider another facet of this issue. All clinicians have observed that patients suffering severe psychopathology tend to come from families with substantial difficulties, often with mothers suffering from grave character pathology. To invoke the metaphor of the modern baby, such severe adult psychopathology is understood to reflect the mother's inability to provide appropriate early infantile maternal care, opportunities for symbiotic fusion, mirroring, holding, and so on. The later pathology is severe, precisely because the mother failed to meet the earliest of the child's needs, thereby blocking further development. All potentially ameliorative later experience is thwarted by the tightly closed circle of the early, primitive psychopathology. Thus, patients suffering from severe psychopathology (or sometimes all of us) are depicted as containing an inner baby, fixed in time (sometimes linked with concepts such as a "psychotic core").

There is ample evidence that children from deprived and disturbed backgrounds and families suffer all sorts of severe later difficulties; however, this does not necessarily imply that it is the earliest years, the earliest developmental needs, that are crucial. Data bearing on this issue, and this issue alone, would be drawn from children who were severely deprived in the first several years of life and then provided with more normal later environments. If developmental reasoning provides a complete explanation, such children should have suffered severe damage in their early years, a warping of personality involving self-perpetuating, pathological internal structures like ego fragmentation, vertical and horizontal splits within the self, false selves, and primitive pathological processes like splitting, projective identification, and so on, making further healthy growth impossible.

Reviews of the literature on such children (including orphaned war refugees, adopted Korean children from impoverished backgrounds, and abused and abandoned children) suggest that despite standard psychoanalytic assumptions, these children, *if* introduced into normal homes sometimes as late as at age ten, suffered minimal ascertainable damage.

> The thing that is most impressive is that with only a few exceptions they do not seem to be suffering either from frozen affect or the indiscriminate friendliness that Bowlby describes. As far as can be determined their relationships to their adopted families are genuinely affectionate . . . The present results indicate that for the child suffering extreme loss the chances for recovery are far better than had previously been expected. (Rathbun, DeVirgilio, and Waldfogel, 1958; quoted in Kagan, 1984, p. 100)

Any psychoanalyst worth his salt can challenge such conclusions. The damage from deprivation of early needs is there, he would argue, merely defended against, hidden. The measures are too behavioral, not subtle enough to pick up the underlying psychopathology. Or, alternatively, he might argue that the subsequent "normal" environments were *more* than normal, that they provided remediation for early deprivation which allowed a thawing of the aborted developmental processes. Both these reinterpretations are relevant, but in my view this kind of data, fairly and nondefensively considered, points to the dangers of putting too much causative weight on the earliest years of life. *What of the studies re: first years of life? (2)*

Parental deprivation is not under most circumstances phase specific. Mothers unable to provide adequate care for infants, who lack warmth, constancy, and so on, often tend to have similar difficulties with the same children as they grow older. The mother who is not attuned to her infant's needs and affects tends to be unable to engage her toddler playfully, to instruct her latency child respectfully, to respond to, yet set limits for, her adolescent joyfully. It is often the same kinds of basic relational issues which are problematic within a family, but in different forms at different ages. *yes.* In longitudinal studies of child-mother dyads from two months to thirty-six months, Stern notes, "the two individuals are conducting their interpersonal business in a similar and recognizable fashion throughout" (1985, p. 186). Developmental reasoning, by searching for early prototypes of later issues, alerts us to the earliest deprivations and pathological integrations. We assign great weight to these, assuming a fixity of developmental processes at this point. By collapsing later versions into earlier prototypes, we assign causal weight to the earliest events. This may very well be arbitrary, as the research discussed above suggests.

Unlike the subjects of this research, many of the patients seen by clinicians had no major discontinuity in parenting. The cast of familial characters during infancy often remains pretty much the same throughout latency and into adolescence. Thus, it seems reasonable to assume that the mother who failed to relate adequately to the infant also posed problems for the child throughout his development, and that the psychopathology of such a child grown to adulthood reflects not simply fixations of earliest developmental needs, but adaptations to and strategies for dealing with a troubled interpersonal environment learned over many years.

Studies of families of severely disturbed adolescents reveal intensely pathological interactions between the parents and their older children. "In families of adolescents who manifest borderline or narcissistic disturbances, we constantly find evidence of a powerful cluster of unconscious assumptions which equate separation-individuation with loss and abandonment. Thinking and action of family members which are not in accord with these assumptions are then perceived and reacted to as destructive attacks" (R. Shapiro, 1979, pp. 130–131). Because the problem has to do with separation, developmental reasoning leads one to locate the origins in the first several years of life. But the data suggest that although the difficulties may have begun in the early years, they are not intrinsic to those precocious interactions, and in fact extend to severely pathological reactions throughout childhood, adolescence, and young adulthood.

The mother who can love only a "lap baby" fails the child at each subsequent developmental stage. Is the constricted adult seeking the freedom to climb onto and get off laps at a three-year-old level, or is he or she seeking ways of being both connected and separate in many different forms and circumstances? From this perspective the *severity* of psychopathology reflects not so much the earliness of the problems, but their rigidity and pervasiveness—not so much parental failure to provide early nurturance, but failure to relate and to allow room for growth across the whole cycle from infancy to adulthood.

Past and Present

One of Freud's most lasting contributions was his discovery of the continuity between childhood experience and adult psychology; the psychodynamics and struggles of later life have reverberating meanings which extend backward into earlier phases of the life cycle. In classical

— are you putting this all on me still?
you can try but... —I won't take it all on!

theory the past is alive in the present because the infantile sexual and aggressive impulses which dominated childhood, the self as beast, still underlie and fuel adult motivation. As Kermode points out, Freud "remained faithful to the principle [derived from nineteenth-century biology and geology] that one best explains how things are by explaining how things came to be that way" (1985, p. 10). There is, in fact, an identity for Freud between how things are and how things got to be that way, because psychological time is layered, the mature is a disguised version of the infantile, the unconscious is timeless, and infantile sexuality and aggression constitute the motivational source throughout life.

Within the developmental-arrest model drive theory has been largely displaced, but some features of the approach to the past have been retained. Here developmental continuity is accounted for in terms of stunted growth. Psychological time moves only if appropriate parental provisions are supplied. Environmental deficiencies result in highly specific developmental arrests, and therefore failures in maternal care in early infancy generate the etiological core of later psychopathology. The modern baby, like Freud's baby, is *inside* the analysand. It is originally an interactive, relational product but, once established, seeks expression and shapes all subsequent experience. The adult becomes a kind of perseverating baby, stuck in developmental time.

A third, more fully interactional option is to regard developmental continuity as a reflection of similarities in the kinds of problems human beings struggle with at all points in the life cycle. Being a self with others entails a constant dialectic between attachment and self-definition, between connection and differentiation, a continual negotiation between one's wishes and will and the wishes and will of others, between one's own subjective reality and a consensual reality of others with whom one lives. In this view the interpersonal environment plays a continuous, crucial role in the creation of experience. The earliest experiences are meaningful not because they lay down structural residues which remain fixed, but because they are the earliest representation of patterns of family structure and interactions which will be repeated over and over in different forms at different developmental stages. Understanding the past is crucial, not because the past lies concealed within or beneath the present, but because understanding the past provides clues to deciphering how and why the present is being approached and shaped the way it is. *yes.*

Looked at in this way, the relational matrix does not have the kind of

I don't think I think in terms of stunted growth as much as learned patterns of adaptation.

fixed, structural properties that developmental-arrest theories attribute to infantilism. The residues of the past do not close out the present; they provide blueprints for negotiating the present. Inevitably the adult is seeking interaction in his *current* interpersonal world, in one form or another, along the lines he considers safest and most desirable.

The probably universal experience of oneself as baby, sometimes with playful delight, sometimes with shame and horror, does not reflect a direct reliving, a contact with one's deepest core, an expression of one's inner structural composition. Rather, the universal experience of self as baby, like the experience of self as beast, reflects a pattern of symbolizing segments and dimensions of adult experience in a form which draws its definition and meanings from past and present relational configurations. As we shall see in the clinical examples presented in the next chapter, the experience of oneself as baby reflects an effort to give voice to dimensions of experience which, both in childhood and in the present, are conflictual and therefore disowned within the predominant configurations of the relational matrix.

It is the predicament of the neurotic that he translates everything into the terms of infantile sexuality; but if the doctor does so too, then where do we get?
—JOSEPH CAMPBELL

6 Clinical Implications of the Developmental Tilt

The relationship between patient and analyst has, from the very beginnings of psychoanalysis, occupied a central place in all theorizing about the analytic situation and its therapeutic action. The manner in which that relationship is conceived, however, has undergone many intricate variations and transformations. Although any generalization about this complex conceptual history runs the risk of oversimplification, it is not at all misleading to note that in recent decades the analytic relationship has been understood more and more as a real and new relationship (Cooper, 1987). For Freud, the relationship with the analyst was a re-creation of past relationships, a new version struck from the original "stereotype place" (Freud, 1912b). The here-and-now relationship was crucial—but as a replication, as a vehicle for the recovery of memories or the filling in of amnesias, and it was this function that was understood to cure the patient. Contemporary relational-model views tend to put more emphasis on what is *new* in the analytic relationship. The past is still important—but as a vehicle for comprehending the meaning of the present relationship with the analyst, and it is in the working through of that relationship that cure resides. (See Racker, 1968, and Gill, 1983, for an extended treatment of this contrast.)

In what does this new relationship consist? There is a wide range of thinking. Fairbairn (1958) puts it this way: in order for the patient to relinquish his tie to bad objects (which is at the core of all psychopa-

151

thology), he must experience the analyst as a "good object." Objectlessness is impossible; one cannot relinquish old attachments unless new ones seem possible and compelling.

That the analyst must become a good object is a formula with which relational theorists of all persuasions would agree. But what does it *mean* to say the analyst becomes a good object? "Good" in what sense? The analyst provides opportunities for relatedness hitherto unavailable to or unutilizable by the patient. What sort of opportunities? It is here that the developmental tilt becomes crucial, because it collapses relational needs in general into the kinds of interactions which characterize the relationship between the small child and the mother.

The Analyst as Good Object

Many relational authors portray the analyst as providing various dimensions of relatedness which characterize intimacy throughout the life cycle: a containment (Bion) or holding (Winnicott) of the other, merger experiences (Mahler), admiration and occasions for idealization (Kohut), a generally caring impact (M. Klein), and so on. Instead of conceptualizing these dimensions of the analytic relationship as providing the patient with a richer, more complex, more *adult* kind of intimacy than his previous psychopathology allowed him to experience, the developmental tilt leads to a view of these dimensions essentially as developmental remediations. Rather than becoming enriched in the present, the patient is seen as having past omissions corrected and developmental gaps plugged up. This lends a regressive cast to the analytic enterprise and seriously distorts the nature of these experiences. Let us consider several examples.

The following is an excerpt from a case discussed by Melanie Klein. The patient is a woman described as aggrieved about every aspect of her life.

> She had been breast-fed, but circumstances had otherwise not been favourable and she was convinced that her babyhood and feeding had been wholly unsatisfactory. Her grievance about the past linked with hopelessness about the present and future . . . The patient telephoned and said that she could not come for treatment because of a pain in her shoulder. On the next day she rang me to say that she was still not well but expected to see me on the following day. When, on the third day, she actually came, she was full of complaints. She had been looked after by her maid, but nobody

else had taken an interest in her. She described to me that at one moment her pain had suddenly increased, together with a sense of extreme coldness. She had felt an impetuous need for somebody to come at once and cover up her shoulder, so that it should get warm, and to go away again as soon as that was done. At that instant it occurred to her that this must be how she had felt as a baby when she wanted to be looked after and nobody came.

It was characteristic of the patient's attitude to people, and threw light on her earliest relation to the breast, that she desired to be looked after but at the same time repelled the very object which was to gratify her. The suspicion of the gift received, together with her impetuous need to be cared for, which ultimately meant a desire to be fed, expressed her ambivalent attitude towards the breast. (1957, p. 204)

Here Klein depicts a woman whose view of her own life and relations with others is characterized by a sense of deprivation, hopelessness, cynicism, and a methodical refusal to allow herself to be given to by anyone. Klein's formulations concerning envy (a deliberate spoiling of the "good") provide a rich metaphorical context for illuminating the patient's dynamics. However, Klein reduces this lifelong refusal of the patient to allow anyone to give her anything, or to allow anyone to become important to her, to her relationship as an infant at the breast. Klein is clear on this point: the breast is not a metaphor for nurturance and hope. Nor is she suggesting that the feelings toward the breast are the first in a series of relationships with others in which the patient deals with hopelessness and anxiety through envious spoiling: "Her impetuous need to be cared for . . . ultimately meant a desire to be fed." Various expressions of the need to be cared for, surely a fundamental relational need throughout the life cycle, are portrayed by Klein as symbolizations and transformations of the earliest longings vis-à-vis the breast.

Balint's writings reveal a similar tilt in his understanding of significant interpersonal events within the analytic process. Balint (1968, p. 128) tells of his work with an "attractive, vivacious, and rather flirtatious girl in her late 20's," who entered treatment complaining of "an inability to achieve anything." Academically successful, she had been unable to complete her final exams; socially popular, she had been unable to become involved with a man.

Gradually, it emerged that her inability to respond was linked with a crippling fear of uncertainty whenever she had to take any risk, that is, take a decision. She had a very close tie to her forceful, rather obsessional, but most reliable father; they understood and appreciated each other; while her relationship to her somewhat intimidated mother, whom she felt to be unreliable, was openly ambivalent.

It took us about two years before these connections made sense to her. At about this time, she was given the interpretation that apparently the most important thing for her was to keep her head safely up, with both feet firmly planted on the ground. In response, she mentioned that ever since her earliest childhood she could never do a somersault; although at various periods she tried desperately to do one. I then said: "What about it now?"—whereupon she got up from the couch and, to her great amazement, did a perfect somersault without any difficulty. (1968, pp. 128–129)

This interaction proved to be an important breakthrough in the treatment; "many changes followed in her emotional, social, and professional life, all towards greater freedom and elasticity" (p. 129).

How does Balint understand the somersault, the "crucial event" in this case? He characterizes it as a regression, which he carefully defines as the "emergence of a primitive childish form of behavior after more mature, more adult, forms have firmly established themselves" (p. 129). This is a peculiar and unpersuasive characterization. Why is turning a somersault childish and primitive? Against what faded and anemic version of adulthood is it being measured? Here is a young woman who lives an adulthood of extreme caution, constriction, and uninvolvement. Given the interpretive context Balint and the patient had developed, and given the patient's subsequent progress, the somersault seems clearly a metaphorical enactment of her new willingness to take risks, to plunge herself into things without knowing exactly how they will turn out, to act in ways other than carefully placing her feet one in front of the other. Why childish and primitive then? The meaning of the act is obviously a progression, not a regression, an expansion of the patient's maturity and potential, not a diminution of them. Is the behavior itself so childish and primitive? Are adults not supposed to make spontaneous physical gestures? to play in this way?

The most striking feature of Balint's characterization of this intriguing clinical moment, however, is his description of it as an emergence. This suggests something that has been contained within this woman, repressed, submerged, pushing for release, as if the somersault and the childlike spontaneity it expressed was *in* her, waiting for the analyst's presence to precipitate its release. Yet, according to Balint's account, this act did not simply emerge—it was invited. It was Balint, the adult analyst, who suggested that the patient try a somersault; what was new was her ability to respond to this invitation.

The patient was closely tied to her obsessional but reliable father. Her analyst of several years, doubtless also obsessional and reliable, acts very differently from the cautious father; he invites her to play, to take a risk, and in so doing takes a risk himself. He seduces her, after a fashion; or, perhaps, he allows himself to respond to her hobbled seductiveness. Here is a man who, despite his respectability, is not bound by convention, is willing to try something very different, the outcome of which is unknown and unknowable. Should we characterize the analyst's invitation as regressive? It seems an extraordinarily misleading way to depict a brilliant and creative piece of clinical work. Patient and analyst have re-created in the transference a powerful attachment mediated through reliability and cautiousness, in which the decorum and professionalism of the analytic situation are symbolic equivalents of the parent's timidity and deep fear of life and spontaneity. Perhaps the crucial event was not the patient's somersault at all, but the analyst's invitation, through which he stepped out of the transferential integration in which he was participating and thereby transformed the relationship.

Balint's clinical data suggest that the patient's psychopathology is strongly bound up with her attachment to her parents and their character pathology. The clarification of that attachment and the mutual development with the analyst of new forms of relationship are ameliorative. The new forms reflect a playfulness, a spontaneity, a willingness to take risks. Balint's way of describing this constructive shift in capacity for relatedness illustrates the two major problems generated by developmental tilt: psychopathology is characterized in terms of missing infantile experiences rather than constricted patterns of relatedness in general, and the missing needs are regarded as residing *in* the patient, pressing to emerge, rather than a function of the interactive relational field the analysand experiences herself as living in. The characterization of the somersault as the emergence, even if benignly, of a piece of childishness strikingly distorts its crucial interactive meaning vis-à-vis the shifting relationship with the analyst.

Developmental tilt is evident not just in the writings of authors from the British school, but also in the work of theorists in the tradition of American ego psychology. Here structural conflict over sexual and aggressive impulses is seen as dominating later childhood and subsequent development. When relational issues are added to the theory, specifically in the contributions of Mahler, Jacobson, and Kernberg, they are introduced as pertaining to the earliest developmental phase; their evidence later in life is regarded as a regressive residue of very early disturbance. Consider this clinical excerpt from Blanck and Blanck, who have synthesized various ego-psychological contributions and applied them to clinical practice.

> *Mrs. Fletcher:* I always feel unwanted. My husband only wanted me for sex, but he never held me just because he liked me.
> *Therapist:* Everyone needs to be held at times, but when do we need it most?
> *Mrs. Fletcher:* You mean when we were babies? You seem to be telling me that when I think of a woman, even if sexually, that it really reflects the way I yearned to be held, cuddled, and loved by my mother.
> *Therapist:* Do you see now why you asked me whether I am a "butch?"
> *Mrs. Fletcher:* Oh, it upsets me. I want a woman.
> *Therapist:* But do you understand why?
> *Mrs. Fletcher:* I need mothering.
> Thus the patient arrives at the realization that her homosexual wishes contain the intense yearning for mothering that was unfulfilled in the age-appropriate symbiotic phase. (1974, p. 306)

Consider the therapist's first intervention. The patient has expressed the view that her husband uses her for sex, without feeling any tenderness or liking for her. The therapist pays lip service to the need for tenderness throughout life, then immediately collapses such a need into the infant's need for tenderness from the mother. Relational needs which might reasonably be regarded as aspects of all adult relationships, the longing to be held and cherished, are depicted as regressive, symbiotic yearnings, unresolved residues from earliest childhood. The introduction of Mahler's concept of symbiosis as prestructural, rather than as a depiction of the tension between autonomy and surrender throughout the life cycle, necessitates the collapsing of the need for tenderness and the longing for fusion into the earliest relationship with the mother. Such yearnings with regard to the mother are not depicted as the first in a series of similar longings in later relationships, but as the only developmental forum in which such needs make sense. (Bergmann, 1971, provides a moving Mahlerian account of adult love as inevitably drawing on symbiotic yearnings, although these are still by definition regressive, even if regressive in the service of romance.)

Whether or not relational issues are tilted toward infancy has important implications in the handling of clinical material, as the following example illustrates.

A young male analysand, a college professor in a discipline related to psychoanalysis who therefore knew much of the psychoanalytic literature, had been struggling with phobic anxiety about presenting his work to his peers. He came from a tight-knit extended family who regarded with high suspicion the external world and particularly people who moved successfully through it. The patient felt strong conflict between his intellectual endeavors and upwardly mobile ambitions and his deep loyalty to the anti-intellectual and paranoid traditions of his family. His mother was a long-suffering daughter-wife-mother who induced great guilt and expected her children to stay with and protect her; his father was a brittle, narcissistic, and grandiose man who was disdainfully and deeply fearful of life outside the narrow confines of his interests. The patient had never felt supported or admired for his accomplishments, which he kept essentially hidden and devalued, convinced that they would destroy both parents and his connections with them—which he both dreaded and longed for.

After working with the analyst on many facets of his phobic anxiety, the patient began one session apologetically reporting a recent success. A long-feared meeting at which he was to present his work had gone very well; in fact, he was exuberant at his display of his powers; he felt that he should be able to go on to other matters, but he still seemed to need to tell the analyst all about it, hoping to elicit approval and praise. He regarded this need for "mirroring" (he had been reading Kohut) as childish and embarrassing, a sign of how deeply he had been damaged in his ability to sustain a sense of self-worth.

What is the nature of this analysand's hesitantly expressed, wished-for interaction? He wants to revel in his success, to crow, to elicit the analyst's admiration, pride, perhaps envy. He regards this wish as childish, and is embarrassed by it. This attitude toward his wish is consistent with the approach taken toward many relational needs generated by object-relations theories through the developmental tilt; it is the position taken by Klein toward her patient's wish for nurturance, by Balint toward the somersault, by Blanck and Blanck toward the patient's wish to be held and cherished. The analyst in this case did not experience the patient's wish to share his success as resembling that of an infant seeking self-recognition in the mother's eyes, or that of a little boy showing off, but rather as that of a man fearfully prideful of his success and newly discovered powers. The analysand's apologetic display asks for reassurance from the analyst (either explicitly or implicitly); it is a request for permission to show his powers, which preserves both the characterological defense of the patient and a subtle protectiveness of the other (who, it is assumed, cannot bear to witness fully the patient's struggles and triumphs). The resultant interaction is a blend of expansive vitality, solicitous protectiveness, deferential obsequiousness, and ultimate secret triumph. Is the prideful man related to the boastful boy or the yearning baby? Of course. These comparisons reflect expressions, at different developmental levels and through different cognitive and symbolic modalities, of the same fundamental relational need. To collapse the various transformations of that need into its earliest manifestation, however, is seriously to distort its meaning and to infantilize the analysand as well.

Conflict and Passivity

The skewing of the relational matrix created by the developmental tilt is often accompanied by two additional clinical emphases: a tendency to minimize the importance of conflict, and a tendency to portray the analysand as essentially passive.

Drive theory is conflict theory—asocial impulses clash with socially inspired defenses against impulses, and it is from this clash that all mental life is generated. Developmental-arrest theorists, who have introduced relational issues via the developmental tilt, tend to present these issues not only as occurring earlier in life, but also as nonconflictual or preconflictual. Relational needs are not asocial, leading inevitably to conflict with the social environment. Relational needs by definition are social; what is sought is some form of relatedness. If the interpersonal environment provides opportunities for that relatedness, there is no conflict; if the interpersonal environment does not provide such opportunities, what results is not conflict but deprivation.

Winnicott expresses the developmental-arrest point of view most clearly, in distinguishing between needs and wishes. Wishes derive from instinctual impulses and eventually clash with social reality; if they are not gratified, they can be repressed, sublimated, transformed into aim-inhibited gratifications. Needs are developmental necessities; the child requires certain kinds of parenting behaviors to gain necessary experiences. If the parent provides them, the child continues to develop; if the parent does not, the child becomes frozen. Similarly, if the analyst does not provide these object-relational opportunities in some manner, nothing else can happen. It is not gratification of impulses; <u>it is a question of reaching the self by providing necessary experiences.</u> Serious psychopathology, in Winnicott's view, is always a result of inadequate provision of needs, always an "environmental deficiency disease," and the simple provision of maternal functions produces in the child nonconflictual experiences and unimpeded unfolding of the self.

Guntrip (1969) similarly operates on the premise that a seamless, conflict-free existence is possible, and certainly desirable.

> If we imagine a perfectly mature person, he would have no endopsychic structure in the sense of permanently opposed drives and controls. He would be a whole unified person whose internal psychic differentiation and organization would simply represent his diversified interest and abilities, within an overall good ego-development, in good object-relationships. (p. 425)

Proper parenting results in perpetual internal harmony and equilibrium.

> Then the grown-up child is free without anxiety or guilt to enter an erotic relationship with an extra-familial partner, and to form other important personal relationships in which there is a genuine meeting of kindred spirits without the erotic element, and further to exercise an active and spontaneous personality free from inhibiting fears. This kind of parental love, which the Greeks called *agape* as distinct from *eros,* is the kind of love the psychotherapist must give his patient because he did not get it from his parents in an adequate way. (p. 357)

In developing his "self psychology in the broad sense," Kohut (1977) takes a very similar position: if parenting is adequate in providing appropriate self-object functions, life proceeds rather simply and easily. Even the peak of the oedipal stage, the climax of instinctual Sturm and Drang in classical theory, is experienced as a joyful exercise of functions. Could it be, asks Kohut, that

> the dramatic conflict-ridden Oedipus complex of classical analysis, with its perception of a child whose aspirations are crumbling under the impact of castration fear, is not a primary maturational necessity but only the frequent result of frequently occurring failures from the side of narcissistically disturbed parents? (p. 247)

Similarly, suggests Kohut, if the analyst avoids subjecting the patient to traumatic failures in empathy as opposed to "optimal empathic failures," the reactions to which are themselves empathized with, the analysis is essentially smooth and nonconflictual.

Some analysts who identify themselves as "orthodox" dismiss relational theories on the ground that such theories necessarily give up the centrality of conflict which these analysts associate with oedipal neuroses. The criticism is a fair one, although the neglect of conflict (like the underemphasis on sexuality) is *not* an inevitable component of a relational perspective, but rather a historical artifact. An underemphasis on conflict results when relational contributions are introduced via the developmental tilt.

To regard conflict as the exclusive property of drive theory and to present relational concepts as fundamentally nonconflictual in nature is seriously to limit the clinical utility of relational contributions. This viewpoint misses the universality of conflicts between and among different relationships and identifications; ties and loyalties to one parent are, to some extent, inevitably experienced as (and in reality may very well be) a threat to ties and loyalties to the other. Also missed is the clinical importance of conflict *within* a single relationship. Intimacy is not a primrose path, but a process which includes risks, choices, and anxieties. Intimacy necessarily entails accommodation which, no matter how freely and willingly undertaken, inevitably generates a pull toward a reclaiming of the self. Intimate relationships, because of their temporal quality, are never static but always entail an active tension and conflict between openness to the other and self-definition, between responsiveness to the other's claims and a need for boundaries. As Winnicott (1963) suggests, each of us needs to remain in some sense "incognito," as the ground for recapturing a sense of personal experience and a renewed capacity for intimacy. *Conflict is inherent in relatedness.*

For analysands whose past efforts at relatedness have been severely dashed, warmth, nurturance, and connection can be a frightening, highly conflictual prospect. As Will notes, for some patients, paradoxically, "closeness to another implies anxiety, separation and death" (1959, p. 213). An analysand's retreat, fragmentation, withdrawal *may* result from a missed connection on the part of the analyst—but not necessarily so. To assume that it is needlessly limits clinical options. It is often not the experience of "empathic failure," but the experience of empathic success that precipitates withdrawal, devaluation, and fragmentation. For someone who has experienced repeated failure of meaningful connection, whose essential attachments are to constricted and painful relationships (in actuality or in fantasy), hope is a very dangerous feeling. It may be precisely the sense of meaningful connection that precipitates the analysand's withdrawal, because the possibility of such connection calls into question the basic premises of the analysand's painfully constricted subjective world. Sullivan's (1953) formulation of the "malevolent transformation," Klein's (1957) concept of envious spoiling, and Bion's (1957) depiction of "attacks on linking" all point to the dangers of hope and the conflictual nature of relational needs. The minimization of the importance of conflict in the developmental-arrest model, in which relational concepts are introduced through the developmental tilt, leads to a view of relational processes which is simplistic and overlooks their essential ambivalence in the psychoanalytic situation.

A CLOSELY related clinical emphasis generated by the developmental tilt is the tendency to portray the patient as passive, detached, and victimized. Psychopathology is a direct product of deprivation, an "environmental failure." Certain kinds of interpersonal experiences are necessary for the growth of the self; when these are lacking, central features of the child remain buried, unevoked, frozen. The patient as he presents himself for treatment is an empty shell vacated by this missing core, which can only be brought to life through the analyst's creation of a more encouraging environment; the passive "true self" of the patient awaits this call. Guntrip states most clearly the premises of this approach to treatment, which might be characterized as the Sleeping Beauty model. Psychotherapy is

> the provision of the possibility of a genuine, reliable, understanding, and respecting, caring personal relationship in which a human being whose true self has been crushed by the manipulative techniques of those who only wanted to make him "not be a nuisance" to them, can begin at last to feel his own true feelings, and think his own spontaneous thoughts, and find himself to be real. (1971, p. 182)

Guntrip sees the neurotic as a "neglected physically grownup child" having been deprived of the "elementary right to the primary supportive relationship that can alone enable him to live" (p. 156). Thus, the analyst brings to the frightened child in the patient missed possibilities for life. "At the deepest level, psychotherapy is replacement therapy, providing for the patient what the mother failed to provide at the beginning of life" (p. 191).

This view of the analysand as an abandoned, deprived, detached infant minimizes the interactive properties of mind vis-à-vis current interpersonal reality. Early mental life is conceived in terms of interaction; but once structured, the mind is perseveratively dominated by vestiges of infantile experience, awaiting appropriate conditions for reemergence. What is overlooked is the extent to which the analysand is involved in an interactive field, trying to shape his current relationships—including his relationship with the analyst—along lines he considers most desirable.

Psychopathology often entails an active, willful clinging to, an insistence on, maladaptive relational patterns, symptomatic behaviors, and painful experiences. Although a fuller treatment of agency and the will is developed in Chapter 9, let me briefly note the importance of active commitment in Fairbairn's object-relations theory, which is somewhat different from a more purely developmental-arrest position.

Fairbairn argues that beneath all forms of psychopathology one finds an attachment to "bad objects," thereby pointing to an active dimension which Guntrip's later formulations lose. Psychopathology is more than an absence or fearful avoidance of good relatedness. We often observe not just an avoidance of the positive, but a fascination with the negative. Analysands with repetitive disturbances in interpersonal relations are drawn, like the moth to the flame, to specific negative types of relations—with sadistic, skittish, withdrawn, debilitated others. This compulsive repetition of painful early experience seems to reflect a detachment from some forms of relationship, and also an attachment to certain others. The masochistic character seeks abuse partially because the violence imparts a fantasy of connection to and caring from others who are experienced as inaccessible in other ways. The depressed character seeks deprivation often because it is a state that makes possible a deep and often fantasied sense of connection with a schizoid or depressed parent, so unavailable in other ways. What the analysand is attached to is often not *actual* attributes of the parent, but fantasied attributes—not satisfying features of their relationship, but precisely the features that are missing. It is the deprivation, the pain, the depression, which serve as vehicles for attachment.

Embedded in much psychopathological experience and behavior are personifications of others, to whom the analysand feels tied through the pathology. The analysand does not simply miss or exclude from consciousness signals which would lead to nurturance and attachment; he looks for *different* cues, which draw him into attachments not based on caring and support but on pain and misery. The danger of the new dimensions of the analytic relationship is that they challenge these allegiances. The analysand must choose between attachments to fantasied images and presences which impart an often subtle sense of safety and connection, and the possibility of attachment to real others along new lines, with all the attendant risks. Thus, analysands often speak of a profound sense of isolation associated with giving up their neuroses. Psychopathology is not a state of aborted, frozen development, but a cocoon actively woven of fantasied ties to significant others. Beneath a seemingly passive detachment is often a secret attachment, largely unconscious, but experienced as necessary and life sustaining.

The relational issues depicted in the contributions of developmental-arrest authors vividly illuminate patients' struggles, both past and present. Yet the tendency to collapse these issues into early infancy and to portray the patient, via the metaphor of the baby, as nonconflictually and passively waiting to reemerge distorts their nature and detracts from a fuller appreciation of the interactive processes through which they are perpetuated.

Neediness and the Self as Baby

Part of the appeal to both analysand and analyst of the reification of the metaphor of the baby is that it corresponds to the experience of many analysands, who *feel* that their wishes and needs are infantile. As they allow themselves to care about and want things from another person, they experience the new desires as overwhelmingly powerful and intense, greedy, demanding—as a bottomless pit. They cannot tolerate not getting what they want from the other person, and not getting it instantly. This "neediness" is experienced as identical to that of the hungry infant or of the clinging toddler. What we are seeing looks like unsatisfied early developmental needs, manifesting themselves inappropriately in an adult context: needs for primitive oral gratification (Freud), infantile dependence (Fairbairn), symbiotic fusion (Mahler), mirroring (Kohut), and so on. These needs have been thwarted for decades and seem to have grown hungry, ravenous, over time. This understanding often makes the analysand's neediness difficult to resolve or work through, because it leads to two equally unappealing options. The choices are an ultimate renunciation of the "infantile" wishes, which are now understood in their proper historical context (classical technique), or an immersion in what is felt to be the gratification of those wishes in the analytic relationship (developmental-arrest technique). The first approach results in what seems to be a kind of resignation, the second in a splitting off of the analytic relationship from the rest of life, as the only domain in which one's desires are truly taken into account.

What the analysand experiences as neediness is often more usefully understood, within a relational-conflict framework, not as reflecting infantile fixations or developmentally arrested needs, but as a complex mixture of perfectly appropriate adult desires interfused with intense anxiety. These analysands often come from families where depending on other people for anything was regarded as weak or babyish (often also as "bad"), leading them to develop character styles organized around either excessive demandingness or its opposite, counterdependent defenses. These analysands probably *were* thwarted as infants. But what they experience as neediness in their adult lives has less to do with thwarted infantile needs and more to do with the ideas and feelings the individuals developed, through these early experiences, regarding desire in general. When such a person experiences any intense wish or longing in relation to another person (the common coinage of adult emotional life), he or she tends to become flooded with anxiety. The desire is felt as weakening them, as making them vulnerable, demanding, bad.

Thus, their experience of early parental reactions to their needs has led to experience of any desire as infused with intense anxiety. The anxiety leads to desire in peremptory, demanding terms, based on the following kind of logic: "I want closeness with you, which makes me feel very anxious and vulnerable, to which I anticipate your reacting with disgust or withdrawal. Therefore, you must give me everything I want, and immediately, to reassure me that you won't leave, to remove me from the experience of my own desire. I must have guarantees." This constellation of feelings and ideas, collapsed into neediness (sometimes as powerful sexual need) is often experienced as infantile, a displacement from the distant developmental past, which leads to limited therapeutic options.

The alternative is to separate the desire from the anxiety with which it is laced, and from the various defensive operations for avoiding that anxiety, all of which are collapsed into the experience of the neediness. This relational-conflict perspective allows the analysand a third option besides renunciation or specially designed gratification: inquiry into the manner in which the inevitable desire for and interdependence upon others have been shaped by early experience in a way which makes these analysands unwilling and unable to sustain current desires and longings long enough to become acquainted with them and negotiate their integration with the needs and desires of others.

Belief in a universal developmental sequence in which affects and behaviors unfold (given proper environmental provisions) on the way to some preconceived vision of maturity, tends to make a good deal of clinical data *look* infantile. The patient who expresses affects, impulses, and wishes in a volatile, unmodulated fashion makes compelling a view of his pathology as reflecting developmental failures in the capacity to regulate affect, tension, excitement. Without such a preconceived developmental scheme, however, one often finds that in some families volatile, unmodulated expression of affect and impulse is a highly developed, familial way of life. There are rules in every family about how needs are to be expressed and experienced. What is it that patients find in analytic treatment? Do they find missed opportunities for the unfolding of prewired capacities, or opportunities for integrating intrapsychic and interpersonal experiences with another person in a *different* fashion, more enriching and adaptive in the world outside their family? Viewing clinical data as arrested development often masks a patient's active belief in and loyalty to his way of living. Although constricted, seemingly infantile feelings and behaviors often still mediate the most important connections with others.

WHILE THE metaphor of the modern baby sometimes sheds considerable light on slowly emerging clinical data gained through painstaking analytic inquiry, with other analysands (where it almost seems demanded by the data) it can be especially misleading. These are patients who in fact see themselves, sometimes consciously, sometimes unconsciously, *as* the image of the modern baby, as having had interrupted, thwarted infancies; they experience a vast longing to become a baby once again. They see themselves as fraudulent adults, unable to feel whole because early needs were unmet. The dynamics in these cases cluster around several recurrent themes. The experience of self as baby is often found to represent not a piece of infantile mental life waiting to emerge, but an active strategy for construing the self so as to make possible various kinds of interactive connections with, and claims on, others.

These analysands often tend to have an ongoing experience of relationships with others characterized by compliance with what they assume are the expectations of others, a willingness to give others whatever they want as the price of connection or approval. Their image of the baby they feel they secretly are (or would like to be) is the opposite of this interpersonal style. They see the essential feature of babies as the freedom not to do or be anything for anyone. Babies are free of responsibility, oblivious to the needs of others, able to be simply centered in their own experience. Within the confines of their compulsive sensitivity and compliance, these patients see babies as the only humans with a right to their own being. The helplessness of the newborn is seen not as a drawback but as an advantage. It is precisely because the baby cannot do anything for himself or others that everything has to be done for him, a state which is romanticized into a blissful euphoria.

A second common feature in the dynamics of patients whose self-image corresponds to the modern baby is that babies, and often damage and helplessness, tend to have special significance within the family ideology, particularly for the mothers. One analysand had a mother who saw herself as a very maternal figure, specifically in the role of feeder of small babies. She felt uncomfortable with older children and seemed almost to resent their relative independence, while she felt most at ease and intimate with infants. This analysand's younger sisters replaced him as the center of his mother's attention and concern. She seemed to dread the total devotion she felt was called for if she had more than one baby, and at the same time to feel guilty of having deprived her son of his privileged status. In the care of a baby this extremely masochistic woman found the only vehicle, albeit a vicarious one, for giving herself anything. As an adult, the analysand was deeply committed to an intense romanticization of childhood and a longing to be a baby. In his family, being a baby and total self-abnegation were the only two possible modes of living.

Another such analysand was the eldest son of parents who were enraptured with the whole concept of babies, specifically *their* babies. The mother had suffered a series of painful losses at an early age. She experienced herself as damaged and trapped, but saw her babies as a chance for an unblemished new life. She spoke of each of her babies, both at the time of their infancy and later on, as perfect creations, physically and intellectually extraordinary, harbingers of a new life form. The analysand grew up with a powerful sense of himself as a disappointment to his mother, as if everything distinctive about himself (and hence human and finite) was not even noticed, as if her gaze in his direction always lighted on the perfect baby she had taken him to be.

The baby the analysand experiences himself as or longs to be is invariably related to familial relationships and values. Another analysand, for example, despite her considerable talents and achievements, experienced herself as a "messy baby inside." This sense of "self as mess" was enacted in various symptomatic behaviors including overeating, a compulsive urge to urinate in sexual situations, and in depressive funks. Analytic inquiry revealed a longstanding sense of each of her parents as a "mess," both literally and metaphorically, in their numerous depressions. Thus, being a messy baby preserved her ties to both parents. Even more relevant was the relationship between her mother and a younger sibling of her mother who had been severely injured in an accident. The mother had shaped her life around her role as caretaker for this "messy" and severely damaged child. The bond between mother and messy, damaged baby seemed to be the closest in the family and became a kind of ideal in this patient's search for relatedness. To be loved as resourceful and appealing was shallow and empty; to be loved unconditionally, as a mess, was the only test of real caring.

THESE VIGNETTES suggest that the metaphor of the modern baby often has great relevance for analysands, in that it serves multiple and complex dynamic ends. The danger of using the metaphor in a concrete and reified fashion, as is often done with the developmental-arrest perspective, is the assumption that this sort of material reflects some generic, universal infantile needs, actual memory traces, and an underlying structural dimension of the analysand's experience. Rather, it functions as a complex construction within the interactional patterns of the analysand's relational matrix, serving to perpetuate conflictual, fantasied ties to significant others and characteristic patterns of interpersonal integration.

It is the quintessential activity of the human mind to generate meaning, to organize isolated and discrete experiences into categories and assign them significance. Meanings are constructed through associating different kinds of experiences with one another, finding common elements, creating connections. The employment of metaphor is therefore a powerful tool of mind. Articulating and elucidating the subtle textures of the analysand's phenomenology dominates the nitty-gritty, day-to-day work of analytic inquiry. The metaphor of the baby, like the metaphor of the beast, is probably universal. We all struggle to make meaningful connections between present and past experience, to segregate the rich complexity of our inner life into motives which seem mature, even "independent" (given the values of Western culture), as opposed to those we associate with memories and longings of childhood. An awareness of the metaphor of the baby as a phenomenological organizer is extremely important in furthering the analytic inquiry.

Yet phenomenology is not all of mental life, nor always an accurate and comprehensive reflector of meaningful psychological processes. Without being fully aware that we do so, we construct our sense of ourselves and our experience with a careful eye toward perpetuating a sense of security and embeddedness within a familiar relational matrix. Metaphorical organizers of meanings become reified, thereby preserving ties to earlier modes of relation and preventing anticipated rebuffs and isolation. Psychoanalytic theories which stress self-organization at the expense of attachment to others and transactional patterns tend to regard these reified interactional metaphors as intact structural and motivational residues of early life, as the true primary ingredients of psychic life, rather than as secondary constructions whose purpose is to hold together a complex relational tapestry.

One of the central skills in the craft of psychoanalysis is the ability to grasp and enter into the analysand's subjective world. How is this person's world put together? What are the dramas? Who are the recurrent characters? What do the words around which the analysand organizes his experience really mean? One learns to see the world in these always highly individualized terms, to become conversant in the analysand's language. In this sense, developmental-arrest theories have been enormously useful in illuminating the clinical utility and evocative power of "baby" and "growth" as important metaphors for symbolizing the process of analytic change. These are universal themes in the mythologies of every known culture, and it is not surprising that they would lend themselves to the representation of analytic experiences of thwarted longings, fresh starts, tentative and delicate beginnings. These metaphors are often a powerful vehicle for articulating and connecting with dissociated aspects of the self. Like the experience of oneself as beast, the experience of oneself as baby can allow access to and help capture intensely passionate, irrational areas of experience not comfortably integrated with conventional rationality and maturity.

As with the metaphor of the beast, however, the metaphor of the baby becomes problematic when reified and confused with explanation. Their clinical utility ultimately rests in the analyst's dual ability to immerse himself in the experiential patterns of the analysand's subjective world, and to discern and convey to the analysand the ways in which that patterning restricts and precludes a greater richness of experience.

To view these experiences as essentially metaphorical does not suggest a technical stance of continually reminding the analysand that he is not *really* a baby. Rather, it suggests that in addition to learning the analysand's own language, the analyst must also learn the context and purposes for which that language was developed and is maintained. The analysand must learn something of that context and those purposes as a prerequisite to the capacity to develop a richer language and live in a more complex world.

As analysts, we know that adult patients continue to re-create their families within their subjective experience long after they are free to leave. The question is whether this pattern is structurally fixed in the first several years of life through deprivation of early needs, or whether it represents adaptation to a social environment fashioned over many years and now actively and loyally maintained. Use of the baby as a metaphor has been so characteristic of psychoanalytic thought from its inception that we tend to assume that explaining adult phenomena in terms of infantile prototypes is actually providing causal accounts, facts, rather than highlighting experiential similarities, which themselves call for further inquiry.

Relational Theories: Arrest or Conflict?

All relational-model theories rest, either explicitly or implicitly, on a broad developmental perspective. Human relations are understood to constitute the basic stuff of experience, and the pursuit and maintenance of relatedness is seen as the essential motivational thrust both in normality and in psychopathology. Relations take different forms across the life cycle—early relationships between infant and caretakers are precursors of later, more complex relationships. A commonly held tenet of all versions of relational-model theories is the premise that disturbances in the earliest relationships with caretakers significantly interfere with subsequent relatedness, and are a predisposing factor in the generation of later psychopathology.

With respect to clinical applications, however, the relational-conflict model and the developmental-arrest model diverge not around the question of what the analysand's problem *was* (that is, what went wrong in his or her early relationships), but around the question of what the problem now *is* and what can best be done about it. This chapter began with the consensus among relational-model theorists that the analyst must become a "good object." What sort of relationship does this imply?

Developmental-arrest authors, who draw on relational-model theory skewed by the developmental tilt, tend to view the patient as an infantile self in an adult body, fixed in developmental time and awaiting interpersonal conditions which will make further development possible. In this view, what was missed is still missing and needs to be provided essentially in the form in which it was missed the first time around. The developmental tilt has collapsed generic relational needs into infantile forms, and the analyst must enter at the point of the so-called environmental failure, providing relational experiences as replacements for those the infant never encountered. It is this view of psychopathology as the encapsulation of past infantile needs that Levenson points to in characterizing object-relations theory as viewing the patient as an adult "stuck with an incorporated infant, like a fishbone in the craw of his maturity" (1983, p. 142).

From a relational-conflict perspective, disturbances in early relationships with caretakers seriously distort subsequent relatedness, not by freezing or fixing infantile needs, but by setting in motion a complex process through which the child creates an interpersonal world (or world of object relations) out of what is available. The child cannot do without relationships, without ties to others, both in terms of real interactions and in terms of a sense of connection, belonging. To be human means to be in relation to others, to be embedded in a relational matrix.

The analysand enters treatment within a narrowed relational matrix; he seeks connections by projecting and re-creating familiar, constricted relational patterns, experiencing all important relationships (especially the one with the analyst) along old lines. He continually reinternalizes and consolidates these relational configurations. The central process in psychoanalytic treatment is the relinquishment of ties to these relational patterns, thereby allowing an openness to new and richer interpersonal relations.

yes, please.
How, indeed!

How do the analyst and the analysand break out of this closed system? Fairbairn's portrayal of the analyst as a "good" object cannot be equated with any of the patient's internal objects or fantasies; the analysand has never known a good object (no wholly available and responsive parent is ever possible); this is why the fragmentation underlying psychopathology has occurred. Surely the "good object" is not equivalent to Fairbairn's "exciting object," the analysand's fantasy of an impossible, unreachable nurturance which sustained him or her in the absence of real relationships. No, Fairbairn's good object operates *outside* the closed system of the patient's internalized object relations (as does Racker's portrayal of the analyst as interpreter); the good object must offer something real, something authentic, which makes possible the leap out of the closed world of the patient's fantasied object ties. The analyst may be experienced by the patient as an exciting object within the latter's closed subjective world, and this is likely to be necessary for the analyst to become important to the patient in any deeply felt way. But the developmental-arrest view that analytic cure lies in the provision of a replacement for missed infantile experience is actually coterminous with the analysand's own infantile fantasy of a magical cure; the analyst attempts to become the exciting object, the "magic helper" (Fromm, 1947, p. 70), to make a reality out of the analysand's "happy thought" (Sullivan, 1956, p. 203).

Some analytic work done under the aegis of object-relations theory via the developmental tilt is thus marred by a collusion between the analysand's fantasy and the analyst's theory. The patient is viewed by both as an exquisitely delicate and brittle infant to be handled in just the right fashion by a uniquely sensitive caretaker, leading to a splitting of the transference and a removal of the analysis from the world of real people, to which it never returns. Other analytic work done under the aegis of object-relations theory via the developmental tilt, such as Balint's invitation to the somersault, seems to be excellent analysis explained in a curious fashion. The analyst interacts with the analysand in a warm, spontaneous, concerned, possibly risk-taking fashion. Dimensions of relatedness are expressed which, in another context, would be regarded as a major component of intimacy throughout the life cycle, including intimacy between adults. Yet the interaction is collapsed into mother-infant terms, translated into the romance of the nursery.

*   *   *

I think this is what I used to do & what KW does.

exciting object → bad object → good enough object.

PSYCHOANALYTIC THEORIZING has swung back and forth dialectically around the issues of guilt and responsibility. Before 1897, parental seducers were seen as the instigators of neurosis, and the child as the innocent victim. Drive theory, drawing heavily on the metaphor of the baby as beast, placed the causal factor of neurosis in the inherent nature of the child, with the parents simply supplying raw material for the child's inevitable constructions. Developmental-arrest theory, drawing heavily on the metaphor of the modern baby, has swung the pendulum back too far, viewing neurosis as frozen, aborted development, with infantile experiences of deprivation and parental failure underlying and predisposing adult experience and psychopathology. It is precisely the polarized quality of these two positions that leads many theorists and clinicians to efforts at model mixing, some eclectic juxtaposition of these two metaphors, these discordant views, so as to find a more balanced position on the complex problem of etiology.

An integrated relational-conflict perspective makes it possible to take into account the crucial input of parental character, while at the same time conceiving the analysand's role in psychopathology as more active. We are not passive victims of experience, but rather active creators and loyal perpetuators of conflictual interactional patterns in a relational world which, if not secure, is at least known. It is not deprivation of generic infantile needs themselves that causes psychopathology, but the child's and the adult's later use of early experiences, memories, and fantasies to establish and maintain ties to significant others, to weave threads of prior events and needs into a tapestry of subjective experience which imparts a sense of familiarity, safety, and connectedness.

Part Four

Narcissism

- how do we negotiate this?

- I'm asking for some responsiveness based of fantasy

- I'm asking for some responsiveness based on what I want in an intimate adult relationship

ALTHOUGH he had been using the term descriptively for some years, it was not until 1914, on the heels of Jung's painful defection from the psychoanalytic community, that Freud formally introduced the concept of narcissism as an important explanatory principle in psychoanalytic theory. Freud was gradually extending drive theory from a theory of the etiology of neurosis to a more general account of human motivations, tracing the entire gamut of human endeavors through complex associative pathways of transformation and disguise, to conflicts over libidinal wishes. Jung objected to what he felt was the narrowness of this account of human motivations, arguing that other kinds of issues, totally independent of sexuality, played a central role in both mental health and psychopathology, particularly in psychotic disturbances such as schizophrenia. To meet Jung's challenge and to rescue his larger ambitions for drive theory, Freud had to account for schizophrenia in libidinal terms, to derive it interpretively from psychosexual wishes and conflicts.

In order to bring schizophrenia within the explanatory sway of drive theory, Freud expanded his view of the nature and developmental course of psychosexuality. Libido does not originate in the array of various infantile component instincts which Freud had unveiled beneath neurotic symptomatology. These wishes constituting infantile psychosexuality are already a secondary phase in the course of libidinal development, in which libido has taken on objects in the external world. Prior to this turn outward, Freud argued, the totality of the infant's desire is directed toward the child's own self, discharged inward. In one of his most evocative metaphors, Freud posits "an original libidinal cathexis of the ego, from which some is later given off to objects, but which fundamentally persists and is related to the object-cathexes much as the body of an amoeba is related to the pseudopodia which it puts out" (1914b, p. 75). By introducing narcissism as a prestage of object relations, Freud was able to generate a plausible account of schizophrenic phenomenology and symptomatology as the product of a libidinal regression beyond infantile parental imagoes (the fixation points for the neuroses), back to an obliviousness regarding the external world and others that is characteristic of an original state of primary narcissism.

The introduction of the concept of narcissism, however, had larger implications than providing a theory of schizophrenia. By granting self-love a position prior to object love and in continual reciprocal relation to it, Freud opened up for psychodynamic consideration the whole realm of issues and phenomena pertaining to self-regard and regulation of self-esteem. While not wholly independent of the fate of object cathexes and the conflicts they generate, self-regard became an area of psychodynamic investigation in its own right. With the subsequent expansion of the role of the ego in Freud's later writings and those of Anna Freud, Hartmann, and others, narcissism remained a crucial conceptual link (along with sublimation and neutralization) through which the ego draws upon libidinal energies to maintain a level of self-regard and to fuel its functions and choices.

The concept of narcissism allowed the drive model to address itself to the kinds of questions which were to become central for subsequent relational-model theorists, questions such as, How does a person come to experience and visualize himself the way he does? How does self-regard develop? How is it maintained? The referent of the term "narcissism" was further and further separated from its original meaning as a form of sexual perversion, or even from more general energic considerations. In drawing on contemporary uses of the concept, Stolorow argued for a "functional" definition of narcissism as essentially equivalent to the maintenance of self-esteem. "Mental activity is narcissistic to the degree that its function is to maintain the structural cohesion, temporal stability, and positive affective coloring of the self-representation (Stolorow and Lachmann, 1980, p. 10). This definition could be used without alteration to depict the functions Sullivan termed the "self system." Over the subsequent history of psychoanalytic ideas the problem of narcissism, the development and maintenance of self-image and self-esteem, has become a common realm into which all psychoanalytic theories—classical, ego psychological, interpersonal, and object relational—have forayed. Although narcissism is often discussed in connection with more severe characterological disturbances, conceptualizations of and technical recommendations for the handling of narcissistic phenomena have had an enormous influence on clinical practice across all diagnostic groupings.

It is the common centrality of the concept of narcissism for all psychoanalytic schools, in terms of both theory and technique, that makes it compelling to use narcissism, following our consideration of sexuality and infantilism, as a major psychoanalytic domain for comparing and integrating different theoretical perspectives. Specific forms of narcissism have been considered *inherent* properties of mind in the drive model and in many relational-model formulations as well. In Chapter 7 I shall consider ways in which the strengths of these formulations can be integrated within a more purely interactional framework. And in Chapter 8 this integrated relational approach will be applied to some extended clinical examples.

*In this world only play, play as artists and children engage in it,
exhibits coming-to-be and passing away, structuring and destroying
. . . And as children and artists play, so plays the everliving fire. It
constructs and destroys, all in innocence . . . Transforming itself into
water and earth, it builds towers of sand like a child at the seashore,
piles them up and tramples them down . . . The ever self-renewing
impulse to play calls new worlds into being. The child throws its toys
away from time to time—and starts again, in innocent caprice. But
when it does build, it combines and joins and forms its structures
regularly, conforming to inner laws.*   —NIETZSCHE

7   The Wings of Icarus

In unveiling narcissism as a powerful undercurrent of human experience,
Freud pointed to the similarities among the megalomania of the schizophrenic, the magical thinking of "primitive" (non-Western) peoples, the
blind infatuation of the lover, and the "childish," doting adulation of
parents toward their offspring. The common element in these states,
Freud argued, is "overvaluation"—whatever is being considered,
whether in oneself or in another, is inflated in importance, its powers
exaggerated, its unique perfections extolled. The narcissistic overvaluations of the schizophrenic, the primitive, the lover, the parent, are all
secondary derivatives of a more fundamental narcissistic condition,
Freud argued, which constitutes the earliest stage of psychic development. Freud portrays the state of primary narcissism as one of total
omnipotence, perfection, completeness. The infant imagines himself as
constituting the entire universe, or certainly all that is good and pleasurable in it.

Illusion as Defense

Although the state of primary narcissism cannot be maintained for long
in a world of inevitable frustrations and increasing parental expectations,
the original narcissistic experience, in Freud's view, is not wholly renounced. Much of narcissistic libido is transformed into object libido,

self-gratification replaced by drive gratifications facilitated by others as libidinal objects. Some of the original narcissism remains intact, however, and self-regard derives from three different forms in which narcissistic libido is preserved.

Some primary narcissism simply remains from its original state and serves, like the protoplasmic body of the amoeba, as a never-wholly-emptied pool of libidinal resources from which pseudopodlike object libidinal cathexes are drawn. Sometimes narcissistic libido is transferred to the sexual object; here the object is not loved in an anaclitic way, modeled after those who provided drive gratifications, but in an idealized, narcissistic fashion, modeled after the inflated self-love of primary narcissism. Some narcissistic libido is set up within the ego ideal. Self-rapture in relation to the child's true attributes is no longer possible; but if the parents' values and expectations can be fulfilled, wholeness and perfection are once again attainable.

The common feature in these three vicissitudes of narcissistic libido is "overvaluation," which Freud identifies as the "narcissistic stigma" (1914b, p. 91). Whether the focus is actually oneself, one's wished-for self, or the beloved, the object is granted positive qualities beyond what is supportable by reality. *Thus, narcissism, in Freud's system, entails the attribution of illusory value.* His metaphor of the amoeba and its oscillatory protoplasm, now extending outward into the world, now retreating backward into the central body, highlights the reciprocal relationship he saw between engagement with reality (and other people) and narcissistic illusions. For Freud, narcissistic illusions (even when they are transferred through idealization onto love objects), ultimately draw one away from real involvements with others and the gratifications they provide.

Although an explorer of the darkest, most irrational dimensions of human experience, Freud was a supreme rationalist in his sense of social, moral, and scientific values. Rationality, fueled by sublimation, represents the highest and most felicitous development of the human mind. The discontents we suffer in civilization are the necessary price of its uplifting advantages. Unless impeded by neurosis, developmental progress is characterized by a movement from primary process to secondary process, from the pleasure principle to the reality principle. Psychoanalysis as a treatment facilitates this process whereby the irrational and fantastic is brought under the sway of the rational and the real—"where id was, there ego shall be" (1933, p. 80).

Kaplan (1985) has described Freud's dedication to rationality in striking terms.

> If people must suffer the loss of their infantile hopes and fantasies, then they should suffer for the fact of this loss rather than for distortions of it in aesthetic bonuses, the empty promises of religion, and the negligible protections of social orders. Unremitting toil in the service of science—naked means toward real ends—was Freud's (1930/1961) alternative in *Civilization and Its Discontents,* at least for himself. Any other kind of life was ensnared by illusion, which was but a small step up from neurosis. (pp. 290–291)

In this larger context, Freud regarded narcissistic illusions as the inevitable residue of the most primitive and infantile state of mind, and therefore as both unavoidable and dangerous. Precisely because narcissism, by definition, entails illusory overvaluation, it runs counter to reality and beckons as an ever-tempting defensive retreat. Withdrawal from reality is always perilous, the ultimate threat being the total loss of connection with the real world (the schizophrenic state) and the less devastating threat posed by the vulnerable loss of self suffered by the unrequited lover, whose narcissism is transferred to the beloved and never returned.

Freud's stress on the defensive function of illusions has been largely maintained in what one might consider the mainstream of contemporary Freudian thought, although exactly what is being defended against varies in different accounts, depending on the larger set of theoretical premises which shape that account. Let us consider, as examples of the traditional approach to illusion as defense, two of the most significant recent contributions to the literature on narcissism from within Freudian ego psychology, those of Kernberg and Rothstein.

ALTHOUGH KERNBERG stresses his loyalties to Mahler, Jacobson, and the ego-psychological tradition, his contributions draw extensively on Melanie Klein's model of mental life, and his approach to narcissistic illusion is greatly informed by her theories. Klein portrays the infant as beset with terrifying anxieties involving the containment of aggression, and sees early development as a movement from paranoid and depressive anxieties toward a more integrated and secure sense of reality. Within Klein's vision, narcissistic illusions operate as defenses and regressive retreats from these frightening early anxieties: idealization is a refuge from persecutory anxiety and murderous rage toward bad objects; grandiosity is a "manic" defense against the depressive anxiety inherent in feeling small, helpless, and abjectly dependent upon another. Kernberg borrows heavily from these conceptualizations.

He distinguishes normal from pathological narcissism, defining the former (following Freud, as amended by Hartmann, 1950, p. 127) as the libidinal investment of the self. What Kernberg means by *normal* narcissism, then, is the resultant of all the processes which bear on self-representation and self-regard. He sees *pathological* narcissism as a particular dynamic mechanism which generates both entitled grandiosity and primitive idealization. Following Klein, Kernberg characterizes these as primitive defense mechanisms, often operating in conjunction with other primitive defense mechanisms such as splitting, denial, and projective identification. Narcissistic illusions are a defense erected within the child's struggle with a "pathologically augmented development of oral aggression" (1975, p. 234), generating paranoid and depressive anxieties; the illusions are constructed from a pathological fusion of ideal self, ideal object, and actual self-image.

How do narcissistic illusions work? In Kernberg's account, the infant is overloaded with primitive aggressive impulses, due to a "constitutionally determined strong aggressive drive, or constitutionally determined lack of anxiety tolerance in regard to aggressive impulses, or severe frustration in their first year of life" (1975, p. 234). He experiences himself and, projectively, other people as well, as essentially sadistic, and this aggressive outlook dominates his early experience. Sticking close to Klein's account of "envy" (1957), Kernberg portrays the narcissistically prone infant as so frustrated and hateful as to be unable to tolerate hope, the possibility of anyone's offering him anything pleasurable or sustaining. So little is forthcoming, the child concludes, and with such ill will toward him, that it is better to expect nothing, to want nothing, to spoil and devalue everything that might be offered. Normal fantasies of self and other as ideal are fused with the child's own realistic self-perceptions, resulting in a "grandiose self" which is experienced as complete, perfect, and self-sustaining. "I am/ have everything. You are/offer nothing." This position serves as both an expression of and a defense against explosive oral aggression, and the only secure solution in a world experienced as treacherous and sinister. Maintenance and protection of the grandiose self becomes the central psychodynamic motive, resulting in a contemptuous character style and disdainful manner of relating to others.

> A narcissistic patient experiences his relationships with other people as being purely exploitative, as if he were "squeezing a lemon and then dropping the remains." People may appear to him either to have some potential food inside, which the patient has to extract, or to be already emptied and therefore valueless. (1975, p. 233)

Primitive idealization of others is also characteristic of personalities organized around a grandiose self, according to Kernberg, but the idealization has little to do with any real valuing of others. Rather, Kernberg's narcissistic patient projects his own grandiose self-image onto others when it becomes impossible to sustain within himself, and also uses idealization as a secondary defense, along with splitting, to ward off and conceal the hateful and contemptuous devaluation of others.

Thus, narcissistic illusions protect the patient from the dreadful state in which he spent much of the first several years of life, depending on others for protection and care, yet perpetually dissatisfied, victimized, and enraged. The establishment of the grandiose self removes the patient from the multifaceted psychic pain of this situation, and, once established, the grandiose self perpetuates the devaluing assumptions about others which made its establishment necessary in the first place. It creates a "vicious circle of self-admiration, depreciation of others, and elimination of all actual dependency. The greatest fear of these patients is to be dependent on anybody else, because to depend means to hate, envy, and expose themselves to the danger of being exploited, mistreated, and frustrated" (Kernberg, 1975, p. 235).

Narcissistic illusions have a perniciously sabotaging effect on psychoanalytic treatment. Based on the illusions of self-sufficiency and perfection of the grandiose self, they undercut the very basis on which the psychoanalytic process rests, the presumption that the analysand might gain something meaningful from someone else (in this case the analyst). Despite what might be considerable psychological suffering and a genuine interest in treatment, the analysand whose character is organized around a grandiose self cannot allow the analyst to become important enough to him to really help him. The analyst and his interpretations must be continually devalued, spoiled, to avoid catapulting the patient into a condition of overpowering longing, abject dependency, and intolerable hatred and envy.

Kernberg's technical recommendations are wholly consistent with this psychodynamic portrait—a methodical and persistent interpretation of the defensive function of grandiosity and idealization as they emerge in the transference (1984, p. 197). Anything else is a waste of time, since the narcissistic illusions systematically destroy the very ground upon which the treatment proceeds. Unless the workings of the grandiose self are continually brought to light and confronted, the impact of the treatment is often subtly but systematically vitiated. "The analyst must continuously focus on the particular quality of the transference in these cases and consistently counteract the patient's efforts toward omnipotent control and devaluation" (1975, p. 246). This traditional emphasis on aggressive interpretation of narcissistic phenomena derives from and is wholly consistent with Freud's early view of "narcissistic neurosis" as unanalyzable and narcissistic defenses as generating the most recalcitrant resistances to the analytic process. (See, for example, Abraham, 1919.)

Rothstein (1984) has presented a rich amalgam of dynamic formulations which he portrays as an "evolutionary" extension of Freud's structural model (from which he has deleted virtually all energic considerations). The result is a psychodynamic account which stresses conflict among various relational motives and puts particular stress on the importance of the actual relationship to significant others. The most pervasive influence on Rothstein's perspective, particularly with regard to more severe disorders, is Mahler's depiction of the process of separation-individuation from an original symbiotic matrix. Rothstein's approach to narcissism is a blend of Freud's original formulations and Mahler's more contemporary view of the child's struggle for relational autonomy.

Rothstein distinguishes Freud's phenomenological portrayal of narcissism as a "felt quality of perfection" from his metapsychological treatment of narcissism (as the libidinal cathexis of the ego). He adds symbiosis to Freud's account of primary narcissism and sees narcissistic illusions as based developmentally on preindividuated experiences of a perfect self fused with a perfect object. The loss of this original state of perfection is a severe narcissistic blow, an inevitable developmental insult which is traversed only by reinstating the lost narcissistic perfection in the ego ideal. By identifying with the narcissistically tinged images of the ego ideal, the child softens the otherwise unbearable pain of separation. "Narcissistically invested identification is the sole condition under which the id can give up its objects and is a fundamental concomitant of primary separation-individuation. The pursuit of narcissistic perfection in one form or another is a defensive distortion that is a ubiquitous characteristic of the ego" (Rothstein, 1983, p. 99).

Thus, like Freud, Rothstein sees some residues of primary narcissism as inevitable, reestablished in the ego ideal. For Rothstein, with his Mahlerian perspective, the loss of infantile narcissism has an additional poignancy, since it represents not just the loss of grandeur and perfection, but the loss of the original symbiotic state. Accordingly, narcissistic illusions operate as defensive retreats not only from disappointments in reality in general, but also from anxiety and dread connected with separation. He holds that "narcissistic perfection is a defensive distortion of reality" (p. 98). Like many defenses within the ego-psychological model, narcissism itself is neither healthy nor pathological; some defenses are necessary and serve adaptive functions within the psychic economy. Although a total relinquishment of narcissistic illusions is impossible, it is the goal of analysis, in Rothstein's view, to identify and work through the salient narcissistic investments.

ALTHOUGH PROCEEDING from a very different set of basic assumptions concerning the motivational and structural underpinnings of emotional life, the major theorists within the interpersonal tradition have taken an approach to the clinical phenomenon of illusions, the implications of which are quite similar to the mainstream Freudian approach from Freud to Kernberg to Rothstein. Sullivan sees idealization as a dangerous, self-depleting security operation and stresses the "cost" to the patient of "thinking the doctor is wonderful" (White, 1952, p. 134). He recommends challenging the patient's assumptions that the analyst is so different from other people, often a product of inexperience in taking risks with others, and sees extended periods of idealization as reflecting a kind of acting out of countertransference. "The effective restriction of idealization is dependent on the physician's own freedom from personality warp. In so far as he is capable of real intimacy in the situation with the patient, to that extent he can inhibit idealization . . . The measure of this capacity [is] intuited or empathized by any patient" (Sullivan, 1972, p. 343).

Similarly, Sullivan regards grandiosity as a dynamic for covering over feelings of insecurity through "invidious comparison" between oneself and others, an accelerating spiral of desperate attempts to prop up a steadily undermined security, with the result that the patient is more and more detested and avoided . . . If the patient will be alert to how small he feels with anybody who seems to be at all contented or successful in any respect, then he may not have need for this hateful superiority—which is hateful in part because he hates himself so much, being unable to be what he claims to be. (quoted in White, 1952, p. 139)

Although Sullivan does not develop an explicit technical procedure for the handling of illusions, one gets the clear impression throughout his writings that the analyst is in no way helpful by failing to address the patient's overvaluation of either himself or the analyst. Both kinds of illusions are seen as self-sabotaging devices propping up a shaky sense of self-esteem, operating as an obstacle to the development of the analysand's own resources and self-respect.

Fromm takes an even dimmer view of the place of illusion in emotional life. He sees psychodynamics in the general context of certain inescapable realities of the human condition, among which are finitude and separateness. To this condition two kinds of responses are possible: progressive, productive responses which accept the existential realities and create meaningful ties to others; and regressive, destructive responses, based on a self-deluding denial of the realities of the human condition. The overvaluing of illusions concerning the self or others from whom one derives some compensatory reassurance are regressive self-deceptions from Fromm's perspective and must be dealt with as such. In fact, at several points Fromm accuses Sullivan, in his emphasis on protecting the analysand's need for security, of being in effect soft on illusions. Anything short of a continual interpretive challenge to the analysand's overvaluing illusions concerning both himself and the analyst would be an expression of countertransferential contempt on the analyst's part, a disrespectful collusion in the analysand's flight from reality and meaning.

THUS, ALTHOUGH deriving from very different psychodynamic traditions and assumptions, the major lines of theorizing within orthodox theory, Freudian ego psychology, and interpersonal theory all converge in an essentially similar technical approach to the clinical phenomenon of narcissistic illusions. The latter are viewed as regressive defenses against frustration, separation, aggression, dependence, and despair.

Transferential illusions concerning either the self or the analyst must be interpreted, their unreality pointed out, and their defensive purpose defined.

Illusion as Creativity

In recent years there has emerged an alternative view of infantile mental states and the narcissistic illusions which are thought to derive from them. This approach is closely connected with the developmental-arrest model of psychopathology and the therapeutic action of psychoanalytic treatment. The most important contributors to this very different perspective have been Winnicott and Kohut, each of whom in his own distinct fashion regards infantile narcissism and subsequent narcissistic illusions in later life as the core of the self and the deepest source of creativity. Here the prototypical "narcissist" is not the child, madman, or savage, but the creative artist, drawing for inspiration on overvaluing illusions.

Although Winnicott did not often write about narcissism per se, his entire opus revolves around the issue which we have seen is central to that domain: the relationship between illusion and reality, between the self and the outside world. For Winnicott, the key process in early development is the establishment of a sense of the self experienced as real. For this to happen, the child requires a very particular sort of relationship with his or her providers, the most distinguishing feature of which is, ironically, that the child must not know of the existence of the relationship, must not know that it is being provided at all.

The essential feature of the necessary "facilitating" environment provided by the mother is her effort to shape the environment around the child's spontaneously arising wishes, to read the child's needs and provide for them. The mother's actualization of the infant's desires makes it possible for the latter to assume that his wishes actually create the objects of his desire—that the breast, in effect his entire world, is the product of his creation. In fact, Winnicott characterizes the child's experience, made possible by the mother's perfect accommodation to his wishes, as the "moment of illusion." The virtual invisibility of Winnicott's "good-enough mother" allows the infant a developmentally crucial immersion in an illusory, megalomaniacal, solipsistic state of "subjective omnipotence."

Eventually the child learns to live in objective reality (introduced largely through the mother's incremental failure to accommodate herself to the child's wishes) as it becomes clear that objects and people have their own independent existence and are only minimally under the child's control. The distinguishing characteristic of the terrain between the original subjective omnipotence and the eventual objective reality, transitional experiencing, is an ambiguity about the status of the other. *Is* the transitional object (the traditional teddy bear, for example) a creation of the child, in some special relation to the child, under his or her control, or is it simply an object within the world of mundane objects, subject to being lost, damaged, discarded, washed? The good-enough parent of the transitional stage allows the child this ambiguity, participating in the child's illusions like the mother whose accommodation makes possible the earlier experience of subjective omnipotence, thereby enabling the child to solidify a sense of self as a consistent source of spontaneous wishes, longings, and resources.

 Freud measured mental health in terms of the capacity to love and work; Winnicott envisions health as the capacity for play, as freedom to move back and forth between the harsh light of objective reality and the soothing ambiguities of lofty self-absorption and grandeur in subjective omnipotence. In fact, Winnicott regards the reimmersion into subjective omnipotence as the ground of creativity, in which one totally disregards external reality and develops one's illusions to the fullest. He originally presented his view of patients with fragmented, aborted (false) selves as a distinct diagnostic group reflecting more severe psychopathology and, employing the developmental tilt, he placed them developmentally as antedating oedipal neuroses. As is often the case with theoretical innovations introduced through the establishment of a new diagnostic category, the category spreads and the formulations take on more and more general relevance. Thus, many varieties of psychopathology came to be viewed by Winnicott as reflecting deficiencies in the establishment of a healthy self, as a consequence of insufficient experience of the illusions of subjective omnipotence and the transitional phase.

This view of the development of the self led Winnicott to redefine both the analytic situation and the analytic process. Whereas Freud saw the analytic situation in terms of abstinence (instinctual wishes emerge and find no gratification), Winnicott sees the analytic situation in terms of satisfaction, not of instinctual impulses per se, but of crucial developmental experiences, missed parental functions. The couch, the constancy of the sessions, the demeanor of the analyst—these become the "holding environment" which was not provided in infancy. Freud saw the analytic process in terms of renunciation; by bringing to light and renouncing infantile wishes and illusions, healthier and more mature forms of libidinal organization become possible. Winnicott sees the analytic process in terms of a kind of revitalization; the frozen, aborted self is able to reawaken and begin to develop as crucial ego needs are met.

Although Winnicott does not apply this model of treatment to the problem of narcissistic illusions per se, its implications are clear. The patient's self has been fractured and crushed by maternal impingement, creating the necessity for a premature adaptation to external reality and a disconnection from one's own subjective reality, the core of the self and the source of all potential creativity. The analyst's task is to fan the embers, to rekindle the spark. He must create an atmosphere as receptive as possible to the patient's subjectivity; he must avoid challenging the patient in any way which could be experienced as an impingement, an insistence once again on compliance with respect to external reality. Narcissistic illusions, in Winnicott's model, are neither defenses nor obstructions. The patient's illusions concerning both himself and the analyst represent the growing edge of the patient's aborted self; as good-enough mothering entails an accommodation of the world to sustain the infant's illusions, good-enough analysis entails an accommodation of the analytic situation to the patient's subjective reality, a "going to meet and match the moment of hope" (1945, p. 309).

The more explicit technical implications of this new understanding of the meaning of narcissistic illusions were developed by Kohut, who, like Winnicott, introduced his innovations in connection with a diagnostic category of greater severity (narcissistic personality disorders), but who expanded those innovations into a broad and novel theory of development, psychic structure, and motivation. In his original 1971 presentation Kohut described two forms of transference, the mirroring transference and the idealizing transference, which, he argued, are very different from ordinary neurotic transferences. Here the patient is not simply transferring infantile impulses and conflicts onto the person of the analyst as a differentiated object. In the mirroring and idealizing transferences, the analyst and his responses function in lieu of missing psychic structures within the patient's own personality. In mirroring transference the patient experiences himself in terms of overvaluing grandiosity and requires the analyst's mirroring responses to avoid a disintegration of self. In idealizing transference the patient experiences the analyst in terms of overvaluing admiration and requires the analyst's allowance of the idealization to avoid a disintegration of self.

In Kohut's account, the appearance of narcissistic illusions within the analytic situation—primitive grandiosity or idealization—represents the patient's attempt to establish crucial developmental opportunities, a self-object relationship unavailable in childhood. These phenomena represent not a defensive retreat from reality (à la Freud, Sullivan, Rothstein, and Kernberg), but the growing edge of an aborted developmental process which was stalled because of parental failure to allow the child sustained experiences of illusions of grandeur and idealization. Thus, the appearance of narcissistic illusions within the analytic relationship constitutes a fragile opportunity for the revitalization of the self. The illusions must be cultivated, warmly received, and certainly not challenged, allowing a reanimation of the normal developmental process through which the illusions will eventually be transformed, by virtue of simple exposure to reality in an emotionally sustaining environment, into more realistic images of self and other.

Kohut stresses throughout that he is recommending an "empathic comprehension" of narcissistic needs and not "play acting" or "wish-fulfillment." But empathic comprehension certainly entails a receptivity to the narcissistic illusions and an avoidance at all costs of anything which would challenge them or suggest that they are unrealistic. "While it is analytically deleterious to bring about an idealization of the analyst by artificial devices, a spontaneously occurring therapeutic mobilization of the idealized parent imago or of the grandiose self is indeed to be welcomed and must not be interfered with" (1971, p. 164). Kohut sees the dangers of interference, analogous to Winnicott's notion of impingement, as very great indeed and warns against even "slight overobjectivity of the analyst's attitude or a coolness in the analyst's voice; or . . . the tendency to be jocular with the admiring patient or to disparage the narcissistic idealization in a humorous and kindly way" (p. 263). Anything short of warm acceptance of narcissistic illusions concerning both the self and the analyst—which illusions are assumed to simply express themselves, independent of the interactional field in which the analyst participates—runs the risk of closing off the delicate, pristine narcissistic longings and thereby eliminating the possibility of the reemergence of healthy self-development.

THERE IS a striking symmetry between these two different traditions of understanding narcissistic illusions; for each, the approach of the other borders on the lunatic. From Kohut's point of view, the kind of methodical interpretive approach to narcissistic transferences recommended by Kernberg is extremely counterproductive, implying a countertransferential acting out. For Kohut, Kernberg's stance suggests great difficulty in tolerating the position in which the narcissistic transferences place the analyst, arousing anxiety concerning his own grandiosity (in the idealizing transference) or envy of the patient's grandiosity (in the mirroring transference). Thus, Atwood and Stolorow argue that the oral rage Kernberg sees in borderline patients is actually an iatrogenic consequence of his technical approach. Methodical interpretation of the transference is experienced by the narcissistically vulnerable patient as an assault and generates intense narcissistic rage, which Kernberg then regards as basic and long-standing, requiring the very procedures which created it in the first place. From the vantage point of self psychology, Kernberg is continually creating the monster he is perpetually slaying.

Similarly, from the more traditional point of view, the Winnicott-Kohut approach is an exercise in futility. An unquestioning acceptance of the patient's illusions with the assumption that they will eventually diminish of their own accord represents a collusion with the patient's defenses; the analytic process is thereby subverted, and the analyst never emerges as a figure who can meaningfully help the patient. From the traditional vantage point, the Winnicott-Kohut approach suggests what Loewald (1973) has termed a countertransferential "overidentification with the patient's narcissistic needs" (p. 346). Loewald further suggests that Kohut's avoidance of any focus on "an affirmation of the positive and enriching aspects of limitations" of self and others constitutes a "subtle kind of seduction of the patient" (p. 349). As Kernberg notes, unresolved narcissistic conflicts in the analyst "may foster excessive acceptance as well as rejection of the patient's idealization . . . To accept the admiration seems to be an abandonment of a neutral position" (1975, p. 298).*

ILLUSION AS defense, illusion as the growing edge of the self—these two approaches derive most broadly from larger divergent perspectives on the relation between the individual and society that have a long history in Western culture. From one perspective (developed to its fullest by the Enlightenment philosophers of the eighteenth century), culture and civilization humanize the individual creature, whose personal subjectivity is beneficially renounced in favor of the higher objectivity and rationality of society. From the other perspective (developed to its fullest in the Romantic movement of the nineteenth century), subjective experience is a higher form of reality; society threatens what is most precious in the individual, and conventional "rationality" is portrayed as an oppressive-repressive force.

These two approaches to illusion have generated an exciting controversy in the analytic literature, particularly because they are dramatically contrasting and mutually exclusive (which is often the case with competing psychoanalytic theories in their polarized swings of the pendulum). This controversy demonstrates dramatically the extent to which concepts like neutrality, countertransference, and empathy are theory bound.

It is a mistake to regard one of these approaches as more empathic than the other. They simply proceed (empathically) from different assumptions about the patient's experience. Kernberg's narcissist lives in an embattled world, in which he and all others are experienced as sadistic, self-serving, and exploitative. The only possible security lies in a devaluation of others, disarming them of their power to hurt him. From this perspective, an empathic response entails an appreciation of his endangered status (see Schafer, 1983) and a delineation of his narcissistic defenses, along with an effort to make some meaningful contact possible. To simply accept the grandiosity would be to empathize only

---

* It should be noted that in Kohut's final, posthumously published work (1984), seemingly in response to criticisms such as Loewald's, he stresses the balance between the reality orientation of the analyst and his encouragement of illusions. The curative factor, for Kohut, still derives from the latter. However objective and limit recognizing an analyst's interpretations may be, he stresses, if they are preceded by understanding and deepen the analysand's recognition that he has been understood, then the "old reassurance of a merger-bond, even on archaic levels, will reverberate, if ever so faintly, with the experience" (p. 191).

with the most superficial level of the patient's defenses and not with what is presumed to be his underlying experience.

Kohut's narcissist, on the other hand, is a brittle creature who lives in a harsh and continually bruising world. The only possible security lies in a splitting off of important segments of the self (either vertically or horizontally) in an effort to protect the deep and tender feelings connected to them, often covered over by bravado or narcissistic rage. From this perspective, an empathic response entails an appreciation of the continual threat of self-dissolution and disintegration, and an encouragement of growth-enhancing illusions. To challenge the patient's illusions would be to perpetuate the repeated traumas of childhood. With narcissistic illusions, as with most analytic phenomena, empathy and countertransference are in the eye of the beholder.

I STRONGLY suspect that the majority of analysts work in neither of these two sharply contrasting ways, that most of us struggle to find some midpoint, undoubtedly reflective of our own personality and style, between challenging and accepting narcissistic illusions. Because subtlety and tone are crucial, it is difficult to formulate such a clinical posture in simple, schematic terms. The following description is offered as a framework for locating such an approach conceptually and in terms of technique, within an integrated relational perspective.

The more traditional approach to narcissism highlights the important ways in which narcissistic illusions are used defensively, but misses their role in health and creativity and in consolidating certain kinds of developmentally crucial relationships with others. The developmental-arrest approach has generated a perspective on narcissism which stresses the growth-enhancing function of narcissistic illusions, but overlooks the extent to which they often constrict and interfere in real engagements between the analysand and other people, including the analyst.

It is possible to draw upon the clinical wisdom in both these contributions by viewing narcissistic illusions in the context of their interactive role in perpetuating the analysand's relational matrix. In viewing narcissism as either only defensive or as fundamentally growth enhancing, both traditions overemphasize what is taken to be the *inherent* nature of narcissistic illusions. What has been neglected is the key function of narcissism throughout the life cycle in perpetuating stereotyped patterns of integrating interpersonal relationships and fantasied ties to significant objects.

An Integrated Relational Approach

All varieties of narcissistic illusions are generated throughout the life cycle, from the exuberance of the toddler to the nostalgic musings of old age: grand estimations of one's own capacities and perfection, infatuation with the larger-than-life qualities of others whom one loves or envies, and fantasies of an exquisite, perfect merger with desirable or dreaded others. The determination of emotional health as opposed to psychopathology, when it comes to narcissistic illusions, has less to do with the actual content of the illusions than with the attitude of the individual about that content. All of us probably experience at various times feelings and thoughts as self-ennobling as the most grandiose narcissist, as devoted as the most star-struck idealizer, as fused as the most boundaryless symbiosis seeker. The problem of narcissism concerns issues of character structure, not mental content; it is not so much what you do and think as your attitude toward what you do and think, how seriously you take yourself. How can this subtle issue of attitude be conceptualized?

Consider Nietzsche's theory of tragedy (1872/1956). Life is lived in two fundamental dimensions, Nietzsche suggests. On the one hand, we live in a world of illusions, continually generating transient forms and meanings with which we play and then quickly discard. This facet of living Nietzsche terms Apollonian, Apollo being the god of the dream, art, and illusion. On the other hand, we are embedded in a larger unity, a universal pool of energy from which we emerge temporarily, articulate ourselves, and into which we once again disappear. This facet of living Nietzsche terms Dionysian, Dionysus representing reimmersion in this undifferentiated oneness and, in Nietzsche's system, the inevitable undoing of all illusions, all individual existence.*

Nietzsche establishes "the tragic" as the fullest, richest model of living, and the truly tragic represents a balance between the Apollonian and Dionysian dimensions. The tragic man (this phrase must be disentangled from all pejorative connotations) is one who is able to

* This is not the later Dionysus of Greek mythology, god of revelry and intoxication, but an earlier, closely related version of the mythological figure representing the undoing and death of the individual.

fully pursue his Apollonian illusions and also is able to relinquish them in the face of the inevitable realities of the human condition. The tragic man regards his life as a work of art, to be conceived, shaped, polished, and inevitably dissolved. The prototypical tragic activity is play, in which new forms are continually created and demolished, in which the individuality of the player is continually articulated, developed, and relinquished. In the passage used as the epigraph for this chapter, Nietzsche uses the building of sandcastles as a metaphor for the dialectic he envisions as the underlying structure of life and the essence of the tragic.

Picture the beach at low tide. Three different approaches are possible. The Apollonian man builds elaborate sandcastles, throwing himself into his activity as if his creations would last forever, totally oblivious to the incoming tide which will demolish his productions. Here is someone who ignores reality and is therefore continually surprised, battered, and bruised by it. The Dionysian man sees the inevitability of the leveling tide and therefore builds no castles. His constant preoccupation with the ephemeral nature of his life and his creations allows him no psychic space in which to live and play. He will only build if his productions are assured of immortality, but unlike the Apollonian man, he suffers no delusions in this regard. Here is someone tyrannized and depleted by reality.

The third option is Nietzsche's tragic man, aware of the tide and the transitory nature of his productions, yet building his sandcastles nevertheless. The inevitable limitations of reality do not dim the passion with which he builds his castles; in fact, the inexorable realities add a poignancy and sweetness to his passion. The tragicomic play in which our third man builds, Nietzsche suggests, is the richest form of life, generating the deepest meaning from the dialectical interplay of illusion and reality.

The very word "illusion," Loewald (1974, p. 354) reminds us, derives from the Latin *ludere*, to play. *Healthy* narcissism reflects Nietzsche's subtle dialectical balance between illusions and reality; illusions concerning oneself and others are generated, playfully enjoyed, and relinquished in the face of disappointments. New illusions are continually created and dissolved. Winnicott (1971) has described the important connections between healthy illusion, play, creativity, and cultural phenomena in general.

In *pathological* narcissism, on the other hand, illusions are taken too seriously, insisted upon. In some narcissistic disturbances, illusions are actively and consciously maintained; reality is sacrificed in order to perpetuate an addictive devotion to self-ennobling, idealizing, or symbiotic fictions. This is the approach of the first man on the beach, blindly building and building. In some narcissistic disturbances, illusions are harbored secretly or repressed; preoccupation with the limitations and risks of reality lead to an absence of joyfulness or liveliness—even a paralysis. Any activity is threatening because it inevitably encounters limitations, and these are felt to be unacceptable. This is the approach of the second man on the beach, holding out for immortality and waiting in despair for the tide.

What is the etiology of such disturbances? What determines whether one will be able to negotiate the delicate balance between illusions and reality in healthy narcissism, or whether one will suffer an addictive devotion to illusions resulting in either a removal from reality or a despair in the face of it? The key factor resides in the interplay of illusions and reality in the character-forming relationships with significant others. What is crucial, therefore, is the interactive function of illusions within the analysand's relational matrix.

The growth of the balance necessary for healthy narcissism requires a particular sort of relationship with a parent, in which the parent is able to comfortably experience both the child and herself in both modes, in playful illusions of grandiosity, idealization, and fusion, and in deflating disappointments and realistic limitations. The child naturally and playfully generates lofty self-overvaluations, glowing overvaluations of the parent, and boundaryless experiences of sameness and fusion. The ideal parental response to these experiences consists in a participation coupled with the capacity to disengage, a capacity to enjoy and play with the child's illusions, to add illusions of his or her own, and to let the illusions go, experiencing the child and herself in more realistic terms. Thus, the parent participates with the child in requisite experiences characterized by shifting idealization and aggrandizements—now the child is elevated, now the parent, now both together. The ideal parental response is neither a total immersion in illusion nor a cynical rationalism, but a capacity to play with illusions while never losing sight of the fact that this *is* a form of play.

Consider the position of the child in relation to a parent who, in one way or another, takes these kinds of illusions extremely seriously, whose own sense of security in fact is contingent upon them. Such a parent insists on specific overvaluations* of the child or herself or both. These illusions have become addictive for the parent, and they become a dominant feature in the possibilities for relatedness which such a parent offers the child. The more addictive the illusions for the parent, the more unavoidable they become for the child, who feels that the only way to connect with the parent, to be engaged with him, is to participate in his illusions. Such a child must regard himself as perfect and extraordinary and be seen by the parent that way, to be seen at all; or he must worship the parent as perfect and extraordinary to become real and important to the parent. Further, children tend to pick up how crucial such illusions are for the parent's shaky sense of self-esteem. Deutsch (1937) long ago noted the role of parental "induction" in cases of "folie à deux," where adoption by the child of the parent's delusion represents "an important part of an attempt to rescue the object through identification with it, or its delusional system" (p. 247). Abandonment of parental illusions thus becomes an emotional equivalent of abandonment of the parents themselves, the avoidance of which, as M. Friedman (1985) has argued, is an underlying feature in many forms of psychopathology.

In such circumstances, sustaining parental illusions becomes the basis for stability and for maintaining connections with others, the vehicle for what Fairbairn repeatedly terms the "tie to bad objects," or what Robbins (1982) more recently has described as pathological efforts at symbiotic bonding. Here illusions are no longer the spontaneously generated, transitory, playful creation of an active mind. Illusions are insisted upon with utmost seriousness by significant others, and they become the necessary price for contact and relation. Ogden (1982) speaks of

> the pressure on an infant to behave in a manner congruent with the mother's pathology, and the ever-present threat that if the infant fails to comply, he would cease to exist for the mother. This threat is the muscle behind the demand for compliance: "If you are not what I need you to be, you don't exist for me." Or in other language, "I can see in you only what I put there. If I don't see that, I see nothing." (p. 16)

This is true not just of infancy, but throughout childhood and later into adulthood. Every analyst is familiar with the dread adult patients

---

* The term "overvaluation" here does not imply some fixed, objective reality against which illusions are measured, but rather a flexible, consensual reality embracing the perceptions and valuations of others.

frequently feel in connection with major characterological change; they anticipate a profound sense of isolation from parents (alive or dead) who related to them, seemed to need so much to relate to them, only through their now-loosened and about-to-be-transcended character pathology (see Searles, 1958).

Thus, addictive parental illusions generate learned modes of contact in the child who will come to develop narcissistic difficulties, modes of contact which are felt to be the only alternative to the impossible option of no contact at all. The more addictive the illusion for the parent, the more unable is the parent to experience the child in any other way; the child necessarily cuts himself off from sources of spontaneously generated fantasies and illusions, and the child's personality becomes brittle, precariously anchored around rigid parental illusions. If the parent is not able to play at illusion building and relinquishment, to offer a full and variegated emotional presence to the child, the latter participates in what *is* provided, and these forms of participation become the learned basis for all future interpersonal relations.

The parent who is mindful only of the incoming tide, who cannot tolerate any play with the child's spontaneously generated fantasies and illusions out of fear or morbid addiction to despair, poses a closely related set of difficulties for the child. Illusions are seen as dangerous, hopefulness and joy as pernicious betrayal of the parent whose sense of security (and, perhaps, specialness) resides in a wooden clinging to a pale and joyless "reality." Here any sense of joy and playfulness in illusion making is deeply repressed and its emergence in the analysis is often accompanied by intense anxiety, shame, or fear of total interpersonal isolation.

THE MYTHOLOGICAL figure of Icarus vividly captures the powerful relationship between the child and the parent's illusions. Daedalus, the builder of the Labyrinth, constructs wings of feathers and wax, so that he and his son Icarus can escape their island prison. The use of such wings requires a true sense of Nietzsche's dialectical balance: flying too high risks a melting of the wings by the sun; flying too low risks a weighing down of the wings from the dampness of the ocean. Icarus does not heed the warning he receives. He flies too close to the sun; his wings melt, and he plunges into the ocean, disappearing beneath a clump of floating feathers.

We have all been born of imperfect parents, with favorite illusions about themselves and their progeny buoying their self-esteem, cherished along a continuum ending with addiction to illusion. We have all come to know ourselves through participation in parental illusions, which have become our own. Like Icarus, therefore, we have all donned Daedalus' wings. It is the subtleties of parental involvement with these illusions which greatly influence the nature of the flight provided by those wings—whether one can fly high enough to enjoy them and truly soar, or whether the sense of ponderous necessity concerning the illusions leads one to fly too high or to never leave the ground.

The myth of Icarus points to another significant feature of generational interaction in the subtleties of narcissistic illusion. In most accounts Daedalus is portrayed as a caring father, at least in his warnings to Icarus to fly neither too high nor too low, and Daedalus himself is able to negotiate a successful flight to safety. Children of illustrious parents are particularly prone to narcissistic difficulties. With parents of distinction of one sort or another, it takes particular sensitivity to be able to help a child sort through and digest parental identifications to generate illusions and ambitions of his or her own.

In both prior approaches to narcissism, pathological grandiosity and pathological idealization are understood largely as forces operating within the internal psychic economy of the individual. They are viewed as internally generated phenomena, either as defensive solutions to anxiety, frustration, and envy, or as spontaneously arising, pristine, early developmental needs. The developmental-arrest approach suffers from this constraint just as much as the more traditional approach. Illusion is treated not as a normal product of mental activity throughout the life cycle, but is located within the earliest developmental phases. And illusions within the psychoanalytic situation are treated as reflective of the early developmental needs, in pure form, rather than as learned modes of connection with others, as the not-at-all-playful, stereotyped, compulsive patterns of integration they have become.

Ever since Freud's abandonment of the theory of infantile seduction, the legacy of drive theory for the subsequent history of psychoanalytic ideas has included an underemphasis of the role of *actual* relationships in the evolution of mental structures and content, and of the residues of actual interactions in fantasied object ties. With respect to narcissism, both traditions isolate the figure within the relational tapestry. In so doing, they overlook the extent to which grandiosity and idealization function as interactional modes, arising as learned patterns of integrating relationships, and maintained as the vehicle for intimate connections (real and imagined) with others. They focus on one dimension of the relational matrix, the self, but not on the self with others; to regard these phenomena solely in terms of self-organization is like working with only half the pieces of a jigsaw puzzle.

The major theorists we have been considering do not completely fail to notice these interactional facets of narcissistic phenomena. They are too astute as clinicians to do so. The problem is that the specifics of parental character and fantasied object ties do not fit into theoretical models emphasizing what are taken to be spontaneously arising, developmental phenomena, so they are noticed clinically and then passed over when major etiological dynamics are assigned or technical approaches developed. The subtleties of the parents' personalities, the ways in which they required the child to maintain narcissistic illusions, are lost; the parents are viewed in a binary fashion, either as gratifying or not gratifying infantile needs (drives or relational).

Freud's paper "On Narcissism," for example, contains a wry and incisive description of parents' narcissistic investment in their children:

> If we look at the attitude of affectionate parents towards their children, we have to recognize that it is a revival and reproduction of their own narcissism, which they have long since abandoned . . . They are under a compulsion to ascribe every perfection to the child—which sober observation would find no occasion to do—and to conceal and forget all his shortcomings . . . They are inclined to suspend in the child's favor the operation of all the cultural acquisitions which their own narcissism has been forced to respect, and to renew on his behalf the claims to privileges which were long ago given up by themselves . . . The child shall fulfill those wishful dreams of the parents which they never carried out—the boy shall become a great man and a hero in his father's place, and the girl shall marry a prince as a tardy compensation for her mother. At the most touchy point in the narcissistic system, the immortality of the ego, which is so hard pressed by reality, security is achieved by taking refuge in the child. Parental love, which is so moving and at bottom so childish, is nothing but the parents' narcissism born again. (1914b, pp. 90–91)

Freud calls our attention to the striking similarity between the parents' attitude toward the child and the child's attitude toward himself. The parent overvalues the child; the child overvalues himself. Freud does not, however, derive the child's narcissism from the parents' attitude! He points to the parents' often-compulsive need to use the child as a magic solution for their own limitations and disappointments. Yet he does not consider how such a set of parental expectations and needs might contribute to the child's sense of who he is and who he needs to be for others. Although parental values, internalized in the ego ideal, become important later on in recapturing the primary narcissistic experience, Freud derives infantile narcissism from the inherent properties of self-directed libido. Infantile grandiosity is an instinctual vicissitude; self-love generates narcissism, apart from the relational matrix. In effect, Freud derives the parents' narcissism from the child's, their *own* unresolved infantile narcissistic longings and the opportunity provided by their child's infantile narcissism to evoke their own. In viewing narcissism as a quality inherent in self-directed libido, Freud underplays the extent to which parental fantasies influence the child's sense of who he is and has to be for the parents. Infantile experience shapes adult character, and adult character through parenting shapes infantile experience, in a continually evolving generational cycle within the relational matrix.

Kernberg similarly provides a vivid portrait of parental narcissism at work in the dynamic interactions within families producing children with later narcissistic difficulties.

> Their histories reveal that each patient possessed some inherent quality which could have objectively aroused the envy or admiration of others. For example, unusual physical attractiveness or some special talent became a refuge against the basic feelings of being unloved and of being the objects of revengeful hatred. Sometimes it was rather the cold hostile mother's narcissistic use of the child which made him "special," set him off on the road in a search for compensatory admiration and greatness, and fostered the characterological defense of spiteful devaluation of others. For example, two patients were used by their mothers as a kind of "object of art," being dressed up and exposed to public admiration in an almost grotesque way, so that fantasies of power and greatness linked with exhibitionistic trends became central in their compensatory efforts against oral rage and envy. These patients often occupy a pivotal point in their family structure, such as being the only child, or the only "brilliant" child, or the one who is supposed to fulfill the family aspirations. (1975, pp. 234–235)

How could a child growing up in such circumstances become anything but narcissistic? become visible to his parents in any form other than as an extraordinary, larger-than-life creature? Why the need to evoke a hypothetical excess of aggression (either constitutional or based on great deprivation in the earliest years) to account for what is more simply and clearly derivable from the relational matrix? Like Freud, Kernberg sees the clinical relevance of parental values and expectations, the constricted forms of relationships they offer to the child; yet this factor is assigned only a peripheral etiological role in shaping later defenses against early conflicts. Kernberg's model of mind, still drawing strongly on the monadic framework of drive theory, regards pathological narcissism as an internally generated mechanism, established in the first years of life in the face of extreme oral rage. The mother is important, not in the subtleties of her character and the particularities of the relational patterns she offers the child, but in her gross role as frustrator of the child's oral needs and as an object for the child's oral rage.

Kohut's clinical reports reflect a similar striking discordance between rich observations of parent-child interactions and a theoretical model of narcissism which assigns the particular content of these interactions to a secondary role. Kohut describes patients who exhibit various forms of grandiosity, some noisily proclaimed, others secretly and shamefully harbored. Kohut considers these to be manifestations of "archaic" grandiosity, which was not allowed to establish itself and undergo normal transmuting internalization because of the parents' failures as self-objects. Thus, his model derives narcissism from the expression of inherent sources. Yet, Kohut often informs us (usually parenthetically) that the parents failed the child in quite specific ways, using that child as a narcissistic extension of themselves in precisely the manner in which the child then constructs his grandiosity.

Within both traditions there has been movement toward granting greater etiological importance to parental character and the specifics of child-parent interactions. From the drive-theory side, Rothstein (1984) has placed increasing emphasis on the role of the actual relationship in the generation and maintenance of narcissistic illusion, and Robbins (1982) has written of the ways in which narcissistic phenomena operate as shared illusions, drawing on grandiose fantasies of idealized objects. From the relational-model side, there has been discussion of the parents, not simply in terms of their failure to provide self-object functions for the child, but also in terms of their use of the child as their own self-object (Atwood and Stolorow, 1984).

I HAVE suggested that in ideal parenting the parent participates with the child in a variable fashion that contains both joyful play with illusions and an affirming embrace of reality. Loewald has depicted the delicate interpenetrability between illusion and consensual reality that can develop from such interactions in a redefinition of the traditional concept of reality testing:

> Reality testing is far more than an intellectual or cognitive function. It may be understood more comprehensively as the experiential testing of fantasy—its potential and suitability for actualization—and the testing of actuality—its potential for encompassing it in, and penetrating it with, one's fantasy life. We deal with the task of a reciprocal transposition. (1974, p. 368)

How does the analyst help the analysand arrive at such a balance between illusion and reality, at the capacity to live in and fuse both realms? Loewald suggests that the analyst's interpretations and demeanor convey a subtle double quality which makes this possible. On the one hand, the analyst's descriptions and interpretations enable the patient to advance his access to his own subjectivity and inner resources. On the other hand,

> There may be at times, in addition, that other quality to the analyst's communications, difficult to describe, which mediates another dimension to the patient's experiences, raising them to a higher, more comprehensively human level of integration and validity while also signaling the transitory nature of human experience. (1974, p. 356)

In the next chapter we turn to this subtle dialectic between articulating and embracing the analysand's illusions, on the one hand, and the provision of a larger context in which they can be experienced, on the other.

If you are vain it is vain to sign your pictures and vain not to sign them. If you are not vain it is not vain to sign them and not vain not to sign them. —FAIRFIELD PORTER

8 A Delicate Balance: The Clinical Play of Illusion

Models attempting to illuminate the meaning and function of narcissistic phenomena necessarily imply a clinical posture by the analyst which best facilitates their resolution; therefore, theories of narcissism tend to appear complete with a recommended technical approach. Narcissism viewed as defense suggests an active, interpretive stance; narcissism viewed as an aborted form of infantile mental life suggests a warmly receptive stance. I have argued that narcissistic illusions are usefully understood neither solely as a defensive solution to an internal psychic threat, nor solely as a pure efflorescence of infantile mental life, but most fundamentally as a form of interaction, of participation with others. From this perspective, grandiosity and idealization sometimes serve defensive purposes and sometimes represent unfulfilled developmental needs; but when they recur in stereotyped form in the analytic situation, their central function is to serve as a gambit, an invitation to a particular form of interaction. What is most important clinically is, as Schwartz (1978, p. 8) has put it, "the 'petition' in the repetition."

Viewing narcissistic illusions as invitations casts the analyst's response in a different sort of perspective. The analysand requires some participation from the analyst to complete the old object tie, to connect with the analyst in a consciously or unconsciously desired fashion. If grandiosity is involved, some expression of admiration or appreciation may be requested, or at least attentive noninterference; if idealization is involved, some expression of pleasure at being adored may be requested, or at least acknowledgment of the analysand's devotion. Often participation in a mutually admiring relationship is requested—both the analyst and the analysand are to be considered truly distinguished, and alike in some unusual fashion. Responding to such an invitation in a way that is analytically constructive is tricky, and difficult to capture in a simple formula. What is most crucial frequently is not the words, but the tone in which they are spoken. The most useful response entails a subtle dialectic between joining the analysand in the narcissistic integration and simultaneously questioning the nature and purpose of that integration, both a playful participation in the analysand's illusions and a puzzled curiosity about how and why they came to be so serious, the sine qua non of the analysand's sense of security and involvement with others.

It is easiest to define the sort of analytic posture I have in mind by locating it between the kinds of recommended positions which have accompanied the major theoretical traditions.

In the classical tradition, narcissistic illusions are ferreted out and exposed to "objective" scrutiny. Such an aggressively interpretive approach (à la Kernberg) misses the *need* of the analysand to establish the narcissistic integration and runs the risk of discouraging the gambit and driving the transference underground. Grandiosity and idealization are efforts to reach the object through familiar, preferred modes of connection and intimacy. In Kernberg's discussion of these issues, for example, narcissistic configurations are understood as *defenses* against anxieties generated by oral aggression in early object relations, rather than as *expressions* of these object relations as entrenched familial patterns throughout childhood.

Kernberg speaks of the manner in which the "pathological grandiose self is utilized in the transference precisely to avoid the emergence of the dissociated, repressed or projected aspects of self and object representations of primitive object relations" (1984, p. 197). He does not consider the possibility that the emergence of the grandiose self within the transference is an effort to re-create actual familial object relations, to re-create early object ties. To interpret grandiosity and idealization simply as defenses risks encouraging resistances to the expression and establishment of these often conflictual and anxiety-filled, yet crucial transferential configurations. It promotes a compliance with what is likely to be experienced as the analyst's insistence on less narcissistic, more "real" perceptions and relations.

In the developmental-arrest tradition, drawing on the metaphor of the analysand as baby, narcissistic illusions in the adult patient are equated with the spontaneous exuberance of childhood, and necessarily encouraged. Such a receptive, unquestioning approach (like that of Winnicott and Kohut) misses the role of the narcissistic integrations in *perpetuating* old object ties, and runs the risk of consolidating them. Atwood and Stolorow, drawing on the self-psychology tradition, regard these narcissistic illusions as the product of the patient's effort "to establish in the analytic transference the requisite facilitating intersubjective context that had been absent or insufficient during the formative years and that now permitted the arrested developmental process to resume" (1984, p. 83). Here narcissistic illusions are reflected, encouraged (as a device for remobilizing a stalled developmental process), and presumed to dissolve of their own accord in the face of reality and the analyst's empathic understanding of the patient's naturally arising disappointments. Yet the analyst's failure to appreciate illusions as vehicles for *preserving* entrenched familial patterns is likely to be experienced by the analysand as the analyst's *own* investment in and encouragement of compulsive narcissistic illusions.

Because they regard narcissistic transferences solely as self-regulation, either in terms of defenses or in terms of the re-creation of infantile states, both prior traditions minimize the interactive complexity of the analyst's response. Both regard the transference as not fundamentally involved in interaction with the *person* of the analyst, so that the analyst can respond to its features from a somewhat detached position, either by challenging or by universally accepting. No attention is paid to the implications of the analyst's response for the analysand's sense of who the analyst is, what the analyst likes, needs, values, and what sort of relatedness is possible between them. A more purely interactive view regards the narcissistic transferences as strategies of engagement, efforts to connect with the person of the analyst according to paradigms of relatedness derived from the past. Such an approach places great importance on the implications of the analyst's response to the analysand's sense of who the analyst is and what can happen between them.

Why can the analyst not simply remain "neutral," neither demanding change nor encouraging perpetuation, but merely silent or descriptively interpretive? If one is invited to a dance, one either attends in some fashion or does not attend in some fashion. Remaining silent and refusing to respond constitute powerful responses and are experienced by the analysand as responses. It is striking in this regard that both Kohut and Kernberg consider their own approach to be neutral, and that of the other to be a departure from neutrality. In my view, each is right about the other, but misses the extent to which his own posture is a form of participation and is inevitably experienced in that way by the analysand. (See Black, 1987, for a discussion of the transferential implications of all technical stances.) As the popular saying goes, "You pay your money and you take your choice."

The most constructive form of analytic participation derives from the discovery of a path between the contrasting dangers of complicity and challenge, a path that reflects a willingness to play, an acceptance of the importance of the narcissistic integration as a special and favored mode of relation, yet also a questioning of why this must be the only way. This posture is similar to the kind of ideal parental response to the child's illusions described in the previous chapter. The parent is receptive to the child's illusions about himself and the parent, but maintains a light touch, conveying a sense of pleasure without the pressure of necessity. The analyst's response to the analysand's transferential gambits should reflect that same openness to playful participation. An ability to play together, including a participation in each other's illusions, is a crucial dimension not only of adult-child relations, but of adult-adult relations as well.

It is not possible to adopt such an analytic posture with any patient at the start and hold it all the way through the analysis. The analyst becomes embroiled in the illusions of each patient, as they manifest themselves in the transferential pushes and pulls. They inevitably arouse conflictual feelings in the analyst about his own narcissistic illusions, and he finds himself sometimes getting too much pleasure out of the patient's attributions, sometimes feeling the need to stop them, sometimes alternatively indulging them and subtly attacking them. The analytic stance I am describing is not a self-conscious posturing, but the result of continually working through narcissistic conflicts in the countertransference to allow for a true spirit of curiosity in the analyst's inquiry into the meaning of the analysand's illusions. Where did the analysand learn this particular pattern of relatedness? What was riding on these illusory notions within the analysand's early significant relations with others?

What were its pleasures? Its costs? The latter question is particularly important.

Analysands who integrate relations with others around grandiose claims tend to believe passionately that this is the best sort of relationship to have. They seek out admirers and discard as uninteresting those who are not admirers. (Analysands who harbor secret grandiose claims believe just as passionately that being the object of devoted admiration is the acme of interpersonal satisfaction, but fear they will never be successful in attaining this goal.) The analytic inquiry into these phenomena opens up important questions. How did this asymmetrical form of relatedness become so highly treasured? One frequently discovers that it was the vehicle for the closest bonds within the family, or for shared familial fantasies about how closer bonds might be achieved. Does the analysand assume that the passion of parental investment in overvaluing him is the most intense sort of connection he can hope for with others? The analysand is generally unaware of what is lost in such asymmetry, that relationships structured around others' admiration of and devotion to him preclude his excitement about and enjoyment of them, his opportunity to take pleasure in them not simply as reflectors of his own glory, but as different, interesting, and admirable in their own right.

It is vital that the analytic inquiry into grandiose illusions and relationships, and what the analysand believes, notices, and does not notice about them, avoid a moralistic tone. Relationships structured around grandiosity are problematic because they truncate the analysand's experience, not because they are unfair or unseemly. The focus should be on what is gained and what is missing in these relationships, and the analysand's limited awareness of both. The analyst's capacity to explore these issues constructively with the analysand is contingent upon an appreciation of this central point. The danger is that the analyst secretly or unconsciously believes that entitlement and grandiose claims are in fact a precious and preferred way of life. This leads either to a more or less subtly conveyed insistence that the patient renounce his claims, motivated by the analyst's envy ("if I can't have this, you certainly can't"), or to a vicarious enjoyment in allowing the analysand an envied and forbidden pleasure denied to himself ("I'm too 'mature' to indulge myself in this precious entitlement, but I can grant it to you").

The analyst's overidentification with the analysand's grandiose claims represents a failure to appreciate how much these claims undermine and sour the analysand's involvements with other people and isolate him in a confusing and often paranoid fashion. The analysand may come to feel more and more that only his analyst is really "sensitive" to him. An additional danger in working with this sort of transference is that the analyst's own conflictual longings to idealize may come to play a role in his admiration of the analysand. This can lead to the analyst's own investment in the analysand's grandiosity and difficulty in allowing him to move past this integration, or to anxiety in the face of the analysand's grandiosity and interference with the unfolding of this narcissistic integration.

ANALYSANDS WHO integrate relations around idealizing others also tend to believe passionately that this is the best sort of relationship to have. Life is seen as extremely complicated and perilous. The easiest and safest strategy for living is to find someone who seems to be secure and successful, who has all the answers, and to apprentice oneself to that person. For the price of considerable devotion, the idealized object will take the disciple under his wing, protecting him, leading him, guiding him along the path they have already cut through the obstacles of life. Analysands who integrate relationships on this basis are convinced that such an idealized bond is a very precious, very special tie. Sullivan would ask of patients idealizing the analyst, "Can they afford it?" It is precisely the cost of idealization which the analysand does not notice.

Feuerbach, the nineteenth-century German philosopher, argued that religion is, by its nature, a form of human self-alienation, that the characteristics and powers attributed to "God" in any religion are inevitably a reflection of human resources which the inhabitants of that culture are frightened to own. God becomes a screen on which are projected dissociated aspects of the self.

Although this is a highly oversimplified account of religion, idealization in human relations does often reflect such a masochistic, projective process. Because of disturbed earlier relationships, there is a terror of individuation and self-development. The analysand fears that finding his own path means isolation, a fear often originating in the context of relationships with parents who demand adoration and deference as the price of involvement. For such an analysand, the only way to ensure human contact is to find someone to go first, to remain always in someone's shadow. The presumption is that all others are as brittle and demanding of deference as the parents, as frightened of the analysand's self-development. They fear that to emerge from the shadow of the parent or the analyst is to lose the parent or analyst. Such an analysand generally fails to appreciate how much mental effort he expends in propping up others, convincing himself that the other is always more advanced along whatever line he himself is pursuing. Despite recurring inevitable disappointments, the analysand does not grasp that life is too idiosyncratic for anyone else's solutions to be a helpful shortcut to reaching his own.

Idealization frequently functions as part of a self-perpetuating cycle, generating the anxiety it then serves to assuage. The idealizing analysand often makes the analyst's interpretations into aphorisms, highly prized possessions which are granted a significance far beyond their actual substance or utility. Rather than working at or digesting the interpretation, the analysand keeps it at a distance, a gift from the idealized analyst, and evokes it at points of anxiety. Preserving the link between the ideas and the analyst protects their magic function in times of doubt or confusion. It also prevents the analysand from transforming the ideas and making them his own. So the lack of self-esteem and confidence in one's own thinking is perpetually undermined by the idealization, which then creates a setting in which the magic from the idealized analyst serves as balm.

As with the analysis of grandiose illusions, the inquiry into idealizing illusions also must avoid a moralistic tone. The problem with idealization is not that it is "childish" (as Freud noted) but that, as an exclusive mode of relation, it strongly limits possibilities. Analysands who compulsively integrate relationships on an idealizing basis remain perpetual disciples and can never fully allow themselves to experience their own strengths and resources. Further, they often secretly harbor the suspicion that the object of their idealization is flawed and brittle, that a close look at the analyst's full humanity would ruin them both. A hazard in the analytic exploration of these issues is that the analyst may overidentify with the analysand's idealizing longings, secretly or unconsciously believing that being under the wing of (or sexually surrendering to) a bigger, more powerful figure is a preferred way of life. This may lead either to a subtly conveyed insistence that the analysand renounce his claims, because of the analyst's envy, or to a vicarious enjoyment in allowing the analysand a forbidden pleasure denied to himself. An additional danger is the analyst's possible overenjoyment of being the object of idealization, so that he has trouble releasing the analysand from the narcissistic integration (or his fear that he *will* enjoy being the object of idealization so much that he cannot allow the analysand this experience).

Analysands manifesting narcissistic transferences generally need to be joined in their self-admiration or idealization in order to feel involved, to feel that something important is happening. The analyst cannot feign this participation. It makes a huge difference to the analysand whether the analyst is genuinely admiring or is patronizing him, whether he is enjoying or is merely tolerating the analysand's admiration. Analysands suffering from rigid narcissistic patterns of integration tend to be extremely sensitive to the genuineness of the analyst's attitude toward them and toward himself. What is called for is not a forced assumption of some prescribed "analytic" demeanor, either "neutral" or "empathic," but a willingness to meet and engage the analysand on his own terms. The analyst has to be able to gradually broaden the repertoire of connections between himself and the analysand, to treat the narcissistic integration as an elective form of play to be enjoyed, rather than as a somber necessity.

The problem with transferential illusions is precisely that they are *not* playful (in the sense of Loewald and Winnicott). They have to be transformed from a desperate prerequisite for connection and security into an enrichment of other forms of engagement. What is called for is an active shift in relatedness on the part of the analyst. This takes time and pacing. The issue of timing is highly complex and determinable only within the complexities of each individual case. Bromberg (1983) has described a shifting "empathy-anxiety balance" as the context within which treatment takes place, and argues that for narcissistic patients the beginning of treatment must be weighted heavily on the side of empathy.

> For certain of these individuals more than others, analytic success depends upon being able to participate in an initial period of undefinable length, in which the analysis partially protects them from stark reality which they cannot integrate, while performing its broader function of mediating their transition to a more mature and differentiated level of self and object representation. (p. 378)

These analysands are apt to be extremely sensitive to the manner in which the analyst reacts to their illusions and gambits. The analytic posture I am describing conveys a willingness to participate as well as a curiosity about the constrictive limits which this form of participation allows. To return to the metaphor of the dance invitation, I do not propose going to the dance and complaining about the music, but enjoying the dance as offered, together with questioning the singularity of the style. How did it come about that the analysand learned no other steps? Why does the analysand believe that this is the only desirable dance there is? Most analysands need to feel that their own dance style is appreciated in order to be open to expanding their repertoire.

One of the great, generally unacknowledged truths about analytic technique is that it is developed on a trial-and-error basis, personally designed in the interaction with each individual analysand. With some analysands, one can question illusions right from the start; with others, this is not possible. There is no way to know beforehand. One tests out different approaches: puzzlement, teasing, probing, intellectual challenge, raised eyebrow (literally and figuratively), until one finds which among the analyst's many voices and positions enables that particular analysand to feel both joined and nudged toward deeper understanding.

Because clinical work with narcissistic illusions is so tailored and subtle, I shall in the remainder of this chapter discuss extended fragments from analyses illustrating the three major kinds of narcissistic illusions: grandiosity, mutual admiration (what Kohut terms "twinship"), and idealization. The purpose is to illustrate the manner in which self-organizations centering on narcissistic illusions concerning self or others have crucial functions in maintaining the analysand's relational matrix, by preserving characteristic patterns of interpersonal integrations and fantasied object ties. The fragments are in no way meant to represent comprehensive case histories. Many dimensions of the work are omitted, to highlight the various aspects I wish to examine. The clinical challenge in each case is how to engage the analysand in immersion in and emergence from narcissistic integrations.

The Company, C'est Moi

John, a man in his early fifties, sought treatment as part of a broader campaign of self-perfection. He was a filmmaker who had turned his passion for adventure and his considerable talent into a successful film company, the management of which had come to dominate his life. The company was nearly always in a state of chaos, which was both a reflection and a direct consequence of his own approach to living. John's willingness to take risks, combined with a considerable business acumen, had enabled him to create the basis for a highly successful operation. Yet his ambitions at any particular time constantly exceeded his resources. His new ventures and overextensions kept the organization on the brink of disaster, and it was often only through his persuasive charm that he was able to keep the company going. Further, none of the individuals he employed in the ever-expanding business were competent to do their job. He invariably hired young, inexperienced people who tended to be creative, idealistic, and devoted to him as a wise benefactor. The threat of calamitous employee mistakes required his continual supervision over all aspects of the company. Despite a series of dazzling successes, he lived in a state of perpetual apprehension and recurrent panic, because a new disaster inevitably seemed to appear just as he had sidestepped the last one. John entered treatment because of extended bouts of depression and anxiety; in part he was looking for help in perfecting his organizational and managerial skills so he would be able to oversee his business operations with greater composure.

The company was his entire life. Still, as we gradually came to understand, the company was really his vehicle for a greater vision and ambition. His view of the business world and of life in general embodied a recurrent dichotomy between stability, organization, and conformity on the one hand and artistic expressiveness, fluidity, and adventure on the other. As John began to give voice to his larger ambitions, he revealed a deep faith in his own ability to achieve a perfect balance between these two poles; the creation of such a balance in his company would result in a radically novel approach to business in general, in which expressiveness and organization would complement each other. This would encourage a larger revolution in business practices, and a more general cultural advance. As we explored these hopes, John would place himself among the great political and cultural figures of contemporary and past societies. He saw himself as a heroic, beleaguered Atlas in a world of incompetents. During business crises, he recalled, he often had repetitive fantasies of himself as Henry Kissinger, negotiating dramatic truces among warring parties, as well as dreams of being in plunging airplanes, grabbing the controls and executing heroic escapes.

John had considerable difficulty in his personal relations, maintaining them only with men and women who regarded him as a guru of one sort or another. He was enormously generous with money and advice, and took great pleasure in helping others along. Although he was available in the moment, his friends all "understood" that his availability could not be anticipated. He was extremely busy, constantly coming and going, and would turn up in their lives in dramatic and compelling fashion, only to disappear again shortly thereafter. He dated rarely, and seemed unbothered by the absence of sexuality in his life. Sex was too complicated and entangling, and his schedule was too unpredictable to plan ahead. His most prolonged relationship had been with a much younger woman whom he regarded as beautiful, full of potential, and fundamentally mishandled by her parents. He took her on as a project, luring her from the control of her overprotective parents and fashioning her, Pygmalion-like, according to his own vision. The relationship collapsed when she turned out to be quite troubled, as well as a recalcitrant student; her increasingly insistent and desperate demands on his time began interfering with his sense of freedom and adventure.

The transference was organized along similar lines. John would talk on and on about his business problems, the enervating lack of dependability of his employees, and the brilliance of his efforts to keep things afloat. He would gather advice from various sources, including self-help books, and regarded the analyst as the ultimate self-help resource and reference. He conveyed a sense of fascination with the contents of his own mind, which he would put on display, arranging and rearranging them for the analyst's appreciation.

Occasional feelings of loneliness would be expressed and quickly avoided by a return to his business worries and dramatic rescues. John and I came to understand that he feared he was unable to sustain any sort of personal relationship, particularly intimate involvement with a woman. He felt he was wonderful on first meeting, but in the long run would have trouble maintaining a level of charm and excitement sufficient to keep a woman interested. He was drawn to women who seemed accomplished and desirable, yet with whom he felt somehow flawed and inadequate. He felt safer in the company of younger, adoring women of high potential, yet he was afraid of their need for him. It became clear that although he felt tormented and enervated by the pressures and worries of his life, he feared that any slackening of the pace would result in emptiness and boredom. Life outside the fast lane would become unbearably tedious and humdrum, and he would lose all his appeal to others. John felt deeply flawed as a person, hovering always on the brink of depression; yet he thought his company was infinitely perfectible and operated as a kind of surrogate self, which he would continue to expand

and perfect. "The company doesn't get depressed or scared. I can always keep changing its public face, and keep changing the parts. When some people fall down, I can just replace them." We uncovered his belief that once his company was flawless and stable, he would be able to emerge as a person in his own right.

John's grandiosity served important defensive functions, the most central of which was its counterdepressive effect. Underneath the glitter, John's sense of living in the world of other people was extremely grim. He saw others as leading desolate lives, as slaves to conventionality, as desperately longing for someone to provide life and excitement for them. He saw himself as able to have a vitalizing, reparative impact on others—but only for a short time. Unable to sustain his counterdepressive efforts, his own depression would emerge and he would be revealed as empty, having nothing to offer, bitterly disappointing to others. The grandiose illusions operated as a powerful defense against this sense of bleakness and personal deficiency.

They also served important functions in the expression and control of aggression. John saw other people as generally worthless and unable to provide him with anything useful or interesting. He felt enraged at their mistakes, almost personally betrayed, as if they were simply demonstrating over and over how little he could count on them. Attributing elevated status to himself expressed his deep contempt for others; it also removed him from the threat of being in a position where he expected anything from anyone. Being uniquely competent and self-sufficient, he did not need to expose himself to vulnerability and rage, or to what he experienced as constant disappointment and betrayal.

Although the grandiose illusions had come to serve secondary defensive functions, their content derived from the structure of relationships within his family, particularly the manner in which he had come to embody his mother's hopes and ambitions. The maternal grandparents had been extremely industrious working-class people, immigrants of Mediterranean extraction, with great aspirations for social advancement. They had worked their way from rather humble conditions into a position which was, for a while, fairly affluent—although eventually a combination of bad business decisions and bad luck once again kept them from attaining the social standing they longed for. John's mother was the younger of two children. Her brother had become a highly successful and renowned lawyer, who occupied an almost mythical status within the family. Although financially well off (which pleased his parents greatly), the brother had chosen to devote himself largely to social causes and public-service projects. He was very much an individualist, had extensive and interesting hobbies, and traveled frequently to exotic places. His wife was a flamboyant and seemingly fascinating person, and their marriage was regarded by most family members as ideal.

John's mother adored her elder brother. Although she too was quite intelligent, much less had been expected of her by their parents, who were mostly concerned that she be taken care of materially. She had attended college briefly, then left to marry John's father, a steady but seemingly dull accountant whom her parents regarded as a "great catch." She worried a great deal about financial stability, at least partially in reaction to her parents' shifting fortunes and the diminished opportunities offered women at that time; her choice of a husband seems to have been dominated by that consideration. John, the firstborn, was followed by three sisters. The mother became very involved with John and one of his sisters, the brightest and most artistic of the children. The other two girls, quieter and more obviously troubled, receded into the background, where dwelt the father.

John's mother placed strong emphasis on nonconventionality and excitement. She saw her husband as hopelessly dull and compared him unfavorably to her brother, who was her model for the good life. She saw John as the heir apparent, not to his father's throne, but to his uncle's. John became his mother's companion in adventure, accompanied his aunt and uncle on their vacations, and developed a wide range of hobbies and exotic tastes, which drew him further into the orbit of his mother and her brother. John's mother gave him lessons in social skills and manners, worked with him to polish his diction and elocution, and even pressured him into cosmetic surgery to "improve" his appearance.

John's father came from an impoverished, Irish-immigrant background. His father had made a meager living. An elder brother led a religious, marginal existence, never managing to leave home or establish any sort of independent existence. A younger sister became a political radical and bohemian. The father was the steadiest of the family and supported the others both financially and emotionally. Having worked at menial jobs to put himself through school, he treasured his hard-earned status as a professional.

In the face of his wife's appropriation of their son, John's father silently and somewhat bitterly retreated. He developed an alliance with the two daughters who were abandoned in disappointment by the mother. The marriage was quite stormy at intervals, and the children were encouraged to take sides. John felt he was often forced to play the judge of his parents' competing claims. Because of their difficulties in reconciling their own differences, the two of them seemed to grant a precocious, Solomon-like wisdom to their son. The marriage eventually broke apart in an atmosphere of mutual hostility and distrust.

Throughout his childhood John felt different from his peers, whom he regarded as conventional and conformistic, yet not good enough to be accepted by the most desirable and popular, in comparison to whom he felt dull and humdrum. His sense of himself had consolidated around his mother's image of him, modeled on her own glittering vision of her brother. He took on positive significance for her only as a reflection of his uncle's brilliance, and his model in all relationships was the one between his uncle and mother, between an all-knowing, infinitely exciting guru and a worshipful disciple. On the other hand, his childhood had been suffused with the continual sense that he had failed his mother, that he never would live up to her ambitions for him, and that her preoccupation with refinement of his behavior and appearance reflected deep disappointment in him. In her sense of herself as compromised and damaged, she seemed to look to him as a vehicle of redemption and justification—which he, of course, could never manage. Success necessitated an escalation of demands, to keep alive the dynamic tension and her hope for a cure of her own depression (through him). The sense of failure also was connected to a secret identification with his father as mediocre and discarded.

The central technical problem in the analysis was the analyst's position vis-à-vis John's grandiosity. On the one hand, systematic interpretation of the defensive functions of the grandiosity, by itself, would probably have driven him out of treatment. His need to display himself and his talents was intense, and the transference was organized around these exhibitionistic needs. In John's view, the analyst was like the mother, needing and enjoying his display, and, in his humble efforts to analyze him, helping him to perfect himself. The analyst's genuine admiration of John's talents and pleasure in him was probably a prerequisite for the analysis to proceed. Merely to interpret the defensive aspects of his grandiosity would have been to miss the importance to him of integrating relationships on that basis, the *only* basis on which he believed he could connect with others. Failure to engage with him in this way would either have made the treatment uninteresting to him or necessitated a submissive, defeated withdrawal (modeled after the father).

On the other hand, allowing John's grandiose claims to stand at face value would not have provided any traction for analytic change. John had a deep conviction that others, including the analyst, led dull and empty lives and that they needed to feed on his vitality. One had the sense that his self-displays could have lasted for years, perhaps decades, that they were not so much opening up something new in him, but perpetuating something old. The analyst's unchallenging participation in this integration could only be experienced as a corroboration of John's belief that this is all that can happen between people: one displays and teaches; the other admires and absorbs.

What seemed most useful was a playful participation in and appreciation of John's grandiose claims, combined with an inquiry into their origins and functions. The analyst's gradually developing ability to enjoy him without needing to take so seriously the demands he placed upon himself, seemed to make it possible for John to begin to laugh at himself, an enormously important positive prognostic sign. Sympathizing with his despair at a business failure, while noting that what was at stake apparently was not just the business venture itself but his role in the evolutionary development of the species, proved useful, as did comparisons between his relation to his company and Louis XIV's relation to the state. We explored his expectations of instant and total rapture in the response of others to him, both within and outside the transference; the selectivity of what he attended to in other people and their response to him; and the alacrity with which he assumed the other to be disinterested and disappointed in him. Particularly startling to him was the analyst's pointing to how little satisfaction he actually expected and obtained in his relations with others. He had a deep conviction that winning appreciation of himself as guru was the ultimate in human affairs. He gradually came to see how much he was missing, and how embittered and angry he was about that lack.

The broader context of the work was an inquiry into the origins and functions of his grandiose claims and ambitions: how they came to be so crucial, how they functioned to preserve his tie to his mother, and his deep fear that to abandon these illusions as compulsive necessities would be to lose forever any possibility of his being important and exciting to anyone. The increasingly collaborative inquiry and jointly constructed interpretations, combined with a lighter, nonaddictive participation in his narcissistic illusions, transformed the analytic relationship into a different sort of integration, making it possible for John to operate increasingly outside his formerly characteristic narcissistic patterns. He learned to enjoy rather than be tormented by his prodigious talents, and to use his ambitions as goals and guidelines rather than as prerequisites to feeling good about himself.

Joined at the Hip

Lucy was a painter in her late twenties who had been in treatment on and off with different therapists for more than ten years. Although she felt vaguely "supported" by these prior therapies in her struggle against depression, she was uninvolved in a deep way in any of them. She had a sense of herself as being very different from other people, and had been unable to connect with her previous therapists. She had been in treatment with her current (female) analyst for eight months, and this time things were quite different. She felt very involved and had an intense sense of importance about what was taking place. The analyst also felt involved in the treatment; in fact, she felt considerable anxiety about what she experienced as overly intense countertransference feelings, which led her to seek consultation on the case.

Lucy was the eldest of five children. Her mother was a strikingly uneven woman, very strong and talented in some respects, yet enormously self-absorbed. The mother had been an adored only child and had a very close relationship with her own mother, who had come to live with the family when Lucy was quite young. The presence of the grandmother had created a breach between the parents, who became increasingly estranged. This apparently was not especially disturbing to Lucy's mother, whose most intense bond seemed to be with her mother. All three generations of women in the family were quite artistic in one way or another, and each was also odd and quirky in her own particular fashion; this was not only tolerated by all, but almost cultivated. The father increasingly removed himself from the family, eventually becoming an alcoholic. He had seemed most fond of Lucy and there was a real bond between them, although it was hard for Lucy to understand the basis for his favoring of her. Their interactions often had an ambiguously sexual quality, even though ritualized and formal.

After her husband's death and the departure of her children, Lucy's mother moved with her own mother into a small cabin in the woods. It was as if extraneous elements had been discarded and a perfect union once again established. Mother and grandmother would sometimes lie in different directions on the same sofa, like two kittens in the sun. The mother would languish about, dabbling in painting and poetry, surrounded by photographs of herself as a young girl, and lost in reverie.

Lucy had been a shy, dreamy, talented, and fearful child who spent a lot of time at home. She ended up marrying her high school boyfriend, a very outgoing young man who was totally devoted to her. They regarded each other as perfect complements: he dealt with the outside world in ways that she could not and arranged the material basis for their existence; she provided the emotional softness and richness he lacked and adorned their life with her rich imagination. She would paint at home, barely leaving the apartment for weeks on end, like a princess in a tower; he would return every evening to fill her in on life in the outside world and to share her exotic realms of fantasy. Her paintings were beautifully executed, but unfashionably representational studies of subjects with highly personal meanings. They seemed to be from another time, and analytic inquiry revealed associations between Lucy's paintings and her mother's dreamy reveries of her own younger days. To the analyst it seemed as if Lucy had become a character in her mother's fantasy life.

Lucy decided almost immediately on meeting her current analyst that the two of them were very much alike, and that conviction had come to dominate much of their work together. Having a very astute eye for detail, Lucy noticed myriad similarities in their tastes, values, and sensibilities. She became convinced that there was a strong, almost spiritual commonality between them. The analyst's interpretive statements frequently evoked a gasp of recognition in her, followed by an amazed "How did you know that?" She felt she had become a very special patient for the analyst because of their kindred spirits, and she searched diligently for clues indicating that this was in fact the case. Lucy became intensely curious about the details of the analyst's personal life. During her hours of solitude she would weave into fantasies of marvelous companionship those facets that she was able to glean. It became imperative to Lucy that the analyst experience their relationship in similar terms. She had decided, for example, that a particular color was the analyst's favorite; it became hers as well and took on significance as a symbol of their special bond. When the analyst wore that color, Lucy would be enormously pleased and comfortable; when the analyst wore a different color, Lucy would feel anxious and betrayed, as if the analyst were deliberately interfering in her well-being, disappointing her in an almost cruel way.

The analyst *did* regard Lucy as a special patient. She too sensed considerable similarity between them, regarding Lucy as, in some ways, a "preanalyzed" version of herself. On the one hand, this was gratifying. She admired Lucy, was flattered by the latter's appreciation of her, and felt a maternal pleasure in helping someone with whom she identified so strongly. On the other hand, she felt increasingly oppressed and trapped by the intensity of the transference and countertransference. She knew that some of the sense of similarity was contrived by Lucy, and that she was not quite as remarkably intuitive as Lucy wanted to think of her as being. Further, it was difficult to know how to respond to Lucy's curiosity, detective work, and confabulations. She knew supplying more details was not called for; yet the pressure Lucy felt to have her confirm their special bond seemed intense. She feared disappointing her, to the point of becoming self-conscious about deciding the color of her clothes on the morning of a session with Lucy. Would she wear the special color and confirm their pact, or wear something different and betray it? She felt increasingly that her hands were tied. The sense of special connection in the transference seemed "precious" for Lucy, both extremely important and especially brittle and delicate.

Early in the analysis Lucy reported dreams in which the analyst appeared—technicolor dreams, with a bright, panoramic quality about them.

> I am walking along the beach with you and my sisters—you and I are walking together—I take off my clothes and go into the water—you remain on the shore—I am frolicking with the fish—I catch a gorgeous blue fish and throw it to you. You catch it deftly. It all seems exquisite and wonderful.

This dream reflects something of the quality of perfect attunement that Lucy, and frequently the analyst, experienced in the transference-countertransference integration at the start of the treatment.

Lucy's experience of herself in relation to other people and to the analyst centered around an illusion of sameness. The only meaningful contact between herself and someone else was contingent upon the symbiotic fantasy that they were identical in some fundamental way, that their psychic content was almost interchangeable. Lucy's life was organized around a search for such relatedness; once she found something akin to it, she clung desperately.

As the analyst's first vacation approached, a second transferential configuration emerged, both in dreams and in fantasies. Lucy began portraying the analyst as "spare," someone who lives a lonely existence, empty of pleasure or joy. The month-long break in the treatment over the vacation proved very difficult for Lucy; she became anxious and regressed, feeling abandoned and somehow helpless. Upon the analyst's return, she reported the following dream.

> You were on vacation—the plan was that I was to follow. I wasn't exactly invited, but I knew you would want me to be there. I arrived at your vacation house. I was very excited. Then I discovered that you were in some kind of trouble, hurt somehow. I could hear or sense you screaming and crying. Then I realized that it was I who was hurt, not you. Then I realized that I was in an isolated place—I couldn't find you—there was no one around—no help. There was a shift in scene to a hospital. You were explaining to me in a very cool way that there was nothing you could do for me. It was a medical problem. You were a doctor in a white coat. You wanted the best for me, but removed yourself from my treatment.

It is clear from the material about the analyst's vacation and the dream following it that illusions of sameness served as a defense, warding off feelings of depression, emptiness, damage, and rejection. Lucy feared the alternative to the special bond of sameness to be a desolate lack of contact, in which she and the other would be face to face with their own pain and inability to reach each other. In that sense, the illusion of sameness was a narcissistic, counterdepressive defense to be interpreted.

We might also regard the illusion of sameness as an expression of a longing for symbiotic union which the mother, in her adhesive tie to her own mother, probably was unable to provide. The mother's eagerness to return to her own fusion with *her* mother made separating seem a precarious business, creating conflicts around the rapprochement crisis and leaving Lucy with a dread of differences and a longing for "oneness" (Silverman, Lachmann, and Milich, 1982). In that sense, the illusion of sameness appeared in the treatment through what Kohut (1971) terms a "twinship" transference, representing a missing developmental experience re-created in the treatment situation, an experience to be encouraged and slowly outgrown.

Both these dimensions of the narcissistic transference are important; as with John's grandiose claims, however, Lucy's illusion of sameness is fully grasped only in the context of the interactive fabric of her early relations with others. This was a family in which there seemed to be very little real involvement with others. Each of the family members was a strong and developed presence, and it was as if each granted to the others the right of self-absorption. Within this armada of ships passing in the night, Lucy seems to have been hungry for contact. The person most involved with her was her father—although the contact was episodic, puzzling, ambiguous, expressed more through rituals than intimacy. The most intense involvement within the family was that between mother and grandmother, and it was a fusion from which Lucy and everyone else was excluded. This relationship became the model for the ultimate form of human contact. Mutual absorption, an identity of values and attributes, the exclusion of others—these became the hallmarks of true intimacy. It was this form of relatedness which Lucy sought in the analytic relationship. When it was not possible to infer its presence, she remained uninvolved; when it was possible, she became intensely absorbed.

What can we say of the analyst's handling of this material? Should the defensive dimensions of this transference have been interpreted aggressively from the beginning? Did gratification in the countertransference lead to the creation of a countertherapeutic folie à deux? Or was the patient's experience of gratification with respect to the illusion of sameness an indication of potential for progress, a developmental growing edge, not to be interfered with in any way?

Lucy's illusion of sameness, consolidated in this transference-countertransference integration, was both essential for treatment to be joined and a retardant to growth that needed to be challenged in some fashion. Based on Lucy's earlier treatment history, it seems reasonable to conclude that the analyst's matching countertransference responses and her willingness to participate in and enjoy the patient's illusions were fortuitous. They made possible a deeper therapeutic engagement than would otherwise have been possible, one that would have been precluded also by early interpretation of the defensive functions of this configuration. Yet, since the illusion of sameness represented not simply potential new growth but also a re-creation of old object ties, allowing this narcissistic configuration to remain unchallenged threatened to become counterproductive.

The analyst began exploring the patient's early relationships as prototypes for the pursuit of identity with others. Simultaneously, she began raising questions about why the patient regarded this form of connection, which (after the patient had introduced the phrase) they referred to as being "joined at the hip," as the ultimate in human relations. She pointed out to Lucy how hard she worked to force an identity when differences might be interesting in their own right. At first, this line of inquiry was strongly resisted; Lucy felt as if the analyst were taking away from her something very precious, and her dreams of exhilarating activities in pure, rarefied mountain air would suddenly change to scenes of muddy, dried-up river basins. This shift was understood as reflecting the patient's fear that the only alternative to shared identity was the desolation she had experienced as a child, a loneliness that she feared was being re-created in the analyst's withdrawal.

Patient and analyst began to work collaboratively on appreciating how contrived many of the illusions of sameness were, based on what they came to call talismanic contact, expressed through rituals and magical signs. One by-product of this work was Lucy's reporting for the first time that she had secret areas of her experience withheld from both her analyst and her husband, the natural counterpart to the forced identity which had seemed to be the price of meaningful connection. Another by-product of this phase of the treatment was an increase in Lucy's freedom to pursue some of her own independent ambitions and activities.

Thus, the analyst's participation in, yet inquiry into, the narcissistic illusions of sameness generated in Lucy a growing awareness of her conflicts over relating through forced identity, and began to transform the analytic relationship into a form of connection more complex in structure and richer in possibilities.

From Good to Pseudoideal

In her discussion of various experiences and fantasies grouped under the developmental organization she terms the paranoid-schizoid position, Melanie Klein speaks variously of "good" objects, "ideal" objects, and "pseudoideal" objects. Although these concepts are not defined and distinguished from one another with much precision, they are all products of splitting, which Klein sees as the central defense mechanism of the earliest months of life, and can be arranged on a continuum of severity. Through splitting the infant keeps separate his good (pleasurable, loving) experiences with others from his bad (painful, hateful) experiences, in order to protect his libidinal relationships from the destructive impact of his aggression. Thus, the good object is a composite of all good experiences with others. The ideal object is the good object elaborated through fantasy, goodness granted magical powers to protect the child and ward off dangers.

But what if the child's experiences with others are nearly all painful and unpleasant—if, in the distribution of experiences, there is no material from which to construct a good or ideal object? Voltaire suggested that if God did not exist, it would be necessary to invent him. Similarly, Klein argues that the child cannot survive without some sense of connection to a loved and loving other, and that if the child does not *experience* the basis for such a relationship, he will imagine it. Thus, the pseudoideal object is not elaborated out of the child's experience, but is created whole cloth.

The distinctions among good, ideal, and pseudoideal objects provide a useful framework for thinking about different kinds of idealization within the transference. Some idealization is based on actual experience with the analyst—interpretations that have been helpful, for example. The illusory element in this sort of idealization is not in the creation of the good qualities or experiences, but in the care taken to prevent recognition and integration of other not-so-good qualities or experiences, such as interpretations that do not help much, or interpretations that feel hurtful. The patient experiences only the dimensions of the relationship with the analyst which he deems acceptable.

Other idealizing transferences are based on actual experiences with the analyst, but are elaborated in more or less fantastic ways. Here some good experience, some actual help, serves as the core around which are woven imaginative attributions of the range and depth of the analyst's powers, the idyllic richness of his personal life, the constancy and purity of his motives, and so on.

A third kind of pseudoidealizing transference is created whole cloth. Here what the analyst says or does seems to matter very little. The analyst's goodness and power are assumed and insisted upon, with scraps of evidence strung together to create the impression of a plausible image. On the pseudoidealizing end of the idealizing continuum, the analyst is likely to have the sometimes uncanny countertransferential experience of not recognizing himself at all in the analysand's experience of him.

*   *   *

DIANE, A YOUNG lawyer and politician, illustrates the workings of an *idealizing transference*.

The significant benchmarks in Diane's emotional development as an adult consisted in a series of intense, idealizing relationships with mentors of various sorts. Choosing men and women who seemed talented and successful at whatever endeavor Diane herself was interested in at the time, she would apprentice herself to them. A talented person in general, she was especially skilled and seductive in the art of discipleship. She was extremely successful at positioning herself beside, behind, and/or underneath (in different contexts, different prepositions apply) the other, whom she would admire, protect, and devote herself to. Analytic inquiry revealed the implicit contract she felt pertained in such relationships. She would place loyalty to her mentor above all else, admiring, defending, and publicly representing him or her as a talented and special disciple, in a way she felt would enhance the mentor's reputation and status. She would speak of the mentor as someone who had attained a lofty, invulnerable pinnacle of existence, with all questions answered, all rough edges smoothed, and no frailties, foibles, or other evidence to the contrary. The mentor in turn was expected to regard her as his special charge, be loyal to her above all others, protect her from the hardships of life, and guide her deftly in a direct, linear fashion to the accomplished, privileged, and invulnerable status he himself had (presumably) attained in life.

The relationships lasted for quite a while and were often mutually satisfying to the two participants, both within and outside the fantasied idealizing pact. Not surprisingly, Diane invariably suffered periods of painful disillusionment and betrayal. Either the adored object exposed clay feet, or he proved less steadfast than Diane. Following periods of intense, smoldering rage and despair, new models would be established. Although very attractive, Diane seemed more girlish than womanly; she had few intense romantic involvements.

Sources for the structure of this idealizing mode were found in Diane's relationships with both her parents, who saw themselves as special, admirable people; they were intensely competitive with each other for recognition in general and for Diane's loyalty in particular. The mother was an extremely tough, overburdened woman, who presented herself as a saintly victim of her husband's failings. She saw Diane as a secret ally who (unlike the father) was sensitive to her plight, yet who, as the father's favorite, could influence him in ways beneficial to herself.

As an older sibling, Diane felt deprived of the affection and nurturance the mother provided for her younger brother and sisters. Demeaning Diane's needs seemed to be in part the mother's way of assuaging her own guilt and despair at not being able to provide fully for everyone. The mother's most intense relationships were with her babies and with damaged relatives of various sorts whom she took care of. Diane could gain access to her only through sympathizing with her, admiring her devotion to others and to herself as a small child, and forgiving her guilt at not constantly providing for Diane as well. Their relationship seemed to center around a deep yearning in both for a perfect mother-infant synchrony.

Diane's father was an extremely volatile, paranoid man who kept his explosive rage and terror in check through an elaborately constructed obsessional devotion to fastidiousness and detail. As a young man, he had been a rather dashing figure, adventurous and successful in sports; but a series of injuries and career disasters left him shaken, somewhat bewildered, and extremely bitter. He had been very involved with Diane, his eldest daughter, especially when she was small. Diane adored her father and loved hearing stories of his bravery and exploits. She became an accomplished student of her father's perfectionism and certainty, a good soldier in her father's army. She believed she had earned his "chosen" status over her siblings, and felt protected and safe under her father's harsh but sure control. It was only as Diane grew older that she realized how fearful and temperamental her father was. There were many disappointments involving her father's refusal to join Diane in activities in the outside world, and frightening outbreaks of sadistic violence. He had enormous difficulty tolerating her accomplishments and would either demean them, claim credit for them, or both. Diane's disillusionment with her father was very gradual; she resisted it strongly. She was frightened at how crazy she feared her father was, but deeply loved the bond she felt as the favorite child of a noble and fearless man.

She developed a strong, conflictual counteridentification with the mother. On the one hand, she felt intense longings to join in what Diane viewed as her mother's masochistic, degraded status; on the other hand, her father was her model for operating effectively in the world. There were intense oedipal yearnings and a sense of herself as an oedipal victor. Surely she would be a better, more submissive, more appreciative wife to her father than her mother was. Furthermore, she felt herself to be like her father in many respects, explosive and rageful.

Although Diane chose a very different life course from either parent and had left the family in many fundamental respects, the structure of her relationship with her father was preserved into adulthood. When she visited, her father would bait her with his political and social prejudices in an effort to reclaim his place as the object of unquestioned loyalty. If Diane (predictably) differed with her father, he would up the ante, his taunts getting more and more bitter. Diane found herself agreeing with her father to "keep him under control." In many respects, she played a central role in the family, operating as a kind of double agent. Her father needed to see Diane as loyal to him, as the repository of his bruised hopes for respect and renewal. Her mother regarded Diane as *her* champion and as leverage with her husband, placating him and thereby enhancing his stability and keeping the family intact. Diane's divided loyalties, as she strove to be each parent's "daughter," made her later career in politics seem uncomplicated; life within the family was a tension-filled juggling act. We came to see that she had taken the common elements in both these relationships, connection through exclusive devotion and through submission, as the basis for her manner of integrating relationships with significant others in general.

The predominant features of the transference were organized around just these lines. The analyst was viewed as someone with ready answers to all of life's important questions, with a perfectly organized and disciplined personal existence. He was seen as demanding total devotion, in terms of solemn dedication to the analytic work and repeatedly expressed loyalty to him as a person. Diane did in fact work very hard, seemed to get a great deal out of the treatment, and tried to be a rewarding patient for the analyst. An early dream, several months into the analysis, provided the first evidence of the doubts Diane unconsciously harbored, an image of the analyst as omnipresent and omniscient.

> I was wandering through some kind of forest. I had to descend a cliff, and had to go very slow, as it was quite steep. It was hard to get a good grip, and I was frightened. I started slipping a little, but then got to a clearing. There were other people there. One was older and wiser. He said that to get down the slope, I'd have to be very careful about bears; sometimes they charge down the mountain. His advice was to take pillows to beat off the

bears. I followed the advice. Then I was beating at the bears frantically with the pillows. I was afraid I would be killed.

Associations to the bears uncovered fears concerning her father's explosive rages and terror of her own rages as well. Her hopes in analysis were for a better idealized father, one who would guide her along a course which would protect her from what she felt was her own bestiality (partially an identification with her experience of her father). It was extremely important to her to see the analyst as perfect and all knowing, as providing a safe route through the dense thicket of her own conflicts, diverse identifications, and divided loyalties. As the dream suggests, she harbored secret fears about the analyst's powers and dependability; the possibility that the analyst was not what he seemed to be provoked extreme anxiety and was difficult for her to sustain in conscious thought.

One of the central dimensions of the analysis entailed an articulation and gradual working through of this erotic-idealizing pattern of integration, both within and outside the transference. The analyst often was pleased and amused by, as well as curious about, the wondrous attributes with which Diane endowed him. It was these countertransferential feelings, combined and expressed in the analyst's participation, which helped to make it possible for Diane to consolidate a relationship with the analyst along necessarily idealizing lines as well as to gradually begin to question and transform that pattern of relating.

Racker (1968) makes the point that a crucial feature of exploration of the transference is inquiry into the patient's fantasies about the countertransference. This was very much the case with Diane. Devotion to the analyst seemed absolutely essential to her, not only because of the security and certainty it seemed to provide, but also because she secretly felt that it was the only sort of relationship the analyst was able to sustain. She was convinced that he, like all people, felt closest to another only when he saw the other as very much like himself, agreeing with all his opinions and prejudices. Differences would surely make the analyst anxious and self-doubting and would be experienced as hostile. Kindness would consist in unquestioning devotion.

Challenging and inquiring into these assumptions began to free Diane of them. She began to see that treating someone else as if they were God might not particularly enhance their self-esteem, and that she regarded other people as shallow, vulnerable, and brittle. She assumed that the analyst would feel he had nothing to offer her as a woman rather than as a baby or small girl. As these beliefs were explored and challenged, the relationship began to open up and become more complex.

If she was not being submissive, Diane feared, competitive feelings might emerge and the relationship would become "messy." There was considerable evidence in her dreams of a longing to dethrone the analyst and other pedestaled icons whom, during her waking life, she was so carefully protecting from herself and others. As she slowly became more competitive, she became aware of fears of retaliation: if you're strong, people "give it to you"; if you appear frightened and confused, kindness and consideration result. She realized how secretly powerful she had come to feel in her passivity, and how little she attended to her considerable prowess and resources as a woman. She both longed for and feared being overwhelmed—as she so often had been, as a child, by her father. Alternatively, she was terrified of how brittle her heroes seemed to be and how easily crushed they might be by her hidden strengths.

The analytic process itself was experienced in the context of this transferential configuration. There was an extraordinary desire to surrender to the analyst sexually and, in a more global way, to be made over according to the image of perfection attributed to the analyst. On the other hand, she deeply resented the submission she felt was demanded of her and struggled resistively against it. A dream midway through the analysis highlighted these issues:

> I had to go for immunization shots. I was very anxious about them, but various people kept telling me it was no big deal. When I got to the doctor's, I had to bend over to get the shots in my rear end. It was very bothersome, but I felt it was a concession I had to make. My primary concern was that they would hurt. The pain was a burning, one in each butt. As it was happening, I tried to concentrate. "It won't burn so much; it will be over quickly." It wasn't nearly so bad as I thought it would be.

The shots in the dream became a central metaphor in Diane's increasing awareness of how much she both desired and resented the (sexual) submission and incorporation she experienced in the analytic relationship. She was supposed to take in the analyst's ideas, look the other way, surrender totally. On the one hand, she felt this act would save her; on the other hand, she felt humiliated and enraged by it.

As these conflictual features of the transference were articulated and questioned, a deep fear of being abandoned and utterly alone emerged. Only gradually was Diane able to sustain a belief in the possibility of the analyst's liking and helping her as her own person rather than as a replica of the image she had fashioned out of the analyst's attributes and her idealizing elaborations of them. She began to realize how much effort was going into convincing herself that the analyst was already far down whatever road she herself was pursuing. She started thinking of admired others not as providing blueprints for living, but as resources to be used, digested, and selectively absorbed.

HENRY WAS born into the kind of familial circumstances which make pseudoidealization an emotional necessity for survival. He was the second of three children born to an extremely poor Jewish family on the lower east side of New York. The father was a remote, highly intellectual man who was only peripherally involved with the family. The mother was a hard-working, long-suffering woman whose experience seemed laced with psychotic terrors and compulsions. She was paralyzed by the outside world, which she experienced as treacherous and forbidding, and felt it necessary to control her children in bizarre and intrusive ways, including forced feedings and rigorous regimes of order and cleanliness. Her first son had been born severely damaged and had died in infancy. Henry's younger sister had become a compliant, seemingly perfect child, surrendering herself to the mother's ministrations. As an adult, this sister suffered from crippling inhibitions and a severely restricted life in close proximity to the mother.

Henry's life centered around an essentially fantastic relationship with his father. He neatly segregated his experience of his parents through splitting: his mother was wholly malevolent and dangerous; his father was benevolent and caring. Everything seemed to depend on being able to preserve this image of the father, which gave Henry at least some hope in an otherwise frightening existence. He portrayed the father to himself as someone extraordinarily wise and in tune with him. The father knew what his son was feeling and secretly joined him in hatred of the mother's oppressive regime. Yet the father knew that it was best for him to remain silent and not interfere. He was with Henry every step of the way, but their secret alliance would have to be denied, for Henry's own good, if he ever attempted to bring it out in the open.

Henry's fantasied bond with his father was mediated largely through the image of the dead elder brother. This loss had been extremely painful for the father and had probably contributed substantially to his withdrawal. He had pictured his eldest son as a renowned rabbi; the birth of the younger children did not begin to compensate for his loss. Henry became very interested in intellectual and religious pursuits; by becoming the father's image of the dead brother, he hoped to consolidate his own tie to his father. It was, ironically, the father's almost-total remoteness which made this fantasy possible. Henry filled in the space vacated by his father's emotional absence with what he needed to protect himself from his fear of and identification with the mother.

Henry was able to draw on his considerable talents and vitality to create a rich and diversified life for himself. Nevertheless, he suffered pervasive anxieties and inhibitions, which had brought him into treatment. He was married to an active, successful woman, in many respects the opposite of both his parents. He felt warm admiration for and dependency upon her, using her as a kind of executive function for any of his own wishes and ambitions in life. Relations with friends and colleagues were integrated along similar deferential lines. The transference was joined on this basis, characterized from the start by extreme idealization divorced from any actual experiences or benefits.

Two dreams, the first about a colleague, the second about his boss, both with clear allusions to the transference, illustrate both the benign and the masochistic dimensions of this type of idealization. The first dream occurred about six months into the treatment.

> I was in an art class with George. We were using special pencils. Every time I went to use mine, it kept breaking off in the sharpener. I began to panic. I couldn't complete the assignment. George walked up to me and showed me his pencil, which was perfect. He was teaching me how to use the sharpener, showing me what I was doing wrong.

This dream captures the hopefulness that is invariably a crucial feature of object ties characterized by idealization and pseudoidealization. By attaching to (and sexually submitting to) a perfect other, a new start is possible; the damaged self (expressed here through the castration imagery) is remediable.

The second dream, reported about a year later, reveals another facet of this sort of integration.

> Harry and I were with some other people in a construction area. We were trapped somehow. Harry figured how to get out. One by one people had to enter a wooden encasement. Harry would push them so they would swing in the encasement out to safety. I was waiting for him to push people

through. Then it was my turn. I got encased and then needed to be pushed through. As I was waiting, I heard Harry walk away. I realized he had forgotten to push me. I felt I would suffocate and started to panic. I told myself, "Don't panic, or you'll use up too much air." Then I awoke.

Once again, the father-boss-analyst is a larger-than-life figure; everything depends on utilizing his powers, on following his lead out of danger. Yet the dread of being let down, the total surrender necessary to be taken care of, the abject dependency required by the other (encased like the dead brother)—these are suffocating.

Both the benign and the masochistic facets of the idealization were prominent in this transference. The analyst and the analytic process were granted wonderful magical powers to heal and to show the way. The relative reticence of the analytic stance made it possible to attribute incredible wisdom to the analyst. His words were coyly sought, captured and savored with great enthusiasm, and transformed into formulas for living, like embroidered homilies hung on the wall. This search for something new and healing had much of the quality that Balint terms "the new beginning," and that Winnicott and Kohut stress in the handling of narcissistic illusions. Henry sought something different within the only framework he knew, through a re-creation of the object tie to the father. Self-abnegation, glorification of and deference to the other, were assumed to be the price of contact, the best way to use the help of another, to capture that person's attention, to sustain his or her interest.

In addition to its reparative features, Henry's idealization served important defensive purposes against his intense rage at the other for what he felt was the deference demanded; his doubts about the other's constancy, resources, and caring; his anxiety about his own capacities and autonomy. Whereas the idealization of his father was a powerful adaptive device during his childhood, saving him from terror and despair, idealization of his wife and the analyst in his adulthood kept him encased in a self-perpetuating cycle of constricted and truncated relations with others. The more he elevated the other as magic savior, the more damaged he felt; the more damaged he felt, the more apprenticeship to the magic savior seemed the only way out.

The most constructive response to Henry's idealizing transference encompassed both acknowledgment and joining of the "new beginning" aspect and questioning and interpretation of the defense aspect. To challenge his idealization vigorously and to interpret it prematurely only as a defense against rage or separation would have been to preclude a deep transferential engagement. Henry's search for a new start was mediated through the old object tie. To refuse to meet him there would have been to drive him out of treatment or into a compliant, superficial adaptation to the analyst's demands. Nonetheless, to avoid interpreting the masochistic and defensive aspects of his idealization would have been to condemn Henry to this and only this mode of integrating relationships with others. One could envision a prolonged, intense devotion to the analyst, helpful in many respects, but without the impetus for Henry to engage others, beginning with the analyst, in a more complex and mutual fashion.

VIEWING NARCISSISTIC illusions as defensive highlights their role in perpetuating internal equilibrium and constrictions in living. Viewing narcissistic illusions as growth enhancing highlights their potential role in enriching self-experience. The defensive and constructive features of narcissistic illusions are integrable; they both are considerably enriched when viewed in the context of a relational matrix, as interactive vehicles for attachments to significant others and as characteristic patterns of interpersonal integration.

In actuality, the analytic relationship is two highly conflictual, simultaneous relationships which continually interpenetrate each other—a neurotic, constricted form of integration (Loewald's "old" object; Fairbairn's "bad" object) that dissolves over time, and a healthier form of integration (Loewald's "new" object; Fairbairn's "good" object) that is slowly opened up and consolidated. The analyst's participation in the analysand's illusions is essential to establishment of the narcissistic integration; the analyst's questioning of illusions is essential to the dissolution of this integration and the establishment of a richer form of relation.

The analyst's descriptions, interpretations, and questions all provide the analysand with a form of participation which operates outside the narcissistic integration. What is provided in this sort of interaction is not an opportunity for the analysand to renounce illusions, but to experience them in a broader context—not as constrictive limits on his relations with others, but as possible forms of enriching interactions. The analyst's own ease in engaging and disengaging in illusions about himself and others is crucial to this process. One might think of it in terms of the analysand's learning or internalizing a kind of "love of life," sustainable without illusions yet continually enriched by them.

Part Five

Continuity and Change

W E HAVE explored the implications of an integrated relational model for several major realms of psychoanalytic theory and technique: sexuality, the traditional province of drive theory; early childhood, the natural focus of developmental-arrest theories; and narcissism, the study of illusion and its relation to self-regard, that crossroad of all currents in contemporary psychoanalytic thought. We conclude with an examination of the most central clinical problems for all practicing clinicians and analytic theorists: Why is it that people perpetuate their psychopathological misery with such consistency? and How does the psychoanalytic process make it possible for them to change?

The first question confronts us directly with the issue of the will or agency, which has shadowed psychodynamic thinking throughout its history, a nagging concern difficult to reconcile with concepts like psychodynamic conflict and repression, yet at the same time impossible to dismiss. In Chapter 9 I identify the will in its key role of preserving the commitments and loyalties of the relational matrix. Then, in the final chapter, I turn to the complex question of the "therapeutic action" of psychoanalysis, the nature of analytic change, to consider how the commitments and loyalties within a constricted relational matrix can open and be enriched through analytic engagement.

Life can only be understood backwards; but it must be lived forwards.

—KIERKEGAARD

9   The Problem of the Will

From its inception psychoanalysis has been plagued by the problem of the will. In one sense, the content of the mind (both normal and pathological) seems to be a *causal product,* shaped by past events, constitutional givens, and current influences. In another sense, the content of the mind seems to be *chosen,* reflecting firm convictions and deep commitments (both conscious and unconscious). How can these two ways of thinking about the mind be reconciled? Is human thought part of a causal chain or is it self-initiating and freely generated?

Freud's early work, following Charcot's lead, demonstrated the poverty of the Victorian concept of "willpower"—the belief that mind consists only in that which is conscious and that the contents of consciousness are controllable by sheer mental forcefulness. Charcot, and later Freud, demonstrated that the hysteric is not a willful malingerer, but the victim of mental processes out of awareness. Conscious thought is merely the tip of the iceberg, Freud argued: the vast majority of mental activity is neither known by nor accessible to consciousness. The choice and control we *seem* to exercise over our conscious mental lives is an illusion, a post hoc rationalization; the real control over mental events lies in unknown and often unknowable psychodynamic forces. All mental events, Freud claimed, are psychically determined.

Yet in characterizing unconscious mental processes, Freud continually employs language which suggests intent, purpose, design. He uses

239

the term "counter-will" (1892a, p. 122) to describe the workings of conflictual motives, and his discussions of "resistances" within analysis draw on military metaphors and clearly suggest active and elaborate sabotage. Freud points to the ultimate responsibility of the dreamer for the dream: "Obviously one must hold oneself responsible for the evil impulses of one's dreams. What else is one to do with them? Unless the content of the dream (rightly understood) is inspired by alien spirits, it is a part of my own being" (1925, p. 133). Further, Freud views the psychoanalytic process as providing an expansion and strengthening of the ego, an extension of the freedom and control which the analysand is able to exercise over his life. The goal of psychoanalysis, Freud suggests, is "to give the patient's ego *freedom* to decide one way or the other" (1923, p. 50n). Thus, the "ego," as a part of the person, or a subset of his or her functions and activities, is designated as the seat of choice and will.

These clinical references to the role of active choice seem particularly difficult to reconcile with Freud's metapsychological vision of the mind as an elaborate apparatus driven by forces and mechanisms in complex quantitative relation to one another. They are also difficult to reconcile with Freud's principle of psychic determinism—each mental event is caused by the mental events and stimuli immediately preceding it. Psychodynamic motivation, according to the principle of psychic determinism, is causally closed. Within this framework the person never generates his or her own causal impact on the sequence of mental events; will and choice have no status. Freud depicts human experience as driven by forces largely unknown, a direct and unwitting product of internal pressures and compromises. Paradoxically, Freud discredits the Victorian concept of willpower, while portraying the mind as a collection of powerful willful designs and intentions; he establishes the principle of psychic determinism, while offering a treatment whose goal is the enhancement of options and responsibility.

The contradictions within Freud's approach to the question of the will are also mirrored within the "classical" literature on analytic technique. Some authors, in some places, stress the patient's assumption of responsibility for his experience and conduct as a prerequisite to analytic cure. Fenichel, for example, emphasizes repeatedly the operation of the "filter of the defensive ego," which strips the patient's experience of his own active wishes and intentions. "I tried to make it clear that . . .

he [the patient] should search within himself and see that this not-having-feelings was really a wish-not-to-have-feelings actually put into play by himself" (1941, p. 7). Fenichel speaks of restoring "ownership" to the ego, and of the importance of the "demonstration of the patient's own responsibility in bringing about experiences that seem merely to happen to him" (pp. 35–36).

On the other hand, the literature is replete with reaffirmations of the principle of psychic determinism, and the dangers of regarding the patient as the creator of his own experience and conduct.

> When we stand back from analysis we can visualize the defensive function of resistance; but when we are actually engaged in analysis the outstanding fact is that the patient's own personality is the mouth-piece through which these defenses are expressed. In short, the general impression given is that the patient is *personally* resisting, instead of being the tool of his unconscious mechanisms and conflicts. (Glover, 1955, p. 80)

The analysand is characterized sometimes as the responsible agent of his actions, and sometimes as the tool and mouthpiece of forces beyond his control.

The Existential Critique and Psychoanalytic Responses

The doctrine of psychic determinism has been the target of a tradition of criticism and subsequent defense of classical psychoanalytic theory that is almost as old as psychoanalytic theory itself. Critics of psychoanalysis, particularly from within the traditions of existential philosophy and existential psychology, have argued that psychoanalytic theory portrays man in a mechanized, dehumanized fashion, as the passive victim of forces beyond his control. Sartre presents the most radical criticism, and our consideration of his position will highlight the basic issues in the debate over this complex problem.

In his early (pre-Marxist), purely existential writings, Sartre argued that the human mind has *no* intrinsic content, no human essence—nothing is given. Being is instead a process, a temporal phenomenon, a consciousness which continually creates and re-creates itself. Because the mind is empty and continually self generating, being hovers always on the brink of nothingness. Because being a person, in Sartre's view, is a lonely and terrifying business, there is a strong temptation to claim for oneself a particularity, an essence, some given and enduring content. In clinical terms, the patient *claims* some structural properties, an enduring diagnostic nature—for example, as a rationale for his or her own choices. "I am an obsessional, borderline hysteric, and so on . . . I am the way I am because my mother was such-and-such a way, or my father did such-and-such to me." For Sartre (as for Fromm, 1941), such claims constitute "bad faith," whose purpose is to remove the subject from the dizzying freedom which human consciousness allows, which the human mind is. For Sartre, Freud's concepts of psychic determinism and repression, his vision of man as lived through by external and internal forces, is a theory in "bad faith," or, in Schafer's language, a theory of "disclaimed actions."

Psychoanalysis itself, in its doctrine of psychic determinism, suffers from the same pathology ("bad faith") it presumes to understand. It characterizes human lives and choices, but leaves out personal responsibility, ascribing those choices, those patterns, to impersonal forces. Sartre does not challenge the *content* of Freud's analysis of motives— Sartre's biographies of Baudelaire (1950), Genet (1963), and Flaubert (1981), and his own autobiography (1964) are filled with depictions of psychodynamic processes and motives and an emphasis on early infantile experiences. What Sartre does challenge is the elimination of personal agency, the failure to recognize the architect of the life in question, the person who chooses to be motivated by this or that event, circumstance, longing. By contrast, existential psychoanalysis as Sartre characterizes it is "a methodology designed to bring to light, in a strictly objective form, the subjective choice by which each living person makes himself a person" (1953, p. 58).

The existential critique of psychic determinism is not limited to classical psychoanalysis, but applies equally to virtually every psychoanalytic school, including those within the relational model. Sullivan's system, for example, is as deterministic as Freud's; in fact, Sullivan goes out of his way at several points to deride the concept of will and to emphasize his belief in the causal determinism of mental phenomena. All behavior, he postulates, is the sum of the various motives impinging on the person at any particular moment. The sense of choosing or personal agency is merely an epiphenomenon, a reflection in awareness of the convergence of various motives pertaining to needs for satisfaction and security, the sum of which is given and not subject to alteration by any deluded sense of willful direction. Sullivan insists:

I know of no evidence of a force or power that may be called a *will,* in contradistinction to the vector addition of integrating tendencies. Situations call out motivation; if there is conflict of motivation outside awareness, a compromise or a temporary domination of behavior and suppression of the weaker motive occurs. If the conflict is within awareness, the self-system is involved, with the corresponding element of insecurity. In these cases, more complex products result, but these too are vector additions, not interventions of some sort of personal willpower. (1940, pp. 191–192)

Sullivan does present a way of understanding the repetitiveness of psychopathological patterns which avoids the mechanical quality of Freud's concept of the repetition compulsion. For Sullivan, the self system operates on the basis of foresight and recall. The self system steers the individual in the direction of the least anxiety; evaluation of the likely level of anxiety resulting from any particular option is based on recall of past similar experiences. Thus, Sullivan describes the *process* of choice; yet, like Freud, he sees these choices as fully determined by necessities. For Sullivan, the person is a product of past interpersonal integrations, preserved in memory and continually restructured through foresight, which is an automatic scanning activity, projecting past situations into the present and future. The crucial question Sullivan does *not* consider is whether one can choose to exercise or not to exercise foresight, or choose to forsee one particular set of circumstances and consequences rather than another.

MIND IS a peculiar, mysterious, and elusive phenomenon, and philosophers and psychologists have tried to grasp its complexities by comparing it to other phenomena. Psychoanalysts have found inadequate the two most prevalent metaphors in our culture—physiological metaphors which equate mind with brain, and religious metaphors which equate mind with a supernaturally derived soul.

Freud and Sullivan both drew on physics for metaphors—Freud on nineteenth-century Newtonian mechanics, Sullivan on twentieth-century field theory. Yet the elusive, insubstantial phenomenon of personhood is not comprehensible in terms of physical laws, so that comparisons drawn from physics seem to lead inevitably to a deterministic frame of reference. Sartre's primary metaphor, by contrast, is political. The most important life experience of his young adulthood was the Nazi occupation of France and Sartre's own role in the French underground. To collaborate, to hide, to resist—these are profound choices—the past referents which seem inconsequential in the face of the choice itself and the chooser's personal responsibility for his action. The central experience of the war for Sartre was dramatic and heroic, which, as he was later to realize, is not necessarily representative of life in general. The political metaphor, although it highlights freedom and the will, leaves unexamined the textured meaning and symbolic referents of choice.

Further, it is not possible to theorize in a vacuum; all theorists, like all analysts, are participant observers, operating in an interpersonal field, a social and intellectual milieu, in which the development of concepts takes shape in dialogue and opposition to others. The predominant scientific theory of mind prior to Freud's day was one in which the mind and consciousness were seen as coterminous. In the nineteenth-century Victorian vision, what I know about myself is all there is to me, and I can shape myself into whatever I want through strength of will and mental discipline. Happiness and the good life are moral achievements; unhappiness and neurosis are moral failings, weakness, a product of bad nerves. Freud saw how little in fact we do know of ourselves, and it was precisely these unknown features to which he gave prominence—hidden motives, unsavory self-perceptions, and so on. He wanted to discount the arrogant claims to self-control of Victorian willpower. Not only is conscious self-control not *all* of the mind, Freud stressed, it does not even maintain hegemony over the mind's other regions.

Sullivan's position with respect to the will was developed in opposition to a similar (if more Americanized) Victorian vision, blended with the Catholic ideal of mind control. Sullivan's vector analysis of motives and stress on the power of circumstances are also steeped in a deep sympathy for the economically and interpersonally impoverished, as are his trenchant jibes at the arrogant claims of the self system to control over the mind.

Sartre's thinking operated in a different context, with different antagonists. For Sartre, Western philosophy has been dominated by various attempts to assign man an essence, and, since the Platonic-Christian tradition has been the dominant influence on our images of ourselves, that essence generally has been negative—man is fallen, bestial, passion driven, and so forth. In this respect, Freud's drive theory is simply the latest version of the Platonic-Christian image of man as a fallen angel corrupted by a lower nature, and Sartre dialectically opposes the determinism of Freud's drive theory as vigorously as he opposes other pre-existential philosophies.

Something of a compromise was struck within ego psychology, where the existentialist criticism was met by an attempt to divide human experience into two realms—a neurotic, conflict-filled realm and a healthy, conflict-free realm—one in which unconscious processes determine all mental events and one in which free, autonomous, and independent choice is possible (Lipton, 1955; Lewy, 1961; Flew, 1970). According to this view (developed from Hartmann's seminal concepts), pathological and conflictual areas within the personality operate under the sway of unconscious drive derivatives and defenses. Infantile, instinctual aims determine experience and behavior, which is secondarily and fallaciously rationalized in conscious experience. In other areas, however, the ego operates with neutralized energy, freed from hidden libidinal and aggressive aims. Here all the relevant information is contained within consciousness—the ego determines its own fate, free from the press of drive and defense. Freud's depiction of the analytic process, "where id was, there ego shall be" (1933, p. 80), characterizes the transition, through the analytic process, from psychopathology to health. Man is both determined and the source of influence and impact in his own right, but in different realms. Rapaport explains this split nature:

> Man has developed an anticipatory apparatus which is far more effective than any other animal's. This apparatus is very effective for outside events and fairly effective (anxiety and other affect signals) for internal events. These events play a causal role in behavior. But man himself (and every organism to some degree) is a source of causes. Man's anticipatory apparatus is a particularly effective mobilizer of man's own causal role. Man isn't freed from internal and external causes by means of his anticipatory apparatus, that is, by dint of his being also a source of causes. But he certainly can within limits avoid, evade, cushion and counteract causes which would determine his behavior. Some of these causes he is less adept at avoiding or cushioning (instinctual drives) but to the extent that he has a relatively autonomous ego, he can do even some of that. (quoted in Lewy, 1961, p. 267)

This solution, although compelling in its balance, ultimately retains an awkward hybrid quality. It posits a radically discontinuous view of human experience: in some areas man is a passive object of interior forces, in some an active creator of his mind and fate. If the will is understood to operate outside causally determined events, if it is put into motion, created through choice by the patient, why should it be restricted to a conflict-free realm? If the mind can choose to exert effort and impact, why not consider the choice of whether or not to exercise the will, and in what direction, a feature of *all* mental events? Are not effort and tenacity also components of much *pathological* behavior? Is not the will often exerted very effectively in the service of neurotic aims? If the capacity to will is an independent factor, not reducible to issues of drive and defense, it seems highly arbitrary to restrict its realm of operation to a healthy, conflict-free sphere. Schafer (1976, p. 113) has termed the claim that certain areas of functioning are free of unconscious meanings "wild ego analysis."

The neat bifurcation of experience into conflictual and conflict-free areas ultimately seems confusing and contrived. For example, Lewy attempts to deal with the thorny problem of the responsibility of the patient for his conduct by suggesting that when the patient experiences his behavior as determined, he is not responsible; and when he experiences his behavior more within the autonomous realm of the ego, he is responsible. "When he can at last see and accept his previously unconscious motivations as his own, as part of himself, we consider him responsible for them; even within the psychoanalytic setting, and from then on we expect him to hold himself responsible" (1961, p. 261). This tautological formulation confuses the analysand's phenomenology with the analyst's understanding, and amounts to saying that the patient is responsible when he assumes responsibility.

Wheelis (1956) developed a similar tautological compromise by arguing that the "will" (defined as "effort") is a crucial factor in psychoanalytic cure, independent of insight, and at the same time reaffirming the principle of "exceptionless determinism" by arguing that the will is part of a larger causal chain and is itself determined. This attempt at compromise again confuses the analysand's phenomenology with our understanding. If the exercise of the will is determined in full by prior events, the experience of the will is an illusion; it makes no sense to speak of "effort" except as a subjective description of a necessary and inevitable process, like a little boy in the first car of a subway train, pretending, with great effort and gusto, to be driving the train, but being carried helplessly along like everyone else.*

TRADITIONALLY, THE analysand has been understood to play an active role in the creation, perpetuation, and cure of his pathology (the existentialists), or to be driven by deterministic causes (the principle of psychic determinism). Ego psychology tries to have it both ways by assigning the will to the rarefied atmosphere of a conflict-free sphere and attempting to meld two models of mental functioning incompatible in their philosophical presuppositions. This solution seems arbitrary and tends to raise more questions than it answers. (See Schafer, 1976, chaps. 4–5, for an incisive critique of the ego-psychological approach to the problem of agency.)

In the face of the existentialist critique and the ego-psychological compromise, the doctrine of psychic determinism has been defended and elaborated by Hanly (1979). Despite Freud's inconsistencies, Hanly argues, the principle of psychic determinism makes sense only if it is understood to pertain to *all* mental events; thus, he rejects the approaches taken by ego psychology as well as by existentialist authors. There is no discontinuity between neurosis and health, Hanly suggests; the vicissitudes of neutralized energy are just as determined as the fate of sexual and aggressive energies. It is only the determinants that are different. Neurotic motivation operates under the causal sway of the pleasure principle; healthy motivation operates under the lawful sway of the reality principle, which supplies its own causal determinants and regulation. The undoing of repressions within the analytic process frees trapped energies for higher-level processes and aims, all exterior to the analysand's activity and control. The fact that man may become aware of his mental life, and that this reflectiveness facilitates the undoing of repressions, should not be confused, Hanly argues, with an impossible "sovereignty over motives" (p. 238). Thus, according to the principle of psychic determinism, "the essential step in defining the concept of freedom psychoanalytically is the recognition that the difference between a free and a compelled act is to be found in the differing nature of their causes, for all acts are caused acts" (p. 268). The existentialist critique of

---

* In a later paper Wheelis (1969) shifts his position and suggests that will and choice are indeed separable from causal determination. His discussion of their role is quite similar to Farber's approach, presented below.

psychoanalysis, Hanly argues, is a return to a preanalytic ignorance of unconscious mental processes, the naive belief that mind is simply coterminous with conscious will.

The problem of the will has been a difficult one for psychoanalysis. The will and psychic determinism have been viewed as alternative explanations, and it has seemed necessary to choose an existentialist disavowal of the concept of unconscious meanings, a classically psychoanalytic disavowal of the meaningfulness of choice and responsibility, or an uneasy juxtaposition of the two views (with each pertaining to different areas of human experience).

A Different Solution

Another approach to this difficult conceptual problem, in many respects prefigured by Rank (see Menaker, 1982), has emerged from several different analytic traditions in the work of Farber, Schafer, and Shapiro.* Farber was trained in the interpersonal tradition; his point of view, anticipated by Fromm's concern with responsibility and freedom, was developed in a series of evocative essays written in the 1960s. Schafer's approach grew out of his work within and eventual dissatisfaction with the tradition of ego psychology, and has been presented in the context of a rigorous and systematic critique of the language and implicit philosophical premises of classical metapsychology. Shapiro's position also emerged from ego psychology and his earlier contributions concerning varieties of neurotic character. Each of these authors, in his own particular fashion and according to his own particular set of concerns, argued that the issue of the will has been incorrectly framed within prior psychoanalytic literature; agency and unconscious motives are not alternative explanations, but simultaneous properties of all mental events.

Farber puts it this way. All nonexistential psychologies have been deterministic, in that they view human experience and behavior as the product of forces (or motives) impinging upon the person; the content of the particular theory supplies the content of the motives. In classical drive theory, man is the product of the interaction between drives and defenses; for Sullivan, man is the product, the vector sum, of needs for security and satisfaction; for Skinner, man is the product of his past

---

* See Hampshire (1962) for an early philosophical presentation of the kind of approach Farber, Schafer, and Shapiro were to develop more fully and strictly psychoanalytically.

history of reinforcement. All deterministic theories, Farber suggests, suffer from the same problem; motive analysis does not provide a complete explanation. A gap exists between the conjunction of motives impinging upon the person (no matter how one conceptualizes the content of those motives) and the activity of the person. This gap, Farber suggests, is the "realm of the will." There is no human activity which is not constituted by *both* motives *and* the will.

At times, Farber suggests, the will is invisible, a silent partner in experiences in which the person acts unselfconsciously, in a seamless unity with spontaneously arising impulses and gestures (as in satisfying lovemaking). At other times, the will disengages itself from the web of motives, standing against them and exerting an influence of its own. (In learning a game like tennis, for instance, one needs a "utilitarian will." Here a disciplined effort is required to keep one's attention on positioning, footwork, grip, and so on; only after considerable mastery has been attained can the will again become invisible in a more fluid and seamless performance.)

For some performances (as in trying to learn tennis), the self-conscious exercise of will is necessary and rewarding. In other areas (as in trying to force intimacy or excitement) the exercise of the will is grandiose and self-defeating. The will claims greater power than it has, in a necessarily futile effort to deny the reality of the complex of motives operating at any given time. (Schafer refers to such efforts as attempts to impose "radical discontinuity.") *This* is the will of Victorian "willpower" and Sartre's effort to grant to consciousness hegemony over all mental events. Much of what takes place within the analytic process, in Farber's view, concerns the sorting out of will and motives and the increasing discrimination between constructive and self-defeating exercise of the will.

> Let me give a few examples: I can will knowledge, but not wisdom; going to bed, but not sleeping; eating, but not hunger; meekness, but not humility; scrupulosity, but not virtue; self-assertion or bravado, but not courage; lust, but not love; commiseration, but not sympathy; congratulations, but not admiration; religiosity, but not faith; reading, but not understanding. I would emphasize that the consequence of willing what cannot be willed is that we fall into the distress we call anxiety. (1976, p. 7)

Traditional psychoanalytic theories have illuminated many features of human motivation; this analysis of motives must, Farber suggests, be complemented by an understanding of the will, if the analysis is not to degenerate into an exercise in post hoc explanations. The explication of motives without recognition of the complicity of the will, either actively or passively, leaves *the person* out of the explanation and hence encourages a self-serving and obfuscating bad faith.

The analysand says, "My trouble with women is due to the fact that my mother treated me badly." Or "My unconscious hostility makes me resistant to analysis." It is not that these explanations are necessarily wrong, Farber argues; they may be partially right. If they are not accompanied by an assumption of responsibility for the actions or feelings involved, however, the possibly correct explanation becomes a disclaimer, an excuse. Instead of opening up understanding and possibilities for change, they cover over, further masking the role of the analysand in perpetuating his own difficulties. The hysteric, Farber claims, is particularly skilled at using explanations to account for *why* he is doing what he is doing, to mask the fact that he *is* doing what he is doing. In Farber's view, the hysteric is often an active and crafty operator (unwittingly) who presents himself as a puppet on a string. Within classical theory too, the hysteric is viewed as a puppet on a string. This confluence between deterministic theory and the hysteric's disclaimed "willfulness," Farber suggests, has had much to do with the difficulty hysterics, from Dora onward, have posed for the traditional psychoanalyst. For Farber, the analysand is not just a puppet acted upon by strings (motives), but is also the puppeteer (the will) who coordinates and chooses among the strings while guiding behavior. Thus, within the framework Farber has developed, one is not asked to choose between psychodynamics and the will. Analysis of motives and the positioning of the will, and an exploration of their relation to each other, are essential to a truly analytic understanding of any activity or experience.

SCHAFER, IN philosophically rigorous and systematic fashion, has taken a similar position. In 1968 he published a codification and critique of psychoanalytic concepts concerning "internalization," with particular emphasis on the processes of identification and introjection. Schafer found much clinical and theoretical utility in these concepts, but was disturbed by the tendency, particularly in Kleinian theory, to attribute to abstract concepts (such as identifications) or fantasied images (such as introjects) properties of real beings—substance, locality, intention, and force. In a manner highly reminiscent of Sullivan, Schafer repeatedly warns against reification, against treating abstract and theoretical concepts as if they were actual entities or beings. The patient may experience himself as inhabited by powerful internal presences; this is symptomatic of his pathology. It is crucial, Schafer argues, for the *theory* to distinguish clearly between what is real and what is not, between the patient himself who has power and does things and his fantasies of others, real or fantastic, whom he imagines as having powers and doing things.

In this early volume Schafer also suggests a radical revision of the concept of drive, again objecting to the traditional practice of ascribing to instincts specific and elaborate attributes. It is not useful to think of energy as having qualities, he argues. Personal motives are libidinal, aggressive, or neutral; it makes no sense to attribute these properties to energies. The concept of psychic energy is necessary only in a quantitative sense, to indicate relative strength of motives. Other aspects of classical theory come under scrutiny as well, such as the assumption of a closed energy system with a finite amount of energy, and Schafer adds personal terms like "motives" and "characteristics" to the more traditional energic and mechanistic terms "functions" and "regulations." Thus, in his 1968 effort to revise classical drive theory, Schafer retains the drive terminology but shifts the emphasis more and more onto the analysand's own activity.

In the early 1970s Schafer produced a series of innovative and provocative articles which he brought together in 1976 under the title *A New Language for Psychoanalysis*. Here Schafer has done with revision and instead presents a detailed, thorough, and brilliantly incisive critique of classical drive-theory metapsychology, proposing a new metatheory and language for psychoanalytic discourse. Classical psychoanalytic theory and language, Schafer suggests, were modeled on Newtonian physics, the prototypical discipline in Freud's intellectual milieu. Mental processes, if they are to be explained "scientifically," must be portrayed in terms of physical events and energic forces. There is no place in the theory for the person as the active agent of his life. Yet psychoanalytic clinical investigation had uncovered a vast array of personal meanings and unconscious intentions that pervaded everyday experience. Therefore, these intentions, these activities were smuggled back into the theory by anthropomorphizing forces, mechanisms, structures. "Sooner or later, these concepts are used, they have to be used, to imply an agency that stands more or less outside the so-called play of forces, the so-called interrelations of functions, the so-called field of determinants . . . There is a gap: between the person on one side and the natural science apparatus on the other" (p. 119). It is not the person who does things, wants things, and so on, but the drive derivatives, the psychic agencies, the mechanisms of defense.

To make matters worse, Schafer argues, the misuse of language within the nineteenth-century scientism of classical metapsychology reproduces exactly the primitive understandings and misuse of language by small children, who picture their mental processes in crude bodily terms, involving places, substances, entrances, expulsions, and so on. The result of this confluence of errors and primitive understanding is a theory whose language portrays the analysand as the passive victim of forces, structures, memories, and mechanisms (which he experiences himself as being when he starts treatment). Metapsychology employs a "psychosexual bodily language inappropriately elevated to the state of theoretical terms" (p. 6). The elimination of active agency within the theory contrasts sharply, Schafer continues, with the actual practice of psychoanalysis, in which the interpretive process is used to make more and more of the patient's life intelligible to him as his own creation, rooted in the active repetition and reenactment of infantile situations and relationships.

Drawing on Wittgenstein, Ryle, and other modern analytic philosophers, Schafer proposes an "action language" for psychoanalytic discourse which eliminates all anthropomorphic and reified concepts and which places the subject as the agent at the center of all activities. All mental events which have meaning, including thinking, feeling, and disclaiming, are most usefully thought of as actions performed by the individual. Actions are performed in many different modes—libidinally, aggressively, consciously, unconsciously. Actions are also taken for "reasons"; reasons do not *cause* the act, but are inseparable *constituents* of the act. For example, one might perform an action for the purpose of seeking pleasure—the pleasure seeking does not cause the act; it does not exist prior to the act as some inherent pressure or intensity. The pleasure seeking is a reason, or one of a family of reasons, for performance of the act. All mental events are constituted both by the subject's activity as agent and by reasons (just as within Farber's system, all events have both will and motives).*

---

* Schafer came to reject the term "motive" as connoting a force separable from action; he would likewise take issue with Farber's description of the will as occupying a "realm."

Subsequent to his critique of the language and the philosophical premises of classical drive theory, Schafer reconceptualized many areas of psychoanalytic theory in terms of his "action language." Much of psychopathology, according to Schafer, entails disclaimed action (as well as "excessively claimed action" or the assumption of responsibility for "happenings" over which one has no control). The psychoanalytic process, as portrayed by Schafer, entails the gradual understanding of reasons and assumptions of agency: "the analysand progressively recognizes, accepts, revises, refines and lives in terms of the idea of self as agent" (1978, p. 180).

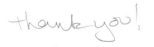

SHAPIRO ARRIVES at a position very similar to that of Farber and Schafer, but via a different route. In his 1965 classic, *Neurotic Styles,* Shapiro demonstrated that neurotic symptoms are not circumscribed, conflict-derived, isolated fragments within the personality, but are natural extensions of particular modes of perception and thought, each with its own distinctive style, advantages for living, and mechanisms of symptom formation under stress. This elimination of the distinction between symptoms and a more general, volitional approach to living led Shapiro to the conclusion that psychopathology derives directly from the patient's world view, that it is in a fundamental sense intended, chosen by the patient. Within the patient's often unrecognized frame of reference, pathological character makes perfect sense, seems to be desirable. This active, intentional quality Shapiro terms "autonomy," and he argues that autonomy is a feature of all behavior, that some degree of impairment of autonomy is a feature of all psychopathology.

He argues against the traditional psychoanalytic view of man as simply need driven. All adults have an active, complex approach to living which is a product of attitudes, beliefs, imaginative processes, all of which combine into a particular characterological style. All of life is expressed in the context of that style; all action is mediated through character. To see psychopathology as an unmediated expression of primitive needs is to miss the crucial sense in which psychopathology is a consequence of an unrecognized state of mind which derives from a particular approach to living. (Weiss and Sampson have proposed a very similar position, emphasizing what they call pathogenic beliefs.)

One major difficulty which has traditionally plagued authors who stress the role of the will has been in establishing the developmental inception of intention and choice. If adults operate with choice and intent, when in the life cycle does this process begin? Do small children operate with intentionality? Do infants? The difficulty of this problem has led most authors of the will, as well as existential philosophers in general, to adopt positions which are essentially nondevelopmental. The will is seen as simply arising, either de nova or through an obscure and unarticulated prehistory.

Shapiro, in contrast, makes great strides in clarifying the developmental and cognitive underpinnings of the will. Drawing on Goldstein's work on organicity, Piaget's model of cognitive development, and an astute depiction of the child's relations with parental authority, Shapiro argues that the capacity for autonomy is predicated upon the the ability to abstract, to separate oneself from others, to "objectify" the world. Thus, he places the development of the will within psychoanalytic developmental theory and cognitive psychology, as a function which becomes possible with the emergence of self-object differentiation and the overcoming of egocentricity.

Shapiro also makes a major contribution to the perennial problem of the confusion of intention with consciousness, as if awareness of the place of the will suggests that all behavior is a product of elaborate deliberation. He distinguishes between consciousness and self-consciousness, arguing that much psychopathological behavior is consistent with consciously held beliefs and attitudes, without being self-consciously thought through. Thus, actions can be guided by conscious aims without being consciously articulated.

In the rigid character, Shapiro argues, conscious intentions have been articulated which do not accurately reflect the state of the patient's subjective experience (Farber's "willfulness"). There is a gap between what the patient claims to want and what he truly wants and strives for. What the patient claims to want represents undigested identifications with parental authority figures, and these unmetabolized identifications, although disowned, strongly influence the analysand's experience and activities. Thus, the rigid character, in his various manifestations, is perpetually at odds with himself, continually trying to superimpose an imperious and impossible mastery over his experience.

Farber, Schafer, and Shapiro each grappled with the problem of the will as an inevitable extension of their own concerns; despite the differences in language and tradition, the kinds of understandings they arrived at are remarkably similar. In the remainder of this chapter we shall consider some of the theoretical and clinical implications of this common solution to the issue of agency, and extend that solution to the processes involved in the creation and regeneration of the relational matrix.

Will and Meaning

Alfred North Whitehead once remarked that the only ideas opposing schools of thought have in common are their tacitly accepted presuppositions, which are fallacious (Langer, 1972, II, 22). One of these tacit and fallacious presuppositions, held by most psychoanalytic and existential schools but avoided by Farber, Schafer, and Shapiro, is that influence and choice are opposed and inversely proportional to each other. Either actions are determined by prior causes, or they are chosen free of constraint. This way of thinking about the problem is poorly framed because the metaphors, drawn from physics and politics, are insufficient to the task. Both Nietzsche and Rank suggested that the processes underlying the patterns which make up a human life are more usefully compared to the creation of a work of art, and the artistic metaphor allows a more balanced and complex vision.

One of the central functions of mind is the generation of a world of subjective meanings, the creation of a textured, symbolic order of representations in which each person locates and identifies himself or herself. I suggest that the basic ingredients of mind are self-organization, attachments to others, and transactional patterns, all of which constitute a complex relational matrix. Where does the content of this subjective world come from? It is neither invented out of thin air nor simply provided by the external world. The creation of a subjective world of meanings is an interactive process; pieces of experience are selected, refashioned, and organized into patterns.

Even in the simplest perception of sensory events, stimuli from the external world are worked over; perceptions are created by an active organism. This is more true of the emotional life in which we reside—our images of self and others, our sense of life and its possibilities, actively assembled from bits of experience, significant others, cultural surroundings, social class values and vistas, and physical sensations. We might say that these are the materials, the media, from which a life, a self, is created, through a whole range of processes both within and outside awareness.

Consider the constituents of artistic creation. If a work of art is to be more than an idea, it must have actuality; that is, it must employ a medium, be made out of materials, derive from some stylistic tradition. The medium, the materials, the tradition, offer possibilities and impose limitations. Beethoven's piano sonatas were created at a particular point in history, at a specific moment in the tradition of Western music, employing the sonata form at an advanced point in its evolution and written for a relatively new and dramatic instrument whose possibilities had barely been tested. A full appreciation of the creative process must take into account both the active imagination of the artist and the constraints and potential of the context and materials with which he or she works.

The error of the determinist is to assume that the product is reducible to, understandable in terms of, the materials, that the choices which constitute a life are the direct, causal product of a particular set of experiences such as drive tensions (Freud), anticipations of anxiety (Sullivan), maternal deprivation (Winnicott), and the like. A deterministic approach to the relational matrix would suggest that the latter simply reflects nonselectively accrued residues of experiences, automatically built up like silt deposits at the mouth of a river.

This deterministic stance tends to be preserved in otherwise innovative contemporary analytic schools such as British object-relations theories and Kohut's self psychology, and is closely tied to the portrayal of the analysand as essentially passive. For these authors, the fate of the individual is generally a simple, direct, inevitable product of that person's experiences; this portrayal is accompanied by a tendency to villainize the parents as the source of psychopathological difficulties. In Fairbairn's system, for example, the developmental transition from infancy to maturity depends on whether the child feels loved in his own right and feels his love is valued. If these conditions are met, he relinquishes his internal objects; if they are not, he holds onto them. Similarly, the therapeutic action of psychoanalysis is understood to entail the relinquishment of attachments to bad objects, wholly contingent upon the analyst's becoming a good object. Nowhere does Fairbairn suggest that choice is part of this process, that the individual has any role in committing himself to a relationship, either internal or external. The ego remains essentially passive with regard to its own fate. Behavior is, for Fairbairn, a direct product of motives (in this case, derived from experiences with others), and thus the classical deterministic assumptions concerning the issue of agency have been preserved.

Through the metaphoric eyes of object-relations theory, we see the patient caught in a web of bad object relations (in the language of self psychology, relations to "self objects"). The parents, because of their own difficulties, have not provided adequate opportunity for healthy, real relationships. Substitutive relations with fantasized others have been established, derived from inaccessible areas of the parents' character. These ties to bad objects are maintained until a good object appears and revives the patient's hidden capacity for connection. What is not reflected in this formulation is that the analysand is not just the fly caught in the web, but is the spider, the designer of the web, as well!

The psychoanalytic deterministic position is comparable to arguing that a work of art is predictable from a thorough analysis of its circumstances and the qualities of the materials—that if one takes into account the features of the piano, the history of music at the end of the classical era, an appreciation of the romantic movement, and the characteristics of the sonata form, one could foresee Beethoven's piano sonatas.

Certainly Beethoven's choices were not limitless; his instrument, form, place in history, personal values, audience, and so on each posed constraints, and our understanding of his work is enriched by an appreciation of those factors. Nevertheless, the work of art is not solely the product of its materials and forms; the artist also contributes. Similarly, the self is created from meanings assigned to experience; one cannot begin to understand a life, a person, without an appreciation of those experiences and what they provide in terms of possibilities and constraints. But the meaning of those experiences is not given; it is composed, created, designed. The self is not produced by motives and causes; there is also the creative will of the individual. Clinical work which does not take this into account becomes an intellectual exercise in explanation and rationalization, rather than providing increased responsibility for one's past and present choices, choices made with clarity and deliberation as well as choices clouded by self-deception and distraction.

On the other hand, writers influenced by the existential tradition emphasize the analysand's activity and responsibility for what she does. The analysand is seen as choosing, creating her own world, then dissembling, concealing her choices from herself and others, by presenting herself as acted upon rather than acting. Alert to the dangers of disclaiming and "bad faith," existential authors tend to avoid analysis of content or motive. The *fact* that the patient chooses and actively creates her world and takes responsibility for her actions is the central focus.

The problem with this approach is that although it is compelling philosophically and ethically, it is not satisfying psychologically and clinically. While placing the responsibility squarely on the patient's shoulders, the emphasis on agency does not provide a persuasive explanation for *why* the patient does what she does. We see this problem most clearly in Sartre, for whom agency, in the form of consciousness, is all. The individual propels herself headlong into the future, creating her past, creating her dynamics. But why *this* choice instead of *that* one? this motivation rather than that? Why maintain this incident as traumatic? that relationship as predominant? Anyone who has struggled with patients and with himself to disentangle from experience the web of meanings, past and present, and who has seen the extraordinary tenacity with which past relationships reappear and permeate one's current world, cannot accept Sartre's view that man is wholly self-created.

The error of the radical existentialist of the Sartrian variety is to assume that the product is *un*constrained by and *un*related to the materials, that the meanings and choices which constitute a life are generated independently of the circumstances and experiences within which that life is lived. Beethoven's sonatas could not have been composed by Bach, nor could they have been written for the dulcimer. Similarly, a life, a self, is a fabric of meanings created out of circumstances and experiences; a deep understanding of that life must include an appreciation of those circumstances and experiences. Clinical work which does not take into account this fabric of meanings becomes an exercise in moral confrontation and blaming, rather than an experience which provides the potential for genuine self-understanding and meaningful change. The analysand is asked to assume responsibility for and alter that which she is clearly doing but which she does not fully understand. No matter how willing the patient is in assuming agency, she is assuming authorship for actions the meaning of which she is at best only dimly aware of. Unless the basic structure of the analysand's relational matrix is brought to light, the *context* within which the analysand operates as agent is missing, and therefore the true meaning of her choices and commitments cannot be fully grasped.

The framework I have sketched makes it possible to view the psychoanalytic exploration of meaning and the Sartrian illumination of freedom and choice not as inevitably mutually exclusive models of mind, but as partial accounts of a process which encompasses both. The psycho-analytic determinist explicates the materials and leaves out the artist; the radical existentialist depicts the artist but leaves out the context and medium. The creation of a work of art constitutes a struggle by the artist *with* her materials. Clichéd art mimics prior work and convention and surrenders to the constraints of the medium; great art challenges conventions and stretches the possibilities of the medium. Similarly, a human life is a synthesis of symbolic meanings from the circumstances of its interpersonal context—conventional lives borrow meanings and constraints from popular culture; creative lives stretch conventions of thought to give birth to new possibilities.

Problems of Consciousness and Repression

Discussions regarding the role of the will often founder on the problem of accounting for unconscious mental processes. This is because the distinction between choice and determinism becomes blurred with the closely related distinction between conscious and unconscious mental events. Proponents of granting the will an important psychodynamic role do sometimes sound like advocates of the Victorian theory of "willpower," regarding mind as transparent and under direct, willful control of consciousness. "I am the master of my fate; I am the captain of my soul," proclaimed William Ernest Henley in what to us today is astounding naiveté regarding the complexities of the mind. For anyone with a modicum of clinical experience, it is evident that none of us has anything approaching total access to, much less control over, his own mental life. The mind is not at all transparent—in fact, it is often quite opaque to itself. The philosopher Daniel Dennett has suggested that pre-nineteenth-century philosophers such as Locke were wrong in assuming that we have privileged access to our own minds. Much of what we are about is more obvious to other people than to ourselves. In fact, Dennett argues, in many respects we have underprivileged access to our own mental life (Miller, 1983, p. 80).

How can this fact be reconciled with theories which grant a crucial place to will, choice, agency? If large portions of mental life are unconscious (for instance, the basic configurations of the relational matrix), does that not mean that processes taking place within those realms are wholly determined by unknown forces, that the agent is passive with regard to these forces, that the will plays no role? How can it be meaningful to speak of choice with respect to unconscious processes?

Part of the difficulty in approaching this problem is the ease with which we have come to make the distinction between conscious and unconscious mental events. Let us look at that distinction more closely.

Freud's topographical model (1900) divides mind according to the criterion of consciousness. All mental life is derivative, Freud thought, of powerful conflicts between unconscious mental forces (impulses) and conscious (and preconscious) mental forces (defenses). The mind is neatly split between that which is accessible to consciousness and that which is unconscious, and these opposing forces are at war.

One of the major reasons Freud replaced this topographical model with the later structural model (1923) was his realization that the earlier model could not really explain how it is that unconscious forces remain unconscious. If conflict operates between unconscious impulses and conscious defenses, the conscious defenses must themselves contain knowledge of the content of the unconscious so that they know what they are repressing. But if the content of the unconscious is contained within conscious defenses, it is not really unconscious. The structural model seems to resolve this dilemma. The defenses themselves are unconscious, Freud suggests. The ego has both a conscious realm and an unconscious realm (which contains the defenses), and it is the latter that keeps unconscious impulses from awareness. Thus, the structural model preserves Freud's neat distinction between conscious and unconscious mental events simply by assigning more of mental life to the unconscious, which now contains not just wishes and impulses, but the complex cognition involved in ego defenses.

However, this new model really does not solve the problem. The ego's defenses must be unconscious, since they keep id impulses from awareness and therefore must contain knowledge of those impulses. But what keeps the ego's defenses from awareness? They too contain forbidden information and therefore must be actively, dynamically barred from awareness. So there must be defenses against the ego's defenses. These cannot operate within the ego's conscious realm, because the defenses against the defenses would also contain knowledge of the forbidden content which those defenses contain. Thus, the defenses against the defenses must themselves be unconscious as well. And what keeps *them* from awareness?

Rather than solving the problem of repression, of providing a persuasive account of how unconscious processes are kept out of awareness, the structural model merely establishes an implicit infinite regress from which there is no escape. Freud conveyed the appearance of a solution only because he arbitrarily stopped his analysis with the first line of defenses. This allowed him to preserve the neatness of the distinction between conscious and unconscious mental processes which he had established with the topographical model; but the structural model really accounts for such a distinction no better than did the earlier topographical model.

Many critics of the psychoanalytic concept of the unconscious have taken the position that there simply is no such thing. They argue that one can categorize various mental processes along a continuum of degrees of vividness and clarity, but that with effort and concentration all these mental contents can be made accessible to consciousness. Freud argues back with one of his brilliant metaphors. The fact that there is a range of different kinds of light, he suggests, does not imply that there is no such thing as darkness. Some mental content is, with varying degrees of effort, accessible to consciousness; other mental content is not. Once again, anyone with a modicum of clinical experience must immediately agree with Freud. True, many areas of experience are potentially accessible to the analysand at the very beginning of the analysis, but are merely overlooked or underutilized; over the course of the analysis, however, new areas of experience are opened up which were simply not available before. Clearly, Freud is right about psychic areas of total darkness; the question is, how are we to understand this darkness— what *happens* in the dark?

The problem with the distinction between conscious and unconscious mental processes is not the contrast between these two different types of mental events, but the neatness and polarization with which the contrast is customarily drawn. Both the topographical and the structural models fail because Freud attempts to portray the boundary between the conscious and the unconscious as a line—on one side is the repressed; on the other, awareness.

The boundary between conscious and unconscious mental content is actually more permeable, shifting, and indistinct. With the introduction of the structural model, Freud assigned sophisticated mental operations to the unconscious. Subsequent developments in psychoanalytic theorizing have extended this view. Fromm, for example, argued that the power and incisiveness of language and metaphor in dreaming often highlight how impoverished an analysand's conscious experience can be in comparison with what he knows, perceives, constructs, outside awareness. And Weiss and Sampson argued that the unconscious consists to a large extent in "pathogenic beliefs," very much like those of conscious mental life. Phenomena like automatic writing and studies of creativity also demonstrate that a great deal of creative thought often takes place outside focal attention. Current thinking about the complexities of the human mind suggests that Freud's concept of a definitive line between conscious and unconscious, of a "dynamic" unconscious in the sense of a realm of unacceptable impulses restrained from access into consciousness by specific defensive forces, is too simplistic; it dramatically underestimates the vast proportion of mental life which operates more or less outside awareness.

Theorists in the field of artificial intelligence, drawing on computer analogies, likewise suggest that the mental activity required for even the simplest and dullest of human thinking is enormous. It would be neither possible nor desirable for such activity to be conscious. This suggests that it is unlikely that mental content lacking consciousness is denied access because of specific defenses directed against it. Rather, we operate, to a greater or lesser degree, obliviously with regard to the meanings of our actions and experiences. The problem is not so much accounting for how parts of mental life become unconscious, but rather how and under what circumstances portions of mental life become conscious.

SULLIVAN INTRODUCED the concept of "selective inattention" to describe the relative inaccessibility of experiences which are not dynamically "repressed" in Freud's sense.

> When things go by rapid transit through awareness into memory without the development of implications, those undeveloped implications are not there for the purpose of recall . . . It is not anywhere near as handy as it might be, because it is not well tied into the general tissue of your life . . . It is susceptible to recall, despite the very great interference with getting the connections that will recall it . . . but it certainly is not facile to recall. (1956, p. 58)

Sullivan is suggesting that as we move along in life we do many, many things, with varying degrees of attentiveness. Accessibility to conscious recall is very strongly contingent on the degree to which we have developed the "implications" of any particular mental event. Further, attending to some mental events (like defensive postures) makes it more difficult to attend to and develop the implications of others (which one might consider the repressed).

This way of thinking about the problem of consciousness and repression, not as discrete forces but in terms of varying degrees of attention, has been picked up by more contemporary authors. Schafer has similarly "operationalized" the unconscious in a fashion strikingly reminiscent of Sullivan.

> Putting the concept of self-deception this way also invites investigation of the modes of action by means of which people can act in selectively inattentive and selectively ignorant modes, especially with regard to personal matters of great moment. The investigation of these reasons and of these actions and their modes is what the metapsychologist would call the investigation of "the dynamic unconscious." (1976, pp. 243–244)

What are the implications for the phenomenon of the will or agency of this way of thinking about unconscious mental processes?

Our lives are made up of a sequence of choices, always within a particular context, always within a complex set of constraints. They are choices nevertheless. As we move through time, the choices we make often have implications for how accessible our past choices will be to our awareness. If I walk through a city in a straight line, I can look back and see the path I have traversed. If I turn corners again and again, looking back no longer allows me access to my past choices. I can retrace my steps, but this now requires considerable effort and time. Similarly, many important character-shaping choices are not instantly recoverable, for subsequent choices obscure their path. The obsessional, who every day chooses to focus on details, because he thinks that is the safest way to live, has no immediate access to the salient, formative emotions of his childhood. The hysteric, who every day chooses to avoid details, because he thinks that is the safest way to live, has no immediate access to the salient, formative events of his childhood. Choices leave behind residues, which can screen out past choices. At any particular moment, the will is free—but free amid the clutter of the derivatives of past choices.

Repression is better understood not as a force but as a state, a condition generated by the obscuring of key past choices by subsequent and current choices. The content of the repressed lies concealed behind other mental content and processes which are granted greater focal attention and visibility. Repressed memories are not accessible, because the analysand, although interested in them, is also *not* interested in them; in some conflictual sense he wants the content of his mind arranged precisely the way it is.

Anxiety plays a key role in both wanting and not wanting to search for conflictual mental content, in both wanting and not wanting to explore current experiences and past choices. As one retraces past actions or lays bare the underlying meanings of current choices and experiences, anxiety rises and falls. Certain mental content may bring with it frightening vistas and implications, at odds with the way one customarily thinks about oneself and one's relations to others. The anxiety makes it harder to look, clouding the vision of even the most sincere analysand. This is one reason why the analytic process takes a long time. Past choices are brought to light, the underlying texture of forgotten or unnoticed meanings is exposed, and it is often necessary to live for a while at this particular vantage point to allow the vision-clouding, dust-spreading effects of anxiety to settle. Thus, the analytic inquiry has an unforced, natural rhythm, not a linear descent, but a sequence of spurts and plateaus. As the analysand makes his way through the analysis, he necessarily pauses for a while to accustom himself to and appreciate the shifting angles on his experience and world which each vantage point provides.

The will thus plays a crucial role in the analytic inquiry, which makes possible a recovery of unconscious mental content. At various critical points the analysand has to decide he *wants* to look. Then, through the analytic inquiry, analysand and analyst collaboratively reverse the process through which the unconscious material was obscured, tracing back the path, removing the screens, and despite anxiety and unfamiliarity eventually reclaiming the memories, feelings, wishes, ideas. From this perspective, the unconscious is composed not of clashing, blind, depersonalized forces, but of all the characteristics of conscious mentation, including strong commitment and effort. The analysand does what he does unconsciously in much the same way that he does what he does consciously. The only difference is the absence of awareness, a lack of clarity, of development—as Sullivan put it, of "implications."

To speak of the analysand's "deciding" to inquire is not meant to suggest conscious, deliberative choice which is sustained throughout. The analysand's posture toward the analytic process is always complex and variable, and inevitably embedded in the shifting transference-countertransference configurations between analysand and analyst.

Much of the analytic process involves being in and eventually grasping and articulating experiences, rather than actively and vigilantly searching. Often the analysand finds himself participating in a process, the nature of which he only dimly understands and the implications of which he had no way of anticipating. Nevertheless, it is always possible and often clinically crucial to locate the position of the analysand vis-à-vis both the analyst and the analytic process, to track the ways in which the will (or the analysand as its agent) is either facilitating or derailing the analytic inquiry, or, as is most common, doing both conflictually and simultaneously.

What keeps the repressed unknown is the combination of the obstacles produced by the residues of past choices and the will that does not want to begin the search. Traditional deterministic psychoanalytic theories, by omitting the role of the will, overlook the analysand's powerful conscious and unconscious commitment to the way in which his mind is arranged. Traditional antipsychodynamic existential theories grant the conscious component of the will too great a power and thereby overlook the serious obstacles and constraints left behind by past choices and unconscious commitments. The analysand cannot will himself to total access to his mental life, but he can inquire into and thereby alter his attitude toward inaccessible mental content; this initiates a process, like searching for a lost object in a cluttered room, whereby greater access can eventually be gained.

Perhaps one of the most significant fruits of the analytic process is that the analysand learns to regard his mind as much more complex than he had ever before imagined. Most people begin analysis with something like the Victorian assumption that they have a fairly wide-ranging access to their mental processes. They end up with an experience of themselves that is multitextured and uneven. Being a person is now understood to be a much more complex business, a dialectic between the "I" that does things, assigns meanings, makes, honors, and betrays commitments and loyalties, and the "I" that *knows* some of the things done, meanings assigned, commitments undertaken, honored, and betrayed.

The concept of unconscious choice seems difficult to grasp. Perhaps a better term would be "design." What seems to make human consciousness (mental life both within and outside awareness) distinctive is its property of reflexivity, the capacity to represent itself to itself, and, as a consequence of that reflexivity, its self-designing capacity. As self concepts are formed, they in turn have considerable impact on the path the individual steers through experience, selectively attending to some features, not attending to others, preserving some aspects of self, disregarding others, in a fashion which in turn determines ways in which self concepts will change or remain the same. The subject of the analytic inquiry is the intricate, subtle, inevitably conflictual, highly textural relational pattern of that design.

Two aspects are crucial: first, the *content* of the choices and patterns discovered, the configurations of the relational matrix, and second, the *experience* of the self as designing and making choices, both within and outside awareness. The analyst holds the analysand accountable for his choices, his design, not for purposes of blame or as a call for conscious, cognitive "reasons," but as a clinical gambit, a demonstration that putting himself in that position begins a process which, over time, opens up access to unconscious meanings and commitments, revealing the structure of the relational matrix which shapes the fabric of his experience.

The Self as Damaged

In previous chapters we have considered evocative metaphors which recur repeatedly in analysis and seem to have a universal quality, such as the self as baby and the self as beast. Another very common metaphorical theme in the phenomenology of many analysands is the image of the self as damaged, the experience of having been traumatized in some irreversible fashion by events in one's past, most frequently in terms of having been crushed in the earliest relationships with caretakers. The forms the sense of damage takes are generally individually styled according to the particulars of earlier interactions and fantasies. The analysand feels he has been crippled, deprived, wounded, hobbled, sabotaged, poisoned, emptied, broken, and so on. These ways of experiencing oneself reflect a particular kind of relationship between past and present in which one's present self is captive to past events, to resources that have been depleted, to potentials that have been cut off.

Schafer (1983, p. 257) has written of the experience of the "imprisoned analysand" as a dynamic configuration which conceals important "disclaimed actions" involving the meanings of the imprisonment and one's own role in maintaining it. Similarly, the many variations on the theme of the damaged self often serve as the centerpiece of an elaborate psychodynamic configuration which provides continuity and connectedness with the analysand's fantasied internal world, and ties to others in the actual interpersonal world as well.

In Chapter 7 we considered the function of the illusion of perfection in maintaining object ties. "I am perfect, and you are part of me." "You are perfect, and I am part of you." "You and I are both perfect together." These are relational configurations all established within early family dynamics and maintained as forms of connection and modes of preserving ties with others. The metaphor of damage is used in parallel ways. The analysand either experiences himself as deeply damaged and needing care, sympathy, or sometimes contempt, or feels he needs to experience another (for example, a child) as severely damaged, so he can care for, sympathize with, or feel contemptuous of him or her. "I am damaged and you take care of me." "You are damaged and I take care of you." "You have damaged me and therefore are bound to me." "I have damaged you and therefore am bound to you." "We are both damaged in the same way and are hence eternally bound together." These are relational configurations, which also are often established very early and operate to maintain and preserve familial ties.

Sometimes images of perfection and damage operate together. There are analysands who aspire to an image of perfection and completeness in connection with an idealized image of a parent or an inherited fantasy of the parents' own. The gap between this perfect image and the inevitable imperfections and incompleteness of the human condition is experienced as a corruption, a "deficit," an "emptiness." Often the child's sense of self as empty and damaged is also borrowed from the parent. Both feel themselves to be inevitably incomplete and damaged in relation to a shared fantasy of perfection and "wholeness."

Manic feelings and experiences often operate in the context of object ties mediated through a sense of damage and depression. The primary connections to others are joined through a shared sense of depletion and constraint, which is generally cultivated and protected. Other relationships and experiences may be structured to represent a defiance of and freedom from these constraints, constituting a manic triumph over the primary object and the sense of deprivation and subjugation required by those ties to the primary object. We saw earlier how the condition Freud termed psychical impotence is often a carefully constructed emotional composition in which some relationships are established and maintained in terms of a surrender to the requirements and wishes of the other, and other relationships are experienced as allowing a flight and freedom from those necessary inhibitions of desire.

Thus, the metaphor of damage is an organizer of experience playing a central role in mediating connections to others—real and imagined, past and present. The sense of damage is often the centerpiece of the analysand's relational matrix.

What is difficult about working clinically with the metaphor of damage is that the analysand does not experience the sense of damage as something desired by him, cultivated and protected because it plays a central role in holding together his sense of connectedness to others. He sees himself as passive in relation to his past, as victimized by it. He sees the damage not as metaphorical but as real. Further, for the process to work psychodynamically, he *has* to see the damage as real. To grasp the metaphorical nature of the sense of damage is, by definition, to consider the possibility of *not* experiencing oneself as damaged, and this assumption of agency threatens to weaken the rigid self-organization, the adhesive ties to others, and the security-maintaining transactional patterns which are mediated through that sense of damage.

The analytic inquiry into these dynamics involves a slow realization, over time, of the analysand's commitment to the experience of himself as damaged, an understanding of how essential that experience is in maintaining his relational matrix, and of how depleted (if also relieved) he would feel without it. The first extended task in the analytic inquiry is reaching and articulating the analysand's experience in precisely the metaphors through which that experience is organized. The metaphor of damage, like the metaphors of the beast and the baby, is central in most analysands' language of experience and has a powerful experiential truth, which the analyst necessarily perceives and identifies with. Most often, it is not until the middle phase of analytic inquiry, the "working-through" phase, that the focus shifts, in a subtle but crucial way: the delineation of the analysand's phenomenology is broadened to include considerations of agency, the role of the analysand's willful commitment to his subjective world. Considerations of agency do not belie or negate the experiential reality of the analysand's subjective organization; they broaden that reality by deepening the context in which it develops and operates. Without this shift in emphasis, analysis can drift along in endlessly expanding interpretations which lack the capacity to generate effective change.

What further complicates the clinical problems associated with the metaphor of damage is the reification of this metaphor in traditional psychoanalytic theorizing. In previous chapters we have seen the manner in which universal experiential metaphors become established as actualities in certain modes of psychoanalytic thought: the metaphor of the baby by developmental reasoning, the metaphor of the beast in the theory of instinctual drive. The metaphor of damage has found its place in current psychoanalytic thought in concepts such as developmental "arrests," structural "deficits," ego "defects," all of which suggest actual substantive damage. Experiences of defectiveness are assigned literal properties, as if the damage resides *in* the mind and itself shapes subsequent experience; they are not regarded as organizational metaphors in an interactional field, serving as paths of connection to others, weaving together past, present, and future in a familiar, sustaining way.

These concepts drawing on the metaphor of damage are extremely useful in their closeness to the phenomenology of many analysands' experience and in highlighting the powerful and pervasive impact of past experiences on present functioning. They are also very misleading in obscuring the role of the will in positioning the analysand in relation to that past, masking the active, albeit conflictual commitment and deep allegiance to past modes of connections which often underlie the most severe psychopathology. Personal ownership of the active and willful dedication to the relational matrix mediated through the metaphor of damage is a crucial prerequisite to expanding that matrix and allowing different kinds of experiences.

SOME CONTEMPORARY philosophers have compared the human mind to an as-yet-uninvented self-designing program, a product created by others which can turn around and redesign itself (Hofstadter, 1979; Dennett, 1985). In Escher's *Drawing Hands,* the fingers of each hand seem to emerge from the paper and draw the wrist of the other hand. The concept of a self-designing program and Escher's image capture something of the kind of approach to the problem of the will developed by Farber, Schafer, and Shapiro. The analysand is "wired" in certain ways, operates within an environmental context, is the inevitable recipient of many experiences and influences of others. Yet these raw materials of experience are shaped, ordered, arranged into an idiosyncratic, inevitably conflictual, relational matrix. Commitments are made to particular forms of relations with others, to a particular world view and self-experience. The analysand's subjective world may be painful, but it is his; and in some deep sense, he wants it just this way (even though he also may not). His conscious, willful commitments and choices support and embellish unconscious commitments and choices—the larger, more complex design which shapes his experience. It is an increased awareness of himself as both the design and the designer that makes possible a richer experience of living.

So every day she wove on the great loom—but every night by torchlight she unwove it.   —HOMER

10 Penelope's Loom: Psychopathology and the Analytic Process

A twenty-year-old student, shortly after beginning analysis, recovers a memory of himself as a nine-year-old boy just back from a camping trip with his father. The latter is a fiercely independent man whose periodic trips out onto the "mountain" provided him with continually sought relief from what he experienced as the suffocating degradation of his domestic captivity. This was the first time he had allowed his son to join him. The trip had been enormously difficult for the eager and spunky boy, as his father eschewed any concessions to convenience or comfort, combining obsessive self-sufficiency with a taunting challenge to his son. The boy felt vast relief at having survived the trip without disappointing his father in any major way.

Later in analysis he recalls speaking with his mother, an anxious, intrusive, overprotective woman, who had waited nervously for his return and then bathed him in effusive sympathy and solicitousness. Although he was usually frightened of his mother's ministrations and therefore tended to avoid them, after the spartan regime of life on the mountain, he was enjoying her interest and concern, telling her details of his trip which were bound to elicit even greater sympathy. In the midst of his account he became aware of his father's presence at the doorway and glanced up to catch a look of surprise and total disgust on the older man's face. Later in analysis he recalls the memory with a dizzying, sickening sense of self-loathing and isolation from both parents.

271

This memory came to play a central role in deciphering and disentangling the strands of this analysand's life. He writes constantly, and his ambition is to be a poet. He works almost completely alone, as if on the mountain, yet with a constant longing for the products of his labors to be loved and taken into people's homes and treasured by them. When a longed-for success in the form of publication or positive critical reaction punctuates a period of dedicated effort, he immediately changes his style of composition. He dreads becoming a panderer for commercial success; the only way to keep his artistic process pure is to abandon immediately any work that gains the approval of others.

His relationships with women are dominated by these same themes. He is drawn to women with deeply depressive longings and helps them in a very sensitive and compelling fashion. He sets them up in a life in which he is the desperately needed emotional center, then constructs realms of escape in which they can only long for but never get to him. There is an aching loneliness for him in these relationships, as he is perpetually struggling to design emotional attachments which, because of their cloying and suffocating quality, he needs always to escape.

Homer in the *Odyssey* depicts Penelope, Odysseus' loyal wife, as besieged by suitors during his many years' absence. They urge her to abandon her missing husband, who has never returned from the battle of Troy, and marry one of them. She is not interested in entering this world of new possibilities and wants to wait for Odysseus' return. In order to keep her ardent suitors at bay, she tells them she cannot think of remarrying until she fulfills her obligations by weaving a shroud for Laertes, her father-in-law. She weaves during the daylight hours and, after the household has gone to sleep, unravels her work by torchlight. She spends years at her endless project, whose seeming futility belies its effective and poignant role in preserving her dedication and holding together her subjective world.

One might regard the relational matrix within which each of us lives as a tapestry woven on Penelope's loom, a tapestry whose design is rich with interacting figures. Some represent images and metaphors around which one's self is experienced; some represent images and phantoms of others, whom one endlessly pursues, or escapes, in a complex choreography of movements, gestures, and arrangements woven together from fragments of experience and the cast of characters in one's early interpersonal world. Like Penelope, each of us weaves and unravels, constructing our relational world to maintain the same dramatic tensions, perpetuating—with many different people as vehicles—the same long-ings, suspense, revenge, surprises, and struggles. Like Penelope in the seeming purposiveness of her daytime labors, we experience our lives as directional and linear; we are trying to get somewhere, to do things, to define ourselves in some fashion. Yet, like Penelope in her nighttime sabotage, we unconsciously counterbalance our efforts, complicate our intended goals, seek out and construct the very restraints and obstacles we struggle against. Psychopathology in its infinite variations reflects our unconscious commitment to stasis, to embeddedness in and deep loyalty to the familiar.

FROM THIS perspective, the life of our student-poet is constructed of conflictual relational strands. Emotional connection to his mother en-tails a bond in which desperate need is met by enveloping solicitousness. He generally plays the role of caretaker, establishing the nurturing environment in which the needfulness of the other can be ministered to. He sometimes (mostly in fantasy) plays the role of the needy child, whose wants will be fulfilled in the warmth of domestic comfort which he can never allow himself to reside in fully. Emotional connection to his father entails accompanying this parent in his heroic isolation, never really "meeting" him, but as powerfully connected as birds in flight along the paths of a parallel formation. He works long hours in self-imposed isolation, setting up repetitive, seemingly impossible challenges for him-self, which he manages barely to overcome at the last moment through cunning and courage.

The father's untamed bestiality is the counterpoint to the mother's domesticity. Each relationship itself is intensely conflictual; the price of connection to each parent is too great. And the two relationships are in intense conflict. Thus, as this young man's personality developed, the conflictual strands of each relationship were teased apart. All the strands were then reassembled in the fabric of his life, which allowed him to maintain powerful connections to these archaic objects, in which each connection was exquisitely balanced by escape routes.

In this analysand's relational matrix, as on Penelope's loom, the action never proceeds to fruition, the dénouement is never reached. This is because conflict and balance are artfully built into the composition itself, and also because (like Penelope) the analysand experiences intense con-flict about the project as a whole. Restrictive difficulties in living operate precisely in this double fashion—delimiting relational configurations are continually restructured *into* daily living, and also struggled *against* in an effort to break free of their constraints. Thus, this analysand is continually finding his mother's furnished rooms and his father's mountain in the content of his daily life, balancing their claims against each other and making monumental efforts to break free of the limits they jointly impose on his life. Unlike Penelope, who knows she both weaves and unravels, the analysand is aware only of his struggles to escape what he experiences as the given structure of experience.

THE METAPHOR of the beast, derived from the drive model, is a recurrent theme in the iconography of many tapestries and the organizational content of the relational world of many analysands. The student, for example, experiences certain features of his sexuality in bestial terms, identifying with his image of his father as powerful and in some sense untamed, in intense conflict with the domesticity represented by his identification with his mother. Still, if we regard the beast as inherent and "instinctual," we fail to grasp the relational configurations and ties which constitute the deeper structure of experience and provide the context within which the experience of the self as beast emerges and operates.

Similarly, the metaphor of the baby, derived from the developmental-arrest model, highlights important early relational issues and needs. The student had a great longing to escape the constant pressure and relentless expectations imposed upon him by his relationship with his father. He yearned to surrender to a nurturing maternal care which, because of the intensity of his divided loyalties and his mother's frightening intrusiveness, he was never able to allow himself to experience fully with his mother or any other woman. Yet if we regard the "baby" as a vestige of the interactional field which becomes actual and takes on invariant properties, we portray the subject as merely a figure in the tapestry rather than also its weaver. The student as baby was a daily re-created product of the continual regeneration of the writer as untamed beast and as solicitous protector, and his daily dedication to accept his mother's never-realizable offer of unconditional love and devotion. The metaphor of the baby reified into theory fails to capture the commitment of the subject to his relational world, a world which is not just the passive residue of experience but is actively woven each day.

Embeddedness and the Relational Matrix

How does one get stuck in a maladaptive relational matrix? Why are human personalities so powerfully shaped by early relationships, and why is the attachment to archaic objects so "adhesive" (to use Freud's term)? We saw in Chapter 3 that Freud had considerable difficulty answering this question and resorted finally to placing explanatory weight on constitutional factors like the inherent antisocial quality of the drives and the workings of the "death instinct." Fixity, for Freud, is built into the instinctual underpinnings of emotional life.

Many relational-model theorists (Fairbairn, Winnicott, and Kohut, for example) shift the responsibility to the environment. The baby is good, not bad, and if properly cared for will be emotionally resilient and free of encumbering attachments. Embeddedness is incompleteness—a failure in provision of essential ingredients for emotional growth. The bestial baby has been replaced by the unempathic parent as the villain of the piece.

In my view, *all* children are bent out of shape (or more accurately, *into* shape) in their early significant relationships, and this is a result neither of inherent bestiality nor of faulty parenting, but of the inevitable emotional conditions of early life. Becoming a particular person is a complex process during which the child, in his "object seeking," searches for and engages other persons to attach to, to shape himself around, to elicit recognition from. Each baby has a wide range of possibilities; the interactions with early significant others contract that range, reduce possibilities to selected channels through which that child can find and be recognized by his significant others. One cannot become a human being in the abstract; one does so only by adopting a highly specific, delimiting shape, and that shape is forged in interaction between the temperamental givens of the baby and the contours of parental character and fantasies.

One of the most profound and universal realizations of later childhood, a realization that probably is never totally integrated, is the discovery that one's parents are not necessarily representative of the human species, that one has grown up in an idiosyncratically structured family with its own peculiarities and dramas. Before that slowly dawning recognition the interpersonal world of one's childhood is the only show in town, and fashioning oneself as part of it is a psychological inevitability.

The prolonged condition of childhood dependency makes the discovery and forging of reliable points of connection not just an emotional necessity but an apparent condition for physical survival. No matter how available the parent, the inevitable confusions and fears of childhood make the parent never seem unconditionally available enough, or available in the right way. The experiences of separation, overstimulation, physical illness and pain, glimpses of human mortality, exclusion from the parental relationship, sibling comparison and competition, childhood dependency, and other travails of early life are certain to make childhood at least intermittently stormy, and early relationships inevitably somewhat insecure. One's position can never be taken for granted. One is always, in some ultimate sense, at the mercy of adults. The parents can never be purely facilitative, simply allowing the child to find his or her own path. The anxieties inherent in childhood make it necessary for the child to employ the parents as specific points of reference, their idiosyncrasies becoming anchors for all subsequent joinings.

Sullivan's concept of the child's sense of "good me" shaped by parental anxiety, Winnicott's depiction of the "false-self" dimension of the child shaped around parental intrusions—these formulations point to the necessity for the child to design himself within the spaces provided by the contours of parental character, to find himself in the points of connection they provide. Reifications in theory of both the metaphor of the beast and the metaphor of the modern baby fail to capture this interactive process, since both posit a preformed content out of which development proceeds: the former, as a wild thing to be tamed; the latter, as an unfolding to be facilitated.

Embeddedness is endemic to the human experience—I become the person I am in interaction with specific others. The way I feel it necessary to be with them is the person I take myself to be. That self-organization becomes my "nature"; those attachments become my sense of the possibilities within the community of others; those transactional patterns become the basis for my sense of interpersonal security and competence to function in the world. Adhesive devotion to the relational matrix reflects a terror of total loss of self and connection with others, as well as a deep loyalty and devotion to the interpersonal world which, no matter how skewed, allowed one to become one's own particular version of human.

ALL IMPORTANT human relationships are necessarily conflictual, since all relationships have complex, simultaneous meanings in terms of self-definition and connection to others, self-regulation and field regulation. As Loewald says, "The deepest root of the ambivalence that appears to pervade all relationships, external as well as internal, seems to be the polarity inherent in individual existence of individuation and 'primary narcissistic' union" (1960b, p. 264). Connection with another always both actualizes and expands the self and also inevitably exacts a price in the narrowing of other options. Accommodation to a particular other, especially of the child to the parent, creates a counterpressure to reclaim what has been given over, to escape the limits of self which serve as the preconditions of any connection. Different channels of connection to the same parent can themselves be in conflict, depending on the continuity or discontinuity of these qualities in the parent.

Each child is likely to develop a deep tie to both conscious and unconscious or disowned currents within the parent's character structure; how well the child can integrate these currents is partially limited by how integrated the parent is, how flexible his or her self-organization is. Further, accommodation and connection to one parent always comes into conflict, in some fashion, with accommodation and connection to the other. How conflictual these different connections and loyalties become is strongly influenced by the family dynamics. Are different kinds of relationships tolerated? sides drawn? exclusive loyalties demanded?

The strands which make up the complexities of personality derive from the inevitable conflicts centering around and between various points of connection and identification with early significant others. Neurotic symptoms are not outcroppings of conflict between wishes and defenses, but loose threads, conflictual relational configurations, unable to be syntonically woven into the dominant themes within the composition of the personality and finding circuitous, displaced, disguised forms of expression.

The foregoing points to the limitations of the so-called medical model as a basis for thinking about the kinds of difficulties in living with which the psychoanalyst deals. The concept of psycho*pathology* implies a normative human mind, analogous to the normative physical functioning of the human body, with psychoanalysis as a treatment for deviations. But if each person is a specifically self-designed creation, styled to fit within a particular interpersonal context, there is no generic standard against which deviations can be measured. Rather, difficulties in living would be regarded with respect to the degree of "adhesion" to one's early relational matrix and, conversely, the relative degree of freedom for new experience which that fixity allows. How rigid is the self-organization forged in early interactions? How much range of experience of oneself does it allow? How adhesive are the attachments to archaic objects? How exclusive are the loyalties demanded by them? How compulsive are the transactional patterns learned in these relationships? How tightly do they delimit actions within a narrow border fringed with anxiety? These interrelated dimensions determine the degree of character pathology.

The universality of accommodation and fixity to original significant relationships suggests that the analytic process is not so much a treatment for psychopathology, but, more broadly, a uniquely structured experience which allows the possibility of loosening the inevitable restraints generated by the residues of early experience. Attachments to archaic objects are not all the same. The more rigid the connection provided by the parents, the more the child is forced to choose between the limited forms of relation or total isolation, and the more compulsive are the residues of those relationships. But conflictual attachments to and identifications with archaic objects are universal. It is the alteration of those ties which constitutes the basic therapeutic action of the analytic process.

Comparing Concepts of Therapeutic Action

Consider the following session in which the analysand expresses bewilderment about how her analysis can possibly move forward.

She begins by noting her pleasure at the previous hour. She had supplied disconnected free associations; the analyst had made some bridging connections the patient had been unaware of. This is something she can rarely let happen, she says, because she cannot trust the analyst enough to allow him to provide her with something she might really need, like organizing her associations. So she generally censors her associations, organizing them herself, and it is precisely this lack of trust and commitment which prevents her from establishing any long-term relationships with others.

For her analysis to really move forward, she goes on, she has to learn to relinquish control, but how can she possibly do that? Her experience with both parents left her feeling very wary of such a surrender. Her mother was a "saintlike" woman who was excessively devoted to her and would do anything for her, in fact insisted on doing most things for her—which, she had come to feel, left her unable to do many things for herself. Her father was a powerful, grandiose, isolated man, totally convinced of his superior wisdom on all of life's major issues. He was also very involved with his daughter, demanding impressive shows of loyalty in returning for his unerring control and direction. Each of the parents, who were very alienated from each other, seemed to look to their only daughter for some sort of contact and completion, offering pleasure and protection at the price of total and exclusive surrender.

She had learned that it was very dangerous to surrender control, to count on anyone else for anything, although she had a great longing to do so and illustrated this through the following metaphor. "It is as if we are in a car with dual controls. I pretend to let you drive, but never *really* relinquish the master control." How can the analysis proceed, she wonders, when to be involved in the process requires precisely the kind of trustful relinquishing of control she feels most unable to do?

What *is* going to help this patient? Clinical psychoanalysis is rife with controversy about exactly this question. Analytic cure is attributed by some to insight, by others to a nurturing relationship, by others to confrontational encounter. The analysand in treatment is viewed by some as pursuing infantile wishes, by others as seeking to fill structural deficits, by others as longing for and also fearing a connection in the present relationship with the analyst. The recommended demeanor of the analyst is described variously as neutral, empathic, aloof, or participatory, and the atmosphere of the analytic setting as abstinent, nurturing, anxiety tinged, or playful.

Proponents of these different positions all tend to regard their own view of the analytic process as correct, making possible a deeper, more emotionally significant experience for their analysands; from each perspective, the other positions appear conceptually flawed and clinically shallow. Each stance is placed at the center of the psychoanalytic universe and the other positions, inevitably located at the periphery, represent a contamination of psychoanalytic truth, and a diminution of the power of the analytic experience.

The problem with the discourse generated by these controversies is the assumption that these different positions operate within the same universe, that their individual, specific components can be meaningfully compared and weighed against each other. This is very misleading. Theories of analytic technique differ not just on specific issues but in fundamental premises regarding the very nature of mind and human interaction. The analytic situation created by practitioners of these various perspectives is not a common phenomenon about which they disagree. Each perspective, by virtue of the manner in which it is structured and the way in which the analysand is initiated into it, creates its own particular analytic situation, which it then explains through its theoretical postulates; each perspective creates its own kind of analytic relationship, which then becomes the vehicle for its own version of analytic cure. In this sense, each perspective *is* at the center of its own conceptual universe. The problem is that there is more than one such universe.

Should the analysand's wishes be gratified or deprived? Should the analyst make many interpretations, or offer them sparingly or not at all? Should the focus of the work be in the transference or outside the transference? Should countertransference be avoided, utilized, expressed? Comparing the approaches to these specific issues leads quickly into a quagmire of semantic confusion. What *is* it that is to be either gratified or denied? What *is* an interpretation and how does it work? Each model understands these phenomena differently, and each position, because of the manner in which it is put into effect, creates different sorts of wishes, interpretations, transference, countertransference. The debate about how these things are to be handled often presumes that they are in fact the same across all models. This is a bit like owners of different models of automobiles arguing about how to get into first gear. For one the gearshift is down in first; for another it is up. For the owners of a car with automatic transmission, first gear is embedded in "drive" (a noninstinctual variety) and takes care of itself. To approach the dimensions of the analytic process without reference to different theoretical models of the nature of mind and the way it changes is like trying to arrive at a consensus about how to get cars into first gear.

THREE BASIC concepts of the therapeutic action of psychoanalysis have dominated psychoanalytic thinking, and they have very different premises, histories, central metaphors, and clinical implications. The contributions of many important contemporary authors (Loewald, Schafer, and Modell, for example) would not fit any one of these models neatly and exclusively. Most of us have come to think of analytic work in a complex combination of ways. But there are three coherent and integrated understandings of analytic change which can be teased out conceptually for purposes of study and comparison; they need to be grasped in the larger historical and theoretical context in which they evolved.

The Drive-Conflict Model

The drive-conflict, or classical, model of psychoanalytic technique was forged in the interaction of two major influences: its prehistory in hypnotism, and the drive-theory premises concerning motivation, development, and psychopathology which provide its basic explanatory framework.

From hypnotism came the emphasis on recovery of memories, which has remained a central feature of classical technique. Eventually the analysis of unconscious derivatives within "free association," and later the analysis of the defenses, replaced hypnotism as the basic instrument for reclaiming memories.

From drive theory came a set of premises regarding the *content* of what is to be remembered. Man's biological heritage and fundamental nature provide him with prepackaged, constitutional, instinctual drives, each component arising at a "source," with an "aim" pressing with a built-in "impetus" toward some predesigned discharge. Man's rationality and capacity for social conscience provide him with capabilities for regulating and sublimating his prehuman and protohuman bestial drives for higher, socially sanctioned purposes. Neurosis represents a grim victory for the drives and irrationality—the libido has withdrawn from useful and pleasurable purposes in the real world to recathect infantile, incestuous images. It is this attachment to infantile parental images and wishes for gratification which fuels neurotic symptoms and lends them durability and tenacity.

The psychoanalytic situation, as conceptualized in the classical psychoanalytic model, is a battleground within the context of this larger vision. The analyst, whose function is to investigate and uncover, is pitted against the resistances, whose function is to protect and keep hidden the infantile wishes and longings. The ultimate aim of psychoanalysis is to overcome the resistance, to flush out the beast, to "track down the libido . . . withdrawn into its hiding place" (Freud, 1912b), to tame the infantile wishes by uncovering them through memory. Freud's favorite genres of metaphor are zoological and military, well suited to delineating this battle between investigation and resistance, between bestial life and intellectual life, between drive gratification and reality.

All the major features of the analytic situation are understood within the context of this mimetic goal and drive-theory premises. The analysand is encouraged to relax the defenses, to allow the derivatives of his wishful impulses to appear uncensored in his free associations. The analyst's function is to cull the infantile wishes and fears from the complexly disguised derivatives in which they are encased. The primary therapeutic tool is "interpretation," in which the conflict between repressed infantile impulses and defenses against those impulses is articulated.

The analyst's interpretations supply, in careful and timely fashion, crucial missing information, which encourages the analysand to remember those pathogenic wishes. The resistance represents the manifestation of the original defenses in this new, highly dangerous situation in which the repressed is being evoked. Wishful, bestial impulses were repressed originally because they posed a grave threat to the peacekeeping purposes of the ego; the analysis itself, in its attempt to uncover libidinal impulses through the analyst's interpretations, poses a similar grave threat.

Resistance, in the classical theory of technique, is the sabotaging of memory and insight, and thus precise understanding is crucial to true analytic change. Analytic interpretations require the precision of the surgeon to uncover and fully delineate pathogenic wishes and conflicts. One does not cut into the *general* area of an abscessed appendix or try to remove *most* of it. Similarly, any interpretation even slightly off the mark is eagerly employed by the resistance to create pseudoinsight and therefore actually strengthens repressions. You are either exactly right or you make things worse, you are either part of the "solution" (as the political slogan of the 1960s phrased it) or part of the problem.*

Transference is the reexperience of the original infantile wishes and fears within the relationship with the analyst, and manifests itself primarily as an obstacle to the required aim of the psychoanalytic process—the recovery of the infantile wishes and fears in their original historical context. In his genius and extraordinary persistence, Freud was able to

---

* In the classical theory of technique *insight* provides the basic leverage for analytic change, loosening repressions, releasing trapped energies, and facilitating the renunciation of infantile wishes. Many contemporary theorists have continued to place central emphasis on insight, even though they have rejected drive theory as an explanatory framework. Removing the drive model from around the clinical concept of "insight" leaves it stranded in a conceptual vacuum. The drive model provides an account of *why* insight cures. Displacing the model necessitates another explanatory framework to perform its functions. Schafer (1983), for example, relocates insight within his hermeneutic-action language perspective, which gives it a crucial role in the assumption of "agency" and the rewriting of narratives, functions very different from those Freud had in mind.

turn transference from an obstacle in the way of analysis to an eventual aid; the displaced feelings and images do provide important data, Freud realized, even though the data are out of context. Instead of remembering what he felt about father and mother, the patient displaces the historical wishes onto the relationship with the analyst. The interpretation of the transference (that is, the setting of those feelings and images back into their original context) thus provides what Glover calls an "affective experience (an affect-bridge) to link the past with the present" (1955, p. 133).

The relationship between analyst and analysand is therefore regarded as a crucial dimension of analysis, stimulating long-buried desires. These are inevitably and necessarily frustrated; the "treatment must be carried out in abstinence" (Freud, 1915b). This is because the transference is employed by the resistance as an alternative to remembering. In the closed-energy system in which the drive-conflict model operates, wishes gratified in the transference are no longer available for "memory work." The same packet of energy cannot be discharged in two different ways. Memory is forced by abstinence and frustration; that which is gratified is perpetually enacted, but never remembered and analytically transformed. Within the drive-conflict model of the psychoanalytic process, analytic change takes place when the transferential experience is converted into memory.

The objectivity and detachment which the drive-conflict model of analytic technique assigns to the demeanor of the analyst is demanded by drive-theory premises. The analysand's neurosis is understood to be a closed system of drives and defenses. The analyst functions to interpret these conflicts, to bring them to light, to reclaim memories and provide insight. As this process unfolds, the patient experiences the analyst in terms of his or her own internal struggles. The resistance uses these transferences to impede the analytic inquiry; the analyst counters by employing these transferences themselves in the service of the memory work.

The transference poses grave dangers, often evoking reactions from the analyst, who, in being exposed to the analysand's transference, is "tried in all directions, his Id stimulated, his ego disparaged and his super-ego affronted" (Glover, 1955, p. 102). In the classical theory of technique the analyst must struggle to resist these pulls. Although Freud urges the analyst to use his own intuition and his own unconscious processes, the analyst's emotional state must always be one of composure, objectivity, and neutrality. The analyst is the bastion of rationality, the major protagonist against the irrationality of the drives. The analyst is present as function, as interpreter, not as person with wishes and fears of his own. He must go about his task deftly and incisively, his equanimity undisturbed by ripples of affect, frustration, or despair. The experience of strong feelings within the analyst regarding the analysand is viewed as a departure, a pathological result of the analyst's own unresolved conflicts and childhood residues. Proper analytic demeanor calls for interpretive, not affective, response. "In what is called 'handling of the transference,' " Fenichel suggests, "not joining in the game is the principal task" (1941, p. 73). Although the minimalism of the analyst's response is extremely difficult for both the analysand and the analyst, it is necessary and in the best interest of the patient.

LET US return to the clinical vignette of the dual-control car, in the perspective of the drive-conflict model. These sessions would be understood to center around the patient's conflict concerning an intense wish for passive surrender, which might be understood in oedipal terms as a sexual surrender to the father, in negative oedipal terms as a homosexual submission to the phallic mother, or, alternatively, as a longing for symbiotic fusion with the preoedipal mother. Both the wish and the fear are currently experienced in the transference to the analyst, even though they need not have anything to do with what the analyst is really like, and would be elicited by any analyst using proper analytic technique. Wish and fear would be allowed to become deeply felt, experiential reality, before the genetic interpretation would reset both in their original context in relation to the parents. It would be crucial for the analyst to remain appropriately neutral, to avoid encouraging surrender in the transference; anything else would be a countertransferential seduction and would obscure the grounds for clarifying the analysand's historically based distortions. Ultimately the longing for and fear of submission to the analyst must be frustrated and *experienced* as intensely frustrating, to allow for the uncovering of the infantile wishes and their eventual renunciation.

The Developmental-Arrest Model

The developmental-arrest model is a relational model which puts the greatest emphasis on the earliest relationship of the infant to the mother. We have seen that it is often used by authors who want to remain loyal to classical theory and technique as appropriate for neurotic patients, while using relational-model concepts and affiliated techniques for patients they consider more disturbed. Object-relations concepts are placed *before* the formation of drives and structural conflict, thereby preserving Freud's theory of the neuroses and forcing the focus to the earliest child-mother relations as the source of all difficulties. In the developmental-arrest model of the analytic process, the therapeutic action works to heal the paralysis and the distortions generated by interferences in that first relationship.

Winnicott, Guntrip, and Kohut have been the major developmental-arrest theorists. Their versions of the analytic process, by no means identical, overlap considerably. Let us consider Winnicott as representative of this approach.

For Winnicott, psychopathology represents a developmental fixation. It is the development of the self, not just of impulses, that unfolds according to a preset course of emotional needs. The caregivers provide certain emotional reactions and an affective ambience necessary for the self to grow and maintain a sense of integrity, continuity, vitality, and coherence. If these responses are not forthcoming, the natural maturational process slows to a stop. The vital center of the person, the "true" core of his or her subjectivity, is stuck in time. "False," shallow psychological structures grow up around this buried core, but they cannot be understood as real or new growth. Winnicott warns the analyst to avoid the "false assumption that the patient really exists" (1950, p. 213). Despite the passage of chronological time, the patient does not age psychologically. Unmet early needs persist in a protected cocoon of defenses; new growth is possible only when and if the missed maternal functions are somehow obtained. While the central narrative of the classical drive-conflict model is the cornering, revelation, and eventual renunciation of the self as beast, the central theme of the developmental-arrest model is the rebirth and reanimation of the self as baby.

Winnicott depicts the analytic process in terms of the rekindling of the subjective omnipotence of the true self. He views the essential dimension of early development as a movement from an initial sense of subjective omnipotence through an ambiguous "transitional" realm, to an eventual tolerance of objective reality. What makes this process possible is a perfectly accommodating mother who, because of her own "primary maternal preoccupation," initially shapes the world to actualize the infant's wishes and fantasies. The mother gradually withdraws from this role of accommodation, making possible an incremental disappointment for the child as he comes to tolerate an objective reality and other subjectivities beyond his control. If the mother does not play this crucial role properly, she is experienced as impinging on the child in a way that he cannot possibly negotiate or integrate with the spontaneous claims of his own subjectivity. The core of his being is blocked, buried, held in abeyance, while a compliant, false accommodation to external impingement is fashioned. Psychological growth has ended. "The mother's failure to adapt in the earliest phase does not produce anything but an annihilation of the infant's self" (1956, p. 304).

Kohut describes, in very similar fashion, a subtle dialectic between narcissistic gratification and inevitable, incremental disappointment, which over time generates a tolerance of more realistic experiences of self and others through a process he terms transmuting internalization. The parent's failure to provide and protect this delicate process results in a forced adaptation to objective reality, very much like Winnicott's description of "impingement," in which various narcissistic sectors of the child's self become split off and are unable to be drawn on in living. The result is a sense of oneself as empty, depleted, fragile, or fragmented.

Winnicott views the analytic process as providing missing parental functions, both in the analytic setting and in the person of the analyst, which makes it possible for the stalled maturation of the self to begin anew. His enormously rich papers describe many examples of different features of the patient-analyst relationship and many different kinds of interactions, all interpreted as enacting facets of the normal infant-mother relationship. A common theme is that the patient structures the analytic situation according to a natural wisdom about what he missed and now needs. Kohut strikes a very similar note: "The interrupted maturational push, the maturational push that was thwarted in childhood, will begin to reassert itself spontaneously as it is reactivated in the analysis in the form of a selfobject transference" (1984, p. 78).

Winnicott's basic injunction to the analyst is, *do not meddle*. The revival of the patient's vital self depends on the analyst's willingness to create an environment structured totally by the patient's subjectivity, in which the analyst, like the good-enough mother, becomes the patient's creation, a subjective object. "The mind has a root, perhaps its most important root, in the need of the individual, at the core of the self, for a perfect environment" (1949a, p. 246). And a perfect environment is one which allows the child-analysand the illusion that the environment is of his own invention, proceeding from "the child's ability to 'think up'—in a way, to *create*—an analyst, a role into which the real analyst can try to fit himself" (1948, p. 169).

What is important for Winnicott is not the insight-generating *content* of interpretation per se, but the way in which the interpretation allows the patient to experience the relationship with the analyst in the necessary mother-child terms. "What matters to the patient is not the accuracy of the interpretation so much as the willingness of the analyst to help" (1958, p. 122). Whereas in the classical model, correct interpretation generates *insight,* which releases the patient from instinctual fixations, for Winnicott correct interpretation facilitates a return to and actualization of *early infantile states.* "Whenever we understand a patient in a deep way and show that we do so by a correct and well-timed interpretation we are in fact holding the patient, and taking part in a relationship in which the patient is in some degree regressed and dependent" (1954b, p. 261). It is important to understand that Winnicott is not speaking of "holding" in metaphorical terms, but as a psychologically "real" event. "A current and well-timed interpretation in an analytic treatment gives a sense of being held physically that is more real (to the non-psychotic) than if a real holding or nursing had taken place" (1988, pp. 61–62).

The analytic process, in Winnicott's vision, is a self-healing in which a corrective environment makes it possible for false, defensive, compensatory adaptations to collapse and thereby allow the stalled development of the true self to begin anew. "The tendency to regression in a patient is now seen as part of the capacity of the individual to bring about self-cure" (1959, p. 128). And crucial to this process of reanimation is the analyst's provision of maternal functions to the patient's nascent self. "The analyst will need to be able to play the part of mother to the patient's infant" (1960, p. 163).

THE BASIC emphases in the drive-conflict model and the developmental-arrest model contrast starkly with one another on certain key issues. In the former, something old is re-created in the analytic relationship— the patient experiences the analyst *as* the object of conflictual longings of the past. New elements in the analytic relationship ("rapport," the "working alliance," and so on) are important as means to get the patient to experience and eventually renounce those old desires. Therefore, frustration provides the key leverage for analytic change; the old is given up to make possible new gratifications outside the essentially abstinent analytic relationship.

In the developmental-arrest model, the patient structures the analytic relationship to provide himself with something new, some essential experiences that were missed early in life. Old elements are there in the form of fears, pessimism, disappointments, and defenses, but the analytic traction derives from the analyst's provision of a novel experience of early developmental states. If the classical model portrays the analysand as bestial and requiring renunciation, the developmental-arrest model views the analysand's authentic self as unformed, awaiting the necessary conditions for further growth. The analyst cannot gratify all the patient's needs, but rage and frustration in the face of inevitable failure and disappointment are responded to with an unruffled empathic understanding, which is starkly different from traumatizing parental reactions. Thus, it is not the frustration of old desires, but the provision of something new (even if not wholly gratifying) that generates the key leverage for analytic change, unleashing the stalled maturational process.*

LET US return now to the clinical vignette (of the dual-control car) from the perspective of the developmental-arrest model. This patient's wish and fear regarding surrender in the transference would be seen not as an expression of infantile libidinal wishes (preoedipal, oedipal, or oral), but as an expression of an ego or self need, a longing for the kind of normal caretaking, parenting function—the containment of the "bits" of her experience in an effective "holding environment," such as was not provided earlier. The patient is experiencing a need, Winnicott would argue, not a wish, and nothing else will happen unless she can feel safe suspending her own self-control sufficiently to trust the analyst to provide a holding environment.

Winnicott would regard both of the parents as impinging in their own way, forcing a precocious reality orientation, and fixating authentic development of the true self. (Kohut would see it in terms of the

---

* In Kohut's posthumous writings, where he was trying to build bridges back to the classical tradition, he emphasized the key structure-building role of frustration, not just in the analyst's "empathy errors," but even in the analyst's correct understanding. "It is *frustrating* because, despite the analyst's *understanding* of what the patient feels and his *acknowledgment* that the patient's upset is legitimate . . . the analyst still does not *act* in accordance with the patient's need" (1984, pp. 102–103; italics in original).

failure to provide appropriate self-object functions with respect to mirroring.) The "need" would be regarded not as pathological in itself, but as the vehicle for cure. The analyst's demeanor should be nurturing and empathic, to allow the analysand to work through her resistance to her hope for a good-enough response from the analyst, to allow a regression to the point of developmental arrest, so that more genuine personality development can be reactivated.

A Relational-Conflict Model

The integrated relational perspective on the therapeutic action of psychoanalysis, which has informed earlier chapters, represents a convergence of interpersonal psychoanalysis, object-relations theories such as those of Fairbairn and Racker, and certain currents of both self psychology and existential psychoanalysis. Writers about this model start from a premise similar to that of developmental-arrest authors, that the pursuit and maintenance of human relatedness is the basic maturational thrust in human experience. But in the relational-conflict view disturbances in early relationships with caretakers are understood to seriously distort subsequent relatedness, not by freezing infantile needs in place, but by setting in motion a complex process through which the child builds an interpersonal world (a world of object relations) from what is available.

While not discounting the importance of the expansion of consciousness and the provision of missed early experiences, this model locates the central mechanism of analytic change in an alteration in the basic structure of the analysand's relational world. Theorists have depicted this process in various ways, focusing on different dimensions of the relational matrix: self-organization, object ties, or transactional patterns.

From the point of view of self-organization, the analytic situation allows the analysand to recover, reconnect with, and fully experience aspects of himself previously disclaimed, hidden, disavowed. The relationship with the analyst is necessarily structured along the old lines. Anxiety and disappointment are anticipated where they were previously experienced, and various areas of self-experience are hidden. The analyst's dogged inquiry into anxiety-ridden areas of the patient's life, and his participation in new forms of interaction, enables the patient to encounter, name, and appreciate facets of his experience unknown before. The analysand can now be a different sort of person in his experience of the analyst and others than he could allow himself to be before.

Other relational-model theorists (Fairbairn and Racker, for instance) describe the same process in terms of alterations in internal object relations. The self here also is formed in complementarity with the character structures of significant others. Areas of deprivation, constriction, and intrusion result in attachments to these qualities in the parents as the form through which contact is made, as vehicles for maintaining a sense of connectedness and relation. Early object ties are maintained as powerful internal presences; current object relations are experienced projectively in terms of those internal object relations and subsequently structured through a reintegration of new experiences into never-changing old configurations. Analytic change entails an alteration of these internal structures and relationships. The analyst, who is inevitably experienced as and transformed into a characteristic bad object, becomes, through the process of interpretation, a different sort of object. The internalization of this experience enables the patient to release his compulsive link to past forms of relation, his ties to bad objects. The intrapsychic domain of his relational matrix is thus transformed. He not only experiences himself as a different sort of person, he experiences himself as residing in a profoundly different human environment.

Other relational-model theorists, particularly those in the interpersonal tradition, have focused on the way in which the analytic process facilitates changes in the analysand's transactional patterns. Anxiety about anxiety has forced the analysand into repetitive, constricted patterns in his interactions with others. From this angle, it is the ritualized action that delimits the experience of *both* self and other, because the continual repetition of stereotyped integrations makes it impossible for the analysand to experience himself or anyone else in other than collapsed, unidimensional ways. By articulating and elucidating these patterns, the analytic process encourages the analysand to try something different, to put himself in a different interpersonal situation in which richer experiences of self and other are possible. These changes in transactional patterns take place both outside the analytic situation as the analytic inquiry continually highlights stereotyped patterns and compulsive enactments, and also in the analytic relationship itself, where analyst and analysand together find ways of being with each other outside those enactments and restraints. (Balint's invitation to the somersault, described in Chapter 6, is an excellent example.)

These three approaches illuminate different facets of the same process. Operating with old illusions and stereotyped patterns reduces anxiety and provides security not simply because the illusions and patterns are *familiar*, but also because they are *familial* and preserve a sense of loyalty and connection. Bad-object ties are adhesive and repetitive not simply because they are *familial*, but also because they are *familiar* and thereby minimize anxiety. The common etymological origin of the words "family" and "familiar" is the Latin *familia*, which originally meant the servants and slaves of a great house, underscoring the close connection between "human bonds and bondage," to use Schecter's phrase (1971). The maintenance of a coherent sense of self and the preservation of secure patterns of interaction are inextricably linked to *securing* connections with others.

How do these different emphases translate into our understanding of clinical data?

From the point of view of self-organization, psychopathology is repeated because it provides the organizational glue that holds the self together. What is new is frightening because it is outside the bounds of experiences in which the analysand recognizes himself to be himself, a cohesive, continuous being.

From the point of view of object ties, psychopathology is repeated because it functions to preserve early connections to significant others. What is new is frightening because it requires what the patient experiences as the abandonment of old loyalties, through which he feels connected and devoted.

From the point of view of transactions, psychopathology is repeated because it works interpersonally; it functions to minimize anxiety. What is new is frightening because it is associated with past parental anxiety. Security operations steer the analysand into familiar channels and away from the anxiety-shrouded unknown.

I regard each of these formulations as useful. The analysand does not know any other way to be, and does not want to know any other way, because of the object loss and guilt, the fear of self-loss and loneliness, that behaving and experiencing oneself differently implies. These approaches enrich one another in illuminating the tenacity and complexity of psychopathology, the tightness and durability of Penelope's weave.

The analysand enters treatment looking for something new *and* for something old. His life is not working in some major respect; he has to determine what is wrong, find a solution, and is hoping for something novel from the analyst—some way to open a door which will expand or transform his experience. No matter how hopeless, defeating, or self-defeating the most pessimistic patient, his presence in treatment is at least a minimal acknowledgment of the possibility of something different, an opening up of his relational world.

Yet the analysand is inevitably looking for something new in old ways. He enters treatment by structuring it along old relational lines, by seeking to engage the analyst according to prestructured notions of how people really connect, really touch each other. The analyst is assigned certain roles or, more generally, a choice of several possible roles. These configurations and roles vary from session to session or even within a single session.

Where does the analyst position himself with respect to these claims and hopes? What does he try to do? How does he help to loosen the tightness of the relational weave?

The classical position places the analyst outside the analysand's relational matrix, pointing his finger at its archaic and conflictual workings and enjoining the patient to renounce its doomed infantile promises. The developmental-arrest position also places the analyst outside the analysand's relational matrix, luring the patient away from its constrictions and offering something better. The third perspective portrays the analyst as discovering himself *within* the structures and strictures of the repetitive configurations of the analysand's relational matrix. The struggle to find his way out, the collaborative effort of analyst and analysand to observe and understand these configurations and to discover other channels through which to engage each other, is the crucible of analytic change.

This way of understanding the analytic situation has emerged from several different theoretical traditions and has been described most persuasively by Levenson, Racker, Gill, and Sandler. For each of these authors, the analyst is regarded as, at least to some degree, embedded within the analysand's relational matrix. There is no way for the analyst to avoid his assigned roles and configurations within the analysand's relational world. The analyst's experience is necessarily shaped by the analysand's relational structures; he plays assigned roles even if he desperately tries to stand outside the patient's system and play no role at all.

His very efforts at disengagement are particular forms of relatedness within the analysand's repertoire of roles and characters. As Hoffman (1987, p. 7) has put it, despite his conscious intentions, the analyst's participation is "relatively uncontrolled at the experiential level." If he is open to the nuances of his experience and the analysand's impact on that experience, he sometimes finds himself enacting the *patient's* old scenarios, speaking in a voice not wholly his, and sometimes enacting his *own* old scenarios, as various parallel or complementary voices from his own past and his own dynamics are evoked within the complexity of the interaction with each analysand.

From this perspective, speaking from within the analysand's subjective world can be regarded as in some sense a precondition for the treatment. Unless the analyst affectively enters the patient's relational matrix or, rather, discovers himself within it—unless the analyst is in some sense charmed by the patient's entreaties, shaped by the patient's projections, antagonized and frustrated by the patient's defenses—the treatment is never fully engaged, and a certain depth within the analytic experience is lost.

This does not grant a license to the analyst to do whatever he feels like. He must always strive to sustain what Schafer has termed the analytic attitude, by continually reflecting on and questioning all the data of the analytic hour and maintaining at all times a concern for the patient's ultimate well-being. But one inevitably and continually loses and regains that attitude; the losses and departures are regarded as interesting and useful in the analyst's struggle to understand what happens between the analysand and other people.

A wonderful story about the composer Stravinsky captures the importance of both dimensions of the dialectic between intent and actuality. "He had written a new piece with a difficult violin passage. After it had been in rehearsal for several weeks, the solo violinist came to Stravinsky and said he was sorry, he had tried his best, the passage was too difficult; no violinist could play it. Stravinsky said, 'I understand that. What I am after is the sound of someone *trying* to play it'" (Powers, 1984, p. 54). Similarly, in characterizing the analyst's presence, two dimensions are crucial: what the analyst is *trying* to do and what he or she *does* do while trying, the inevitable engagement in various configurations within the analysand's relational world. The relational-conflict model places much greater importance on the content of the analyst's unintended forms of participation.

If the analyst is caught in the patient's "affective net" (L. Friedman), if he comes to experience himself as the patient's archaic objects, and if the patient inevitably experiences the analyst according to the old categories anyway, how is it possible for the analyst, even when interpreting, to step outside the patient's system and be experienced by the patient as offering a different sort of relatedness? If the transference-countertransference configuration is sadomasochistic, will the analysand not *hear* the analyst's interpretations as either sadistic assaults or pitiful surrenders? If the basic transference-countertransference configuration concerns symbiotic merger, will the analysand not experience the analyst's interpretive activities as either seductive fusions or remote detachments? Altering the analysand's relational matrix seems to require a kind of bootstrapping operation in which analyst and analysand in a quantum leap lift themselves from one kind of interpersonal engagement to another.

The analyst must not simply *understand* the analysand, he must also find a voice to communicate that understanding; to be heard by the analysand, he needs to somehow find a way out of the analysand's conventional patterns of hearing and experiencing. This process involves the art of interpretation and the struggle with countertransference, both complex and closely intertwined processes.

Interpretation, Transference, Countertransference

Interpretation has always been regarded as the quintessential activity of the analyst, the basic lever to generate analytic change. But important differences have emerged in the efforts to understand what happens when the analyst interprets, what it is in the interpretive process that allows for change. In the classical model, the interpretation has its effect in the internal psychic economy of the analysand; the information conveyed by the interpretation reveals hidden content, lifts repression barriers, and thereby shifts the internal balance of psychic forces. In the developmental-arrest model, the interpretation has its effect in the *experience* it generates in the patient, who feels deeply cared about and understood; it is not the content, the information conveyed, but the affective tone and its emotional impact that restimulate the stalled developmental process.

In the relational-conflict model, both the informational content and the affective tone are regarded as crucial, but their effects are understood somewhat differently—in terms of their role in *positioning* the analyst relative to the analysand. An interpretation is a *complex relational event,* not primarily because it alters something inside the analysand, not because it releases a stalled developmental process, but because it says something very important about where the analyst stands vis-à-vis the analysand, about what sort of relatedness is possible between the two of them. As Levenson puts it,

> When we talk with someone, we also act with him. This action or behavior is, in the semiotic sense, coded like a language. *The language of speech and the language of action will be transforms of each other;* that is, they will be, in musical terms, harmonic variations on the same theme. The resultant behavior of the dyad will emerge out of this semiotic discourse. (1983, p. 81; italics in original)

Finding a voice with which to make useful interpretations itself involves a struggle to emerge from the strictures of the jointly created transference-countertransference configurations. Levenson characterizes this process as "resisting transformation"; Racker calls it "mastering the countertransference." This is a two-stage process. The analysand necessarily must get into the transference (overcoming what Gill, 1982, terms "resistance to the awareness of the transference") before he can get out of it (overcoming "resistances to the working through of the transference"). Similarly, the analyst must first *experience* the countertransference, or rather discover himself within it, before he can begin to find his way out of it. One cannot resist or master something one has not first been transformed by.

The analyst discovers himself a coactor in a passionate drama involving love and hate, sexuality and murder, intrusion and abandonment, victims and executioners. Whichever path he chooses, he falls into one of the patient's predesigned categories and is experienced by the patient in that way. The struggle is toward a new way of experiencing both himself and the patient, a different way of being with the analysand, in which one is neither fused nor detached, seductive nor rejecting, victim nor executioner. The struggle is to find an authentic voice in which to speak to the analysand, a voice more fully one's own, less shaped by the configurations and limited options of the analysand's relational matrix, and, in so doing, offering the analysand a chance to broaden and expand that matrix.

Kohut argues repeatedly that there are two options in approaching the analysand's material, particularly transferential needs and attributions. One either empathically accepts them as developmentally appropriate or "censoriously" judges them as inappropriate and immature; one either accepts and shapes oneself according to the patient's subjectivity, or imposes one's own version of objective reality. This dichotomy (forged in Kohut's dialectical reaction to his experience of the classical stance) omits a third option—genuine curiosity. How did we get into this? Why do you experience differences between us as assaultive and disrespectful? Why do I often find myself assaulting (or wanting to assault) you? How can we together find a way of talking with each other which allows you your self-respect and me some possibility of being and using myself more authentically in a way that might be helpful to you? Not all these questions are asked explicitly, and certainly not all at once, but they frame the kind of inquiring stance the analyst strives to establish and invites the analysand to join.

In this view of the analytic process, change is brought about neither by exploring and mirroring or "holding" the analysand's subjective experience, nor by entreating the analysand to realign his hopes and wishes according to the analyst's sense of appropriateness (presented as "reality" or "maturity"). Rather, analytic change entails a struggle by both participants to overcome precisely these kinds of imbalances, which characterize pathological patterns of integration and in which differences in experience threaten the interpersonal connection rather than enrich it. As Schwartz has put it, "In the analytic setting, the work of interpretation is not to exchange illusion for reality but to establish a boundary between the patient's experience and the analyst's and to bridge it simultaneously" (1978, p. 9).

The problem with techniques which suggest a specific analytic demeanor and position from which the analyst delivers interpretations, such as concepts of "neutrality," "working alliance," the "empathic stance," is that in addition to undermining the genuineness of the analytic interaction, they presuppose that from the beginning the analysand sees the analyst as speaking from outside the analysand's transferential configurations. Rather, the analyst becomes the various figures in the analysand's relational matrix, taking on their attributes and assuming their voices; the analyst and the analysand gradually rewrite the narrative, transforming those characters in a direction which will allow greater intimacy and more possibilities for varied experience and relatedness. One never stands completely outside the transference-countertransference configurations; instead, one struggles continually to emerge from them. As constricting transferential constraints are clarified through interpretive activity, the newly won relational positions themselves take on new transferential meanings which carry with them their own constraints. (See in this connection Black, 1987.)

CONSIDER THE differences among the three models with regard to understanding and engaging transference. Does the analysand experience the analyst in terms of the past (what Freud called "earlier editions"), or is the transference at least partially a response to input from the analyst?

Arlow (1985) highlights drive-conflict premises when he argues that the actuality of the analyst operates like the day residue in the dream, an inconsequential trigger allowing a smuggled access to the preconscious, making possible the emergence of unconscious fantasy. "The persistent influence of unconscious fantasy creates the mental set against which the data of perception are perceived, registered, integrated, remembered and responded to." The patient literally is blinded to, misses the actual, or what we might call the "interpersonal," because he is living subjectively in the past. "The neurotic process and transference may be understood as representing how the individual misperceives, misintegrates, and misresponds to, the data of perception, in terms of the mental set created by persistent unconscious fantasies" (p. 526).

Hoffman (1983) has contrasted this approach with what he terms a relativistic-social view of the analytic situation, our third model. Here the analysand is regarded as building subjective reality in the transference out of the "plausible" (to use Gill's term) interpretation of what is actually going on. One can understand the analyst's participation in various ways: as bringing to the field his own character and individuality; or as transformed, through induced countertransference, by the analysand's transference. What these approaches have in common is the assumption that the analysand's subjective experience of the analyst is open to and to a large extent shaped by the interactions with the analyst.

Abrams and Shengold (1978) contrast this view of the analytic situation as an "encounter" with the view of it as an examination of intrapsychic processes. From the traditional drive-conflict point of view, there is no encountering the analyst except as a screen for the patient to encounter himself. From the point of view of our third model, there is no examination of intrapsychic processes except as they are transformed and in a sense uniquely created in the encounter with the analyst.

The developmental-arrest point of view tends to emphasize the importance of *past* interpersonal experience, but not the particularities of the *present* interaction with the analyst. The child's early experience is regarded as heavily influenced by his or her interpersonal world, resulting in a developmental arrest, which is reexperienced *as emerging* in the analytic situation. But the patient's experience of the analyst is understood to be largely intrapsychically determined and merely *released* by the nurturing presence of the analyst. Goldberg notes the contrast between this and a more fully interactive position:

> Self psychology struggles hard not to be an interpersonal psychology not only because it wishes to avoid the social psychological connotations of the phrase but also because it wishes to minimize the input of the analyst into the mix . . . Since self psychology is so preeminently a developmental psychology, it is based on the idea of a developmental program (one that may be innate or pre-wired if you wish) that will reconstitute itself under certain conditions. (1986, p. 387)

Here again is the assumption that there is an "inside" to the patient which can manifest itself more or less independently of the interactive situation in which it appears. The analyst's responses are meaningful, but in a generic, binary sort of way. They are either empathically attuned enough to release the stalled developmental process, or they miss and thereby perpetuate the stalemate. Gill (1983) has noted that in such formulations, the analyst is not so much a fully interpersonal "participant-observer" but rather a "precipitant-observer," a simple trigger for processes inside the patient.

All experience, whether in childhood or in the analytic situation, is composed of a complex mixture of what the subject brings to the experience, either constitutionally or from past interactions, and what he encounters in real transactions with others. Psychoanalytic theories of technique differ in how they conceive the ratio of these ingredients. Gill has argued for an integration which grants centrality to both sets of determinants.

> The individual sees the world not only as his intrapsychic patterns dictate, but also as he veridically assesses it. Furthermore, the two kinds of determinants mutually influence each other. The intrapsychic patterns not only determine selective attention to those aspects of the external world which

conform to them, but the individual behaves in such a way as to enhance the likelihood that the responses he meets will indeed confirm the views with which he sets out. This external validation in turn is necessary for the maintenance of those patterns . . . The unique contribution of psychoanalysis is the demonstration of the power and persistence of the intrapsychic determinants. But these determinants become only artificial abstractions if they are dealt with in isolation from the interpersonal context in which they find expression. (1982, p. 92)

Which model of the analytic situation is correct? Is the analysand playing out intrapsychically determined structures regardless of the particularities of the analyst's participation? Is the analysand patterning the analytic situation to find missing parental experiences to unlock his frozen growth? Or is the analysand structuring the analytic situation in an effort to reach and engage the analyst, the particular analyst with all his idiosyncrasies and individually styled presence, in the only ways he knows? It is probably not useful to ask about the relative truths of these perspectives, since they can never be compared in empirically controlled fashion. It is more useful to ask about the implications of each model for the analytic process, the way in which each understanding of the analytic situation structures the process itself and creates a distinctive sort of analytic relationship.

In the classical model, as Arlow's description makes clear, the patient *misses*—"misperceives, misintegrates, and misresponds" (1985, p. 526). The analyst provides an "objective" perspective; nothing in the patient's perceptions sticks to him. This is a model of the analytic situation composed of one subject and one observer, both studying the mind of the patient, and the analytic relationship is structured in hierarchical fashion.

In the developmental-arrest model, the analysand, like the proverbial "customer," is always right. The analyst attempts to melt into the background; the focus is on articulation of the analysand's phenomenology, with particular emphasis on organizations concerning the self as baby and the self as damaged. This is a model of the analytic situation composed of one subject and one facilitator, the latter allowing the mind of the patient to resume interrupted growth; the analytic relationship is structured in a benevolently protective fashion.

In the relational-conflict model, there is a continual oscillation between old and new relational configurations, between the articulation of the passions and organizational structures of the analysand's phenomenology and the introduction of the analyst's perspective (as neither more "real" nor more "mature," but as different and possibly useful). The analyst is constantly in the midst of the transference-countertransference integrations, shaped by the analysand's relational configurations and struggling to understand and thereby reshape them from within. The aim is to broaden the analytic relationship, and by extension the analysand's other relationships as well, into richer, more dialectical exchanges.

The implications of the distinction between the premise of mind as monadic and the premise of mind as interactive are nowhere so clear as they are in approaching the complexities of the analytic situation. If one views the analysand's experience of the analysis and the analyst as fundamentally monadic, the analyst is outside that experience and should *stay* outside it. Ultimately it has nothing to do with him. The analysand's free associations and transferential experiences unfold in his presence, and would do so (the same in all fundamental respects) with any analyst employing "proper" technique. Efforts to relate the material to himself would make the analyst an intruder, a contaminant, whether one regards the process as an unfolding of infantile wishes or of developmental needs.

If one views the analysand's experience of the analysis and the analyst as fundamentally interactive, as an encounter between two *persons,* the analysand is struggling to reach *this* analyst. Familiar timeworn strategies are employed, to be sure, but as pathways to connect with what the analysand has experienced about this particular analyst as a person. The problem is no longer past significant others, but how to connect with, surrender to, dominate, fuse with, control, love, be loved by, use, be used by, *this* person.

From a monadic standpoint, the analyst finds the patient, as the patient transposes past experience into the neutral medium of the analytic situation. From an interactive standpoint, the patient also finds the analyst, and it is crucial that the analyst recognize this finding as an encounter, not just a transposition to him of something foreign. Within this framework, for the analyst to view the analytic situation as monadic and the analysand's experience of him as by definition distorted—this is a powerful and destructive form of interaction indeed.

HOW WOULD one view the clinical vignette of the dual-control car from the perspective of the relational-conflict model? The wish to surrender would not be regarded as emerging from inside the patient, either as an instinctual derivative to be renounced or as the cutting edge of authentic growth to be nourished. Rather, the wish would be seen as the patient's effort to connect with the analyst in the way she connected with the parents. Although conflictual, she regards such a surrender as the most precious human bond, and as the price of a promise of total, protective care. The patient longs for and in fact spends her life seeking to make good on this bad promise, while at the same time dimly recognizing its fraudulence and danger. In this view, one never gives up the master control, and the lure of doing so is part of the illusory solution to life offered by the parents.

The analytic relationship will be organized around the patient's conflictual longing and fear; the analysis itself (and the process of free association) will be experienced as submission to an illusory total care, provided by the analyst's interpretations. The therapeutic action will reside in the analyst's discovering himself in this integration, in the traces of his own claims to omnipotence and his own impinging dominance, and in finding a voice with which to describe their relationship to the patient which involves neither submission, detachment, nor assumption of control. The gambit is gradually declined. What is therapeutic is not a surrender to the analyst's illusory wisdom and control, but a gradual restructuring of the relationship on more collaborative terms.

Authenticity on the part of the analyst does not imply impulsivity or compulsive confession, but a struggle first to experience himself and the patient outside the predesigned categories into which all interpersonal experience is slotted. There is generally no grand revelation: what happens is a gradual process of disentanglement, through the analyst's interpretive activity. The progress of the analytic relationship is not like a hatching, in which new life breaks free of its shell once and for all; it is more like a series of moltings, in which new life emerges from old skin, becomes greatly facilitative for a time, and eventually itself becomes constraining and must be discarded so that further growth can occur.

Return to the Mainland

The following vignette illustrates the way the analytic process might be thought of as a broadening of the relational matrix to allow new experiences of self in relation to others, and shows the central role of the analytic relationship in facilitating that change.

Sam came to treatment because of compulsive overeating, recurrent depressions, and a long-standing romantic involvement with a woman considerably more overweight and depressed than himself—whom he wanted to leave but could not. The most striking feature of his life was its unevenness. He was an extremely capable and creative person, highly successful and respected in his career, yet he experienced himself as depressed, deeply flawed, fundamentally damaged; his most intimate relationships had been adhesive, joyless attachments to women seen as disadvantaged in some important respect. A considerable portion of the time he and his lover were physically separated would be spent on the telephone with each other, not talking, but listening to the other breathe, keeping alive the contact.

Sam was the elder of two children born to second-generation Italian parents who both felt crushed by life. His mother's family had been impoverished and dominated by her tyrannical, repressive father. She, frightened and terribly shy, led an isolated and sheltered life, finally marrying, quite late, a man who seemed to offer some hope of escape. Sam's father, in his younger years, was a vital, expansive, somewhat manic character, who offered Sam a lively and crucially important alternative to his mother's anxious attempts to control and protect him. When Sam was four, a sister was born, who came to represent all the mother's hopes and dreams. Although the parents denied it for years, it slowly became apparent that a traumatic birth had left the girl severely brain damaged. This blow, in addition to several business failures and illnesses, led to a deep, depressive withdrawal by both parents. They would take hot baths for hours, lie around in bed, often with the damaged child, and find joy only in gluttonous eating. Except for Sam, the family members became slovenly and inactive. Sam was viewed ambivalently: on the one hand, he was the family's emissary to the real world—he would take care of them and save them; on the other hand, his involvement with life was viewed suspiciously, as an abandonment and a betrayal.

Analytic inquiry revealed that Sam's deep sense of self-as-damaged and his depression functioned as a mechanism for maintaining his attachment to his family. Sam and his family, it gradually became clear, had made depression a credo, a way of life. They saw the world as a painful place, filled with suffering. People who enjoyed life were shallow, intellectually and morally deficient, by definition frivolous and uninteresting. He was drawn to people who seemed to suffer greatly, was extremely empathic with and helpful to them, then would feel ensnared. The closest possible experience for people, he felt, was to cry together; joy and pleasure were private, disconnecting, almost shameful.

Sam and his analyst considered how this form of connection affected his relationship with the analyst. They explored various fantasies pertaining to the analyst's suffering, Sam's anticipated solicitous ministrations, and their languishing together forever in misery. In a much more subtle way, Sam's deeply sensitive, warmly sympathetic presence contributed to a sad but cozy atmosphere in the sessions that the analyst found himself enjoying. Sam's capacity to offer this kind of connection was both eminently soothing and somehow disquieting. The analyst came to see that this cozy ambience was contingent on Sam's belief that in some way he was being profoundly helpful to the analyst. The latter was the mighty healer, the one who needed care. This evoked what the analyst came to identify as a strong countertransferential appeal to surrender to Sam's attentive ministrations, which alternated with equally powerful resistances to that pull, involving detachment, manic reversals, and so on. The mechanism of Sam's self-perpetuated depression and the crucial struggle in the countertransference to find a different form of connection was expressed most clearly in one particular session.

He came in one day feeling good, after some exciting career and social successes. As it happened, on that day the analyst *was* feeling depressed. Although, as far as he could tell, the origins of his mood were unrelated to Sam, Sam's ready solicitations and concern were, as always, a genuine comfort. Early into the session, Sam's mood dropped precipitously as he began to speak of various areas of painful experience and a hopeless sense of himself as deeply defective. The analyst stopped him, wondering about the mood shift. They were able to reconstruct what had happened, to trace his depressive response back to the point of anxiety. With hawklike acuity he had perceived the analyst's depression. He had been horrified to find himself feeling elated and excited in the presence of another's suffering. An immediate depressive plunge was called for. To feel vital and alive when someone else is hurting seemed a barbaric crime, risking hateful retaliation and total destruction of the relationship. His approach to all people he cared about, they came to understand, was to lower his mood to the lowest common denominator. To simply enjoy himself and his life, without constantly toning himself down and checking the depressive pulse of others, meant he hazarded being seen as a traitorous villain and, as a consequence, ending up in total isolation. The analyst asked him in that session whether it had occurred to him that the analyst might *not* resent his good mood, but might actually feel cheered by Sam's enthusiasm and vitality (which was in fact the case that day). This never had occurred to him, seemed totally incredible, and provoked considerable reflection. Through this and similar exchanges their relationship gradually changed, as they articulated old patterns of integration and explored new possibilities. Sam began to feel entitled to his own experience, regardless of the affective state of others.

Thus, Sam's sense of self-as-damaged, which was the core of his depression, eventually was understood as a vehicle for the perpetuation of old object ties and his characteristic mode of integrating relationships with others, as well as a means for controlling anxiety. The members of his family felt connected through psychic pain, inadequacy, and defeat. The depressive fusion of the parents, and the despondent caretaking of their damaged daughter, became Sam's model of human intimacy. To relate in other ways and to assume full ownership of his resources and successes was to be pervaded by intense anxiety, the anxiety of the unfamiliar and of options incompatible with the familial mode of contact.

In one session after several years of treatment, Sam experienced for the first time a strong sense of euphoria—which precipitated an anxiety attack. He moved from feeling intensely joyful and buoyant to feeling lighter and lighter, less and less substantial, to feeling in terror of floating off into space, losing touch with others altogether. To feel joy placed him, experientially, outside the family, outside the realm of deep human connection. What was most deeply repressed in Sam was precisely his capacity for joy, which posed the severest threat to his characterological pattern of living.

Sam presented the following dream toward the end of treatment, during a period when he had been experiencing himself and his relationships with others in a more positive way. Like all important experiences which stretch the boundaries of character, these changes made him anxious. He feared that it was his depression and sensitivity to depression in others that made him a desirable person.

> I am on a small island off the mainland with my parents and sister. I take a boat to the mainland to pick up some things or do some errand. There is a carnival going on. I walk around, watching the people, participating, having a great time. Then I remember that I must return to the island. I get

in the boat and try to go back, but insects come and sting me. If I move back and stop rowing, they stop. I start to move toward the island and they sting again. I stop; they stop. I am very conflicted about what to do. After a long time of trying and stopping, I give up with a sense of relief and rejoin the activities on the mainland.

The dream seemed to capture Sam's experience at this point in treatment. He had begun to feel a sense of rich possibilities which life and other people offer. Yet he also felt bound by his loyalties to his family and their ways. The connection to them was maintained through a stinging pain. As long as he suffered as they had, experiencing himself as irreversibly damaged and isolated from others, he was bound up with them. To live more fully would be to abandon them and the security provided by the tie to them.

THE RE-CREATION of the constricted self-organization, internal object ties, and rigid interpersonal patterns which constitute the relational matrix is an active, often obstinately willful process. Deep characterological alteration through the analytic process is not simply a change in psychic economy, but a profound change in the inhabitants populating the world in which the patient lives. As bad-object ties are slowly given up and risks are taken for other sorts of relationships, the cast of characters in one's subjective world changes—the possibility of a new kind of life emerges. To endure this, and to tolerate the new sense of aloneness that comes with giving up the fantasied contact with parents which psychopathology often provides, the analysand must begin to *believe* that another world is possible. Even so, analytic change requires great courage.

If the deepest, most fundamental levels of the analysand's pathology are to be reached, the relationship with the analyst becomes the vehicle for the establishment and articulation of bad-object relations. The analyst cannot enter the analysand's world in any form other than as a familiar (that is, "bad," or less than gratifying, object). This is true even though there often are elaborate resistances to the experience of the transference (Gill, 1982). Otherwise the analysis does not touch the analysand deeply, offers no promise, no hope for connection and transformation.

The analysand insists that the analyst remain a transferential, unsatisfying object; the analyst, in his internal struggle to grasp and free himself of this role, and in his interpretive effort to clarify and understand the patient's insistence, offers something different, something new, another form of engagement and relation. It is left to the analysand to choose, and that choice is not a single event but a continual process. Just as the island in Sam's dream is always there, calling him back, old relational configurations do not disappear but continue to exist as a perpetual possibility. In this sense, psychoanalytic models that depict health in terms of structural change can be as misleading as the metaphor of damage in explaining psychopathology, as if some vast adaptive machinery has fallen into place or some massive internal foundation has been set in concrete. Postanalytic residues of constricted self-organization, old object ties, and rigid transactional patterns all exist as perpetual possibilities. Constructive, creative living necessitates continual choice.

References
Index

References

Abraham, K. 1919. A particular form of neurotic resistance against the psycho-analytic method. In *The evolution of psychoanalytic technique,* ed. M. Bergmann and F. Hartman. New York: Basic Books, 1976.

———— 1921. Contributions to the theory of the anal character. In *Selected papers on psycho-analysis.* London: Hogarth Press, 1973.

Abrams, S., and L. Shengold. 1978. Some reflexions on the topic of the 30th Congress: "affects and the psychoanalytic situation." *International Journal of Psychoanalysis,* 59:395–407.

Arlow, J. 1985. The concept of psychic reality and related problems. *Journal of the American Psychoanalytic Association,* 33:521–535.

Aron, L. 1988. Dreams, narrative and the psychoanalytic method. *Contemporary Psychoanalysis* (in press).

Atwood, G., and R. Stolorow. 1984. *Structures of subjectivity: explorations in psychoanalytic phenomenology.* Hillsdale, N.J.: Analytic Press.

Balint, M. 1968. *The basic fault: therapeutic aspects of regression.* London: Tavistock.

Bergmann, M. 1971. Psychoanalytic observations on the capacity to love. In *Separation-individuation: essays in honor of Margaret S. Mahler,* ed. J. McDevitt and C. Settlage. New York: International Universities Press.

Berlin, I. 1953. *The hedgehog and the fox: an essay on Tolstoy's view of history.* New York: Simon and Schuster.

Bion, W. R. 1957. Differentiation of the psychotic from the nonpsychotic personalities. In *Second thoughts: selected papers on psycho-analysis.* New York: Jason Aronson, 1967.

Black, M. 1987. The analyst's stance: transferential implications of technical orientation. In *The annual of psychoanalysis*. Chicago: University of Chicago Press.

Blanck, G., and R. Blanck. 1974. *Ego psychology: theory and practice*. New York: Columbia University Press.

Bloom, H. 1986. Freud, the greatest modern writer. *New York Times Book Review*. March 23.

Bowlby, J. 1969. *Attachment*. New York: Basic Books.

———1973. *Separation: anxiety and anger*. New York: Basic Books.

———1975. *Loss: sadness and depression*. New York: Basic Books.

Braudel, F. 1949. *The Mediterranean and the Mediterranean world in the age of Philip II*, trans. S. Reynolds. New York: Harper.

Brenner, C. 1982. *The mind in conflict*. New York: International Universities Press.

Bridgeman, P. W. 1927. *The logic of modern physics*. New York: Macmillan.

Bromberg, P. 1983. The mirror and the mask: on narcissism and psychoanalytic growth. *Contemporary Psychoanalysis*, 19:349–387.

Campbell, J. 1959. *The masks of God: primitive mythology*. New York: Viking Press.

Cooper, A. 1987. Changes in psychoanalytic ideas: transference interpretation. *Journal of the American Psychoanalytic Association*, 35:77–98.

Dennett, D. 1985. *Elbow room: the varieties of free will worth wanting*. Cambridge, Mass.: MIT Press.

Deutsch, H. 1937. Folie à deux. In *Neuroses and character types*. New York: International Universities Press, 1965.

Eagle, M. 1984. *Recent developments in psychoanalysis*. New York: McGraw-Hill.

Eagleton, T. 1983. *Literary theory: an introduction*. Minneapolis: University of Minnesota Press.

Ellenberger, H. 1970. *The discovery of the unconscious: the history and evolution of dynamic psychiatry*. New York: Basic Books.

Erikson, E. 1950. *Childhood and society*. New York: Norton.

Escher, M. C. 1967. *The graphic work of M. C. Escher*. New York: Hawthorn/Balantine.

Fairbairn, W. R. D. 1952. *An object-relations theory of the personality*. New York: Basic Books.

——— 1958. On the nature and aims of psycho-analytical treatment. *International Journal of Psychoanalysis*, 39:374–385.

Farber, L. 1976. *Lying, despair, jealousy, envy, sex, suicide, drugs, and the good life*. New York: Basic Books.

Fenichel, O. 1927. Identification. In *The collected papers of Otto Fenichel*. New York: David Lewis.

——— 1941. *Problems in psychoanalytic technique*. New York: Psychoanalytic Quarterly.

——— 1945. *The psychoanalytic theory of neurosis*. New York: Norton.

Flew, A. 1970. Psychoanalysis and free will. In *Psychoanalysis and philosophy*, ed. C. Hanly and M. Lazerowitz. New York: International Universities Press.

Freud, S. All references are to *The standard edition of the complete psychological works of Sigmund Freud*, vols. 1–24. London: Hogarth Press, 1953–1974. *(SE)*

—— 1892a. A case of successful treatment by hypnotism. *SE*, 1:117–128.

—— 1892b. Preface and footnotes to Charcot's *Tuesday lectures*. *SE*, 1:131–146.

—— 1894. The neuro-psychoses of defense. *SE*, 3:43–61.

—— 1895. Project for a scientific psychology. *SE*, 1:283–387.

—— 1896. Further remarks on the neuro-psychoses of defense. *SE*, 3:159–185.

—— 1900. *The interpretation of dreams*. *SE*, 4 and 5.

—— 1905a. *Three essays on the theory of sexuality*. *SE*, 7:125–245.

—— 1905b. Fragment of an analysis of a case of hysteria. *SE*, 7:1–122.

—— 1906. My views on the part played by sexuality in the aetiology of the neuroses. *SE*, 7:269–279.

—— 1907. Delusions and dreams in Jensen's *Gradiva*. *SE*, 9:7–96.

—— 1910. A special type of choice of object made by men. *SE*, 11:163–175.

—— 1911. Formulations on the two principles of mental functioning. *SE*, 12:218–226.

—— 1912a. On the universal tendency to debasement in the sphere of love. *SE*, 11:177–190.

—— 1912b. The dynamics of transference. *SE*, 12:99–108.

—— 1912–13. *Totem and taboo*. *SE*, 13:1–162.

—— 1914a. On the history of the psycho-analytic movement. *SE*, 14:1–66.

—— 1914b. On narcissism: an introduction. *SE*, 14:67–102.

—— 1915a. Instincts and their vicissitudes. *SE*, 14:117–140.

—— 1915b. Observations on transference-love. *SE*, 12:157–171.

—— 1916–17. Introductory lectures on psycho-analysis. *SE*, 15 and 16.

—— 1917. Mourning and melancholia. *SE*, 14:237–258.

—— 1918. From the history of an infantile neurosis. *SE*, 14:3–122.

—— 1920a. *Beyond the pleasure principle*. *SE*, 18:3–64.

—— 1920b. The psychogenesis of a case of homosexuality in a woman. *SE*, 18:147–172.

—— 1921. *Group psychology and the analysis of the ego*. *SE*, 18:65–143.

—— 1923. *The ego and the id*. *SE*, 19:1–66.

—— 1924a. The economic problem of masochism. *SE*, 19:155–170.

—— 1924b. The dissolution of the Oedipus complex. *SE*, 19:173–179.

—— 1925. Some additional notes on dream-interpretation as a whole. *SE*, 19:127–138.

—— 1927. Fetishism. *SE*, 21:147–157.

—— 1930. *Civilization and its discontents*. *SE*, 21:59–145.

—— 1933. *New introductory lectures on psycho-analysis*. *SE*, 22:1–182.

—— 1940. *An outline of psycho-analysis*. *SE*, 23:139–207.

—— 1950. Extracts from the Fliess papers. *SE*, 1:173–280.

—— 1985. *The complete letters of Sigmund Freud to Wilhelm Fliess, 1887–1904,* trans. and ed. J. M. Masson. Cambridge, Mass.: Belknap Press, Harvard University Press.

———— 1987. *A phylogenetic fantasy: overview of the transference neuroses.* Cambridge, Mass.: Belknap Press, Harvard University Press.

Freud, S., and J. Breuer. 1893. On the psychical mechanism of hysterical phenomena: a preliminary communication. *SE*, 2:1–13.

Friedman, L. 1978. Trends in the psychoanalytic theory of treatment. *Psychoanalytic Quarterly,* 47:524–567.

Friedman, M. 1985. Toward a reconceptualization of guilt. *Contemporary Psychoanalysis,* 21:501–547.

Fromm, E. 1941. *Escape from freedom.* New York: Avon.

———— 1947. *Man for himself.* Greenwich, Conn.: Fawcett.

———— 1964. *The heart of man.* New York: Harper and Row.

———— 1970. *The crisis of psychoanalysis.* Greenwich, Conn.: Fawcett.

Gay, P. 1969. *The Enlightenment: an interpretation.* New York: Norton.

Gedo, J. 1979. *Beyond interpretation.* New York: International Universities Press.

Gedo, J., and A. Goldberg. 1973. *Models of the mind.* Chicago: University of Chicago Press.

Gill, M. 1982. *Analysis of transference,* vol. 1. New York: International Universities Press.

———— 1983. The interpersonal paradigm and the degree of the therapist's involvement. *Contemporary Psychoanalysis,* 19:200–237.

Gilligan, C. 1982. *In a different voice.* Cambridge, Mass.: Harvard University Press.

Glover, E. 1955. *The technique of psycho-analysis.* New York: International Universities Press.

Goldberg, A. 1986. Reply to discussion of P. Bromberg of "The wishy-washy personality." *Contemporary Psychoanalysis,* 22:387–388.

————, ed. 1983. *The future of psychoanalysis.* New York: International Universities Press.

Gould, S. J. 1977. *Ontogeny and phylogeny.* Cambridge, Mass.: Belknap Press, Harvard University Press.

———— 1985. *The flamingo's smile: reflections in natural history.* New York: Norton.

———— 1987a. *Time's arrow, time's cycle.* Cambridge, Mass.: Harvard University Press.

———— 1987b. *An urchin in the storm.* New York: Norton.

Greenberg, J. In preparation. *Psychoanalytic theory in clinical practice.*

Greenberg, J., and S. Mitchell. 1983. *Object relations in psychoanalytic theory.* Cambridge, Mass.: Harvard University Press.

Guntrip, H. 1969. *Schizoid phenomena, object relations and the self.* New York: International Universities Press.

———— 1971. *Psychoanalytic theory, therapy and the self.* New York: Basic Books.

Hampshire, S. 1962. Disposition and memory. *International Journal of Psychoanalysis,* 43:59–68.

Hanly, C. 1979. *Existentialism and psychoanalysis.* New York: International Universities Press.

Hartmann, H. 1939. *Ego psychology and the problem of adaptation.* New York: International Universities Press.

———— 1950. Comments on the psychoanalysis of the ego. In *Essays on ego psychology.* New York: International Universities Press, 1964.

Hoffman, I. 1983. The patient as interpreter of the analyst's experience. *Contemporary Psychoanalysis,* 19:389–422.

———— 1987. Discussion of "The intrapsychic and the interpersonal" by Stephen A. Mitchell. Meeting of the Chicago Association for Psychoanalytic Psychology, December 5.

Hofstadter, D. 1979. *Gödel, Escher, Bach: an eternal golden braid.* New York: Vintage.

Holt, R. 1976. Drive or wish? A reconsideration of the psychoanalytic theory of motivation. In *Psychology versus metapsychology: psychoanalytic essays in memory of George S. Klein,* ed. M. Gill and P. Holzman. *Psychological Issues,* Monograph 36. New York: International Universities Press.

Homer. *The odyssey,* trans. R. Fitzgerald. New York: Doubleday, 1961.

Jacobson, E. 1964. *The self and the object world.* New York: International Universities Press.

Jones, E. 1957. *The life and work of Sigmund Freud,* vol. 3, *The last phase, 1919–1939.* London: Hogarth Press; New York: Basic Books.

Kagan, J. 1984. *The nature of the child.* New York: Basic Books.

Kaplan, D. 1985. Cultural affairs. *Contemporary Psychology,* 30:290–291.

Kermode, F. 1985. Freud and interpretation. *International Journal of Psychoanalysis,* 12:3–12.

Kernberg, O. 1975. *Borderline conditions and pathological narcissism.* New York: Jason Aronson.

———— 1980. *Internal world and external reality.* New York: Jason Aronson.

———— 1984. *Severe personality disorders: psychotherapeutic strategies.* New Haven: Yale University Press.

Khan, M. 1979. *Alienation in perversions.* New York: International Universities Press.

Klein, G. 1976. Freud's two theories of sexuality. In *Psychology vs. metapsychology,* ed. M. Gill and P. Holzman. New York: International Universities Press.

Klein, M. 1935. A contribution to the psychogenesis of manic-depressive states. In *Contributions to psychoanalysis, 1921–1945.* New York: McGraw-Hill, 1964.

———— 1940. Mourning and its relation to manic-depressive states. In *Contributions to psychoanalysis, 1921–1945.* New York: McGraw-Hill, 1964.

———— 1945. The Oedipus complex in light of early anxieties. In *Contributions to psychoanalysis, 1921–1945.* New York: McGraw-Hill, 1964.

—— 1957. Envy and gratitude. In *Envy and gratitude and other works, 1946–1963*. New York: Delacorte Press, 1975.

Kohut, H. 1971. *The analysis of the self.* New York: International Universities Press.

—— 1977. *The restoration of the self.* New York: International Universities Press.

—— 1979. The two analyses of Mr. Z. *International Journal of Psychoanalysis,* 60:3–27.

—— 1984. *How does analysis cure?* Chicago: University of Chicago Press.

Kuhn, T. 1962. *The structure of scientific revolutions,* 2nd ed. Chicago: University of Chicago Press.

Kundera, M. 1984. *The unbearable lightness of being.* New York: Harper.

Lachmann, F. 1985. Discussion of "New directions in psychoanalysis" by Michael Franz Basch. *Psychoanalytic Psychology,* 2:15–20.

Laing, R. D. 1976. *The facts of life: an essay in feeling, facts and fantasy.* New York: Pantheon.

Langer, S. 1972. *Mind: an essay on human feeling,* vol. 2. Baltimore: Johns Hopkins University Press.

Levenson, E. 1983. *The ambiguity of change.* New York: Basic Books.

—— 1985. The interpersonal (Sullivanian) model. In *Models of the mind,* ed. A. Rothstein. New York: International Universities Press.

Lewy, E. 1961. Responsibility, free will and ego psychology. *International Journal of Psychoanalysis,* 42:260–270.

Lichtenberg, J. 1983. *Psychoanalysis and infant research.* Hillsdale, N.J.: Analytic Press.

Lichtenstein, H. 1961. Identity and sexuality: a study of their interrelationship in man. *Journal of the American Psychoanalytic Association,* 9:179–260.

Lipton, S. 1955. A note on the compatibility of psychic determinism and freedom of will. *International Journal of Psychoanalysis,* 36:355–356.

Loewald, H. 1960a. On the therapeutic action of psychoanalysis. *International Journal of Psychoanalysis,* 58:463–472.

—— 1960b. Internalization, separation, mourning, and the superego. In *Papers on psychoanalysis.* New Haven: Yale University Press, 1980.

—— 1973. *Heinz Kohut: the analysis of the self.* In *Papers on psychoanalysis.* New Haven: Yale University Press, 1980.

—— 1974. Psychoanalysis as an art and the fantasy character of the psychoanalytic situation. In *Papers on psychoanalysis.* New Haven: Yale University Press, 1980.

—— 1976. Primary process, secondary process, and language. In *Papers on psychoanalysis.* New Haven: Yale University Press, 1980.

—— 1978. The waning of the Oedipus complex. In *Papers on psychoanalysis.* New Haven: Yale University Press, 1980.

Loisel, G. 1912. *History of the menagerie in antiquity.* Paris: Dion et Laurens.

Mahler, M. 1967. *On human symbiosis and the vicissitudes of individuation,* vol. 1, *Infantile psychosis.* New York: International Universities Press.

Mahler, M., F. Pine, and A. Bergman. 1975. *The psychological birth of the human infant: symbiosis and individuation.* New York: Basic Books.

Masson, J. 1984. *The assault on truth.* New York: Farrar, Straus and Giroux.

McDougall, J. 1980. *Plea for a measure of abnormality.* New York: International Universities Press.

McPhee, J. 1980. *Basin and range.* New York: Farrar, Straus and Giroux.

Menaker, E. 1982. *Otto Rank, a rediscovered legend.* New York: Columbia University Press.

Miller, J. 1983. *States of mind.* New York: Pantheon.

Mitchell, S. 1981. Twilight of the idols. *Contemporary Psychoanalysis,* 15:170–189.

Modell, A. 1984. *Psychoanalysis in a new context.* New York: International Universities Press.

Nietzsche, F. 1872. *The birth of tragedy.* In *The birth of tragedy and genealogy of morals,* trans. F. Golffing. New York: Doubleday Anchor, 1956.

————— 1876. *Philosophy in the tragic age of the Greeks.* Chicago: Gateway, 1962.

Ogden, T. 1982. *Projective identification and psychotherapeutic technique.* New York: Jason Aronson.

Person, E. 1980. Sexuality as the mainstay of identity: psychoanalytic perspectives. *Sigma,* 5:605–630.

Pine, F. 1985. *Developmental theory and clinical process.* New Haven: Yale University Press.

Porter, F. 1979. *Art in its own terms: selected criticisms,* ed. R. Downes. New York: Taplinger.

Powers, T. 1984. What's it about? *Atlantic Monthly.* January.

Racker, H. 1968. *Transference and countertransference.* New York: International Universities Press.

Rank, O. 1932. *Art and artist.* New York: Knopf, 1958.

Rapaport, D. 1960. *The structure of psychoanalytic theory: a systematizing attempt. Psychological Issues,* 2, #2, monograph 6.

Rathbun, C., L. DeVirgilio, and S. Waldvogel. 1958. A restitutive process in children following radical separation from family and culture. *American Journal of Orthopsychiatry,* 28:408–415.

Rickman, J. 1957. *Selected contributions to psychoanalysis.* New York: Basic Books.

Robbins, M. 1982. Narcissistic personality as a symbiotic character disorder. *International Journal of Psychoanalysis,* 63:457–474.

Rothstein, A. 1983. *The structural hypothesis: an evolutionary perspective.* New York: International Universities Press.

————— 1984. *The narcissistic pursuit of perfection.* New York: International Universities Press.

Rutter, M. 1979. Maternal deprivation, 1972–1978: new findings, new concepts, new approaches. *Child Development,* 50:283–305.

Sandler, J. 1987. *From safety to superego: selected papers of Joseph Sandler.* New York: Guilford Press.

Sartre, J.-P. 1950. *Baudelaire.* New York: New Directions.

————— 1953. *Existential psychoanalysis.* Chicago: Gateway.

—— 1963. *Saint Genet: actor and martyr*. New York: Braziller.

—— 1964. *The words*. New York: Fawcett.

—— 1981. *The family idiot: Gustave Flaubert*, vol. 1. Chicago: University of Chicago Press.

Schafer, R. 1968. *Aspects of internalization*. New York: International Universities Press.

—— 1976. *A new language for psychoanalysis*. New Haven: Yale University Press.

—— 1978. *Language and insight*. New Haven: Yale University Press.

—— 1983. *The analytic attitude*. New York: Basic Books.

Schecter, D. 1971. Of human bonds and bondage. In *In the name of life: essays in honor of Erich Fromm*, ed. B. Landis and E. Tauber. New York: Holt, Rinehart and Winston.

Schimel, J. 1972. The power theme in the obsessional. *Contemporary Psychoanalysis*, 9:1–16.

Schwartz, M. 1978. Critic, define thyself. In *Psychoanalysis and the question of the text*, ed. G. Hartmann. Baltimore: Johns Hopkins University Press.

Searles, H. 1958. Positive feelings in the relationship between the schizophrenic and his mother. In *Collected papers on schizophrenia and related subjects*. New York: International Universities Press.

Shapiro, D. 1965. *Neurotic styles*. New York: Basic Books.

—— 1981. *Autonomy and rigid character*. New York: Basic Books.

Shapiro, R. 1979. Family dynamics and object-relations theory: an analytic group-integrative approach to family therapy. In *Adolescent psychiatry*, vol. 7, ed. S. Feinstein and P. Giovacchini. Chicago: University of Chicago Press.

Silverman, D. 1987. What are little girls made of? *Psychoanalytic Psychology*, 4:315–335.

Silverman, L., F. Lachmann, and R. Milich. 1982. *The search for oneness*. New York: International Universities Press.

Simon, J., and W. Gagnon. 1973. *Sexual conduct*. Chicago: Aldine.

Spence, D. 1982. *Narrative truth and historical truth: meaning and interpretation in psychoanalysis*. New York: Norton.

Stern, D. 1977. *The first relationship: mother and infant*. Cambridge, Mass.: Harvard University Press.

—— 1985. *The interpersonal world of the infant*. New York: Basic Books.

Stoller, R. 1985. *Observing the erotic imagination*. New Haven: Yale University Press.

Stolorow, R., and F. Lachmann. 1980. *Psychoanalysis of developmental arrests*. New York: International Universities Press.

Sullivan, H. S. 1940. *Conceptions of modern psychiatry*. New York: Norton.

—— 1953. *The interpersonal theory of psychiatry*. New York: Norton.

—— 1956. *Clinical studies in psychiatry*. New York: Norton.

—— 1972. *Personal psychopathology*. New York: Norton.

Sulloway, F. 1979. *Freud: biologist of the mind*. New York: Basic Books.

Tronick, E., and L. Adamson. 1980. *Babies as people.* New York: Collier.

Veltre, T. 1987. Menagerie, metaphor and communication. Unpublished.

Wachtel, P. 1982. Vicious circles: the self and the rhetoric of emerging and unfolding. *Contemporary Psychoanalysis,* 13:259–273.

Waelder, R. 1936. The principle of multiple function. *Psychoanalytic Quarterly,* 35:45–62.

Weiss, J., and H. Sampson. 1986. *The psychoanalytic process: theory, clinical observation, and empirical research.* New York: Guilford Press.

Wheelis, A. 1956. Will and psychoanalysis. *Journal of the American Psychoanalytic Association,* 4:285–303.

—— 1969. How people change. *Commentary.* May.

White, M. 1952. Sullivan and treatment. In *The contributions of Harry Stack Sullivan: a symposium,* ed. Patrick Mullahy. New York: Hermitage House.

Will, O. 1959. Human relatedness of the schizophrenic reaction. *Psychiatry,* 22:205–223.

Winnicott, D. W. Unless otherwise noted, references are from *Through paediatrics to psycho-analysis.* London: Hogarth Press, 1958 (*TPP*), or from *The maturational process and the facilitating environment.* New York: International Universities Press, 1965 (*MPFE*).

—— 1945. Primitive emotional development. *TPP.*

—— 1948. Paediatrics and psychiatry. *TPP.*

—— 1949a. Mind and its relation to the psyche-soma. *TPP.*

—— 1949b. Birth memories, birth trauma, and anxiety. *TPP.*

—— 1950. Aggression in relation to emotional development. *TPP.*

—— 1951. Transitional objects and transitional phenomena. *TPP.*

—— 1954a. Metapsychological and clinical aspects of regression within the psycho-analytical setup. *TPP.*

—— 1954b. Withdrawal and regression. *TPP.*

—— 1956. Primary maternal preoccupation. *TPP.*

—— 1958. Child analysis in the latency period. *MPFE.*

—— 1959. Classification: is there a psycho-analytic contribution to psychiatric classification? *MPFE.*

—— 1960. Counter-transference. *MPFE.*

—— 1963. Communicating and not communicating leading to a study of certain opposites. *MPFE.*

—— 1971. *Playing and reality.* Middlesex, England: Penguin.

—— 1988. *Human nature.* New York: Schocken Books.

Index